MOOD AND TEMPERAMENT

EMOTIONS AND SOCIAL BEHAVIOR

Series Editor: Peter Salovey, Yale University

MOOD
and
TEMPERAMENT

David Watson

THE GUILFORD PRESS
New York   London

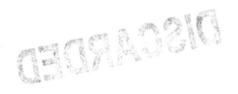

For my parents,
Dick and Lois Watson

© 2000 The Guilford Press
A Division of Guilford Publications, Inc.
72 Spring Street, New York, NY 10012
www.guilford.com

Printed in the United States of America

This book is printed on acid-free paper.

Last digit is print number: 9   8   7   6   5   4   3   2   1

Library of Congress Cataloging-in-Publication Data
Watson, David.
    Mood and temperament / David Watson.
        p. cm. — (Emotions and social behavior)
    Includes bibliographical references and index.
    ISBN 1-57230-526-6 (hardcover : alk. paper)
    1. Personality and emotions. I. Title. II. Series.
BF698.9.E45 W38 2000
152.4—dc21   99-054213

ABOUT THE AUTHOR

David Watson, PhD, is Professor of Psychology and head of the Personality and Social Psychology Training Program at the University of Iowa. He received his doctorate in Personality Research and Assessment from the University of Minnesota in 1982, followed by two years of postdoctoral training in the Psychiatry Department of the Washington University School of Medicine. Dr. Watson has broad interests in personality, health, and clinical psychology and has published widely in the top journals in these fields. He has also served on the editorial boards of numerous journals and since 1994 has been the Associate Editor of the *Journal of Abnormal Psychology.*

SERIES EDITOR'S NOTE

*M*ood and *Temperament* represents the latest volume in The Guilford Press series, Emotions and Social Behavior. No one in the area of mood and emotions research has contributed more to our understanding of the experience of naturally occurring feelings than David Watson. This volume, as a reflection of Dr. Watson's research program, touches on the cyclical aspects of our moods, individual differences in the tendency to experience different kinds of moods, the situational inducers of affect, and the relationship of these processes to human development and physical and mental well-being. Interwoven through this discussion is the tricky issue of how best to measure feelings, that is, translating subjective, highly personal experiences into some kind of objective representation. More generally, *Mood and Temperament* is a notable example of how to conduct programmatic research. Dr. Watson takes a fascinating area of study and explores it from every possible angle. Readers will find this volume enormously helpful; I know I have.

PETER SALOVEY, PHD
*Professor of Psychology
and of Epidemiology and Public Health
Yale University*

PREFACE

When I began graduate school in 1975, scientific psychology still focused primarily on the study of behavior. The topics of mood, emotion, and temperament attracted very little attention from researchers; indeed, many psychologists believed that they were of little real importance and did not merit serious scientific scrutiny. The situation had not changed much in late 1979, when I began my first major study of daily mood. I therefore approached this study (which also was the basis for my doctoral dissertation) with more than a little apprehension, wondering if I was consigning my career to a peripheral domain that never would be valued highly by my colleagues.

Fortunately, things have worked out much better than I feared. Indeed, since that time, there has been an "affective explosion" within psychology, which finally has acknowledged the central importance of affect in human experience. During the 1980s and 1990s, thousands of articles, books, and book chapters have examined various aspects of short-term mood fluctuations and longer-term individual differences in temperament and emotionality. The purpose of this book is to summarize the key findings from this newly emerging literature, using my own ongoing 20-year research program as an organizing framework. In doing so, I have attempted to give the reader a basic overview of this immense body of scientific evidence.

I felt it was particularly important to present theory and research related to both mood and temperament in the same volume. For whatever reason, these topics have given rise to largely distinct literatures that remain relatively disconnected from one another. Previous books in this area have reflected this schism: Several have examined mood and several have discussed temperament, but no book has integrated these two topics within the same framework. This is unfortunate, because (as will become quite clear to the readers of this book) many of the same constructs and processes are centrally implicated in both domains. Most notably, in the chapters that follow I explore the nature and significance of two general biobehavioral systems—one that regulates the experience of negative moods (such as fear and anger) and the other that is associated with positive mood states (such as enthusiasm and delight). I show how these two systems are important in understanding short-term mood fluctuations, circadian and seasonal cycles, long-term individual differences in temperament and emotionality, and physical and psychological health.

The topics discussed in this book should be of considerable interest to clinicians and to a broad range of serious psychological researchers. These individuals, however, will not be satisfied with pat conclusions; rather, they will insist on seeing the relevant evidence so that they can draw their own inferences from the data. To satisfy these scholars, the book presents an enormous amount of empirical data (much of it drawn from my own intensive studies in this area), including numerous tables and figures. I encourage readers to study these data carefully and draw their own conclusions.

I also hope that readers may gain some knowledge and insight into their own affective lives. I must emphasize, however, that this is not a self-help book that is designed to teach people how to be truly happy. At the same time, however, I have tried to make the book accessible to a broad audience by avoiding lengthy presentations of complex, technical material. Although the book discusses many complex methodological and data analytic issues, it does so in a straightforward and nontechnical manner. Consequently, the book can be read by anyone (including both undergraduate and graduate students) with a reasonable background in basic psychological research.

This book—and the research reported in it—would not have been possible without the help of numerous people. I would like to acknowledge four individuals in particular. First, my wife, Lee Anna Clark, who has been my valued collaborator over the past 20 years; she worked with me on my very first mood project (which relied heavily on her fluency in Japanese) and has been an invaluable resource ever since. Second, my graduate mentor, Auke Tellegen, who began to study mood long before the topic became fashionable. He was the one who first suggested to me that it might be an area worth pursuing. As always, he gave me good advice. Third, James Pennebaker, who was instrumental in getting me my first research position at Southern Methodist University (SMU). More than anyone else, he helped to get my research career started; he also taught me that research can be fun. Finally, Cathey Soutter, who was a key collaborator in the daily mood studies we conducted at SMU. Much of the evidence I present in this volume would not exist except for her relentless, indefatigable pursuit of data.

In addition to these individuals, I would like to acknowledge the valuable help of my many research collaborators, including Jana Smith Assenheimer, Mary Dieffenwierth, Elizabeth Gray, Allen Harkness, Julie Harrison, Paul Hook, Brock Hubbard, Philip Kendall, Jay Leeka, Paul Marshall, Rene Martin, Richard McCormick, Curt McIntyre, Susan Mineka, Ann Slack, Milton Strauss, Jatin Vaidya, Lori McKee Walker, Kris Weber, and David Wiese. I also have benefited from the advice and support of numerous colleagues, including Michael Best, Rebecca Eder, Laura King, Don Fowles, and Jerry Suls. Finally, I would like to thank the thousands of people who participated in our studies, particularly the hundreds of individuals who completed our demanding, longitudinal studies of momentary and daily mood. I have always seen them as collaborators in this fascinating, never-ending enterprise.

DAVID WATSON, PHD

CONTENTS

1

AN INTRODUCTION TO THE STUDY OF MOOD AND TEMPERAMENT

We remain profoundly ignorant of the universe and of ourselves. Nevertheless, the 20th century has witnessed a remarkable lessening of this ignorance. In the past several decades we have split the atom and have begun to unlock the heretofore secret code of genetic transmission. We have brought all of humanity closer through the development of powerful new means of transportation and communication. We have made great progress in improving health and in increasing the average human lifespan. For the first time, we even have managed to venture beyond the confines of our home planet.

Scientific psychology clearly has not produced any dramatic breakthroughs of this same magnitude during the century. This should not be construed, however, as indicating that psychology has stalled or stagnated during this period. On the contrary, psychologists have made enormous advances in a number of areas, advances that have important implications for our understanding of ourselves and how we live our lives. The purpose of this book is to bring together contemporary thinking and evidence in an area that has seen tremendous advancement in the past decade or so: the study of the moods and feelings that color our daily lives.

Of course, people have been fascinated by the vicissitudes of mood for thousands of years. We all experience obvious fluctuations in our mood state, and it is natural to be curious about the underlying causes of these fluctuations. Because of this, moods and emotions long have been a favorite topic of poets and philosophers. Unfortunately, until quite recently mood fluctuations could only be studied through careful introspection, a notoriously unreliable and scientifically unsatisfactory approach (e.g., Stagner, 1988). Accordingly, scientific progress in this area was extremely slow; indeed, the whole topic of "mood" gradually acquired an aura of mystery—or perhaps better, whimsy—that appeared to put it beyond the grasp of human understanding. To a considerable extent, this sense of the unexplainable mystery of emotion has persisted to the present day. In contemporary society, people still are likely to attribute a negative mood to "getting up on the wrong side of the bed," or having a "bad hair day," or even "El Niño"; this is tantamount to admitting that one's behavior is powerfully influenced by widely fluctuating and ultimately incomprehensible forces.

In actuality, these forces no longer are completely incomprehensible. Starting in the late 1970s, there was an explosion of scientific research on mood that has continued unabated to the present. Thayer (1989), in fact, was able to identify approximately 1,000 papers that had been published in the previous decade that dealt directly or indirectly with mood. This vigorous and flourishing line of research has—in a relatively brief time—produced tremendous advances in our understanding of the vicissitudes of mood.

We can identify two basic reasons for this "affective explosion," one theoretical and the other technological. The theoretical reason was the gradual decline of behaviorism as a dominant force in psychology (see Lazarus, 1991a; Thayer, 1989). Radical behaviorists generally were opposed to the use of intraorganismic concepts and explanations, and they specifically viewed moods and feelings as uninteresting epiphenomena (i.e., mere by-products of more fundamental processes of conditioning) that could—and should—be completely ignored by psychologists (e.g., Skinner, 1971). Accordingly, during the long ascendance of behaviorism, research on moods and emotions was widely perceived to be scientifically disreputable; not surprisingly, this intellectual climate produced few serious investigations of these phenomena.

The second, technological reason was the rapid emergence and ready availability of high-speed computers that could analyze vast amounts of data quickly and easily. To understand the ebb and flow of ongoing daily experience, one must conduct intensive investigations of individuals under more naturalistic conditions. Accordingly, mood researchers have made extensive use of within-subject designs in which individuals rate their moods (either how they feel "right now," or how they have felt "to-day" or the "past few days") repeatedly over a period of several days, weeks, or months. For example, using these intensive within-subject de-signs, my colleagues and I have collected more than 45,000 mood assess-ments (representing a total of more than 2 million ratings of individual mood terms) from approximately 1,000 individuals. Data of this sort are extraordinarily rich and informative, and they can be used to address is-sues that cannot be examined using more traditional research designs. For these reasons, I make heavy use of within-subject data in the chapters that follow. Clearly, however, it was virtually impossible to analyze data sets of this size and complexity before the advent of the computer.

CONTRASTING "MOODS" AND "EMOTIONS"

Defining "Emotions"

I have assumed thus far that readers are generally familiar with the con-cept of "mood," and that they have at least a vague sense of what this term means. At this point, however, it is necessary to go beyond this vague familiarity and to define the concept of mood more precisely.

In doing so, it may be helpful to begin by examining the extremely influential and closely related concept of "emotion." Several prominent models of emotion have been proposed in recent decades, including those of Ekman and Friesen (Ekman, 1982; Ekman & Friesen, 1975), Izard (1971, 1972, 1977, 1991), Plutchik (1962, 1980), Tomkins (1962, 1963). These theo-ries differ in many significant ways, but they all emphasize the impor-tance of a relatively small number of discrete, fundamental emotions. Furthermore, a core set of emotions—joy, interest, surprise, fear, anger, sadness, and disgust—are recognized by all of these theorists (see Ekman & Davidson, 1994).

What, then, is an emotion? Extrapolating from the writings of these theorists, we can define an emotion as a distinct, integrated, psycho-physiological response system; in essence, an emotion represents an orga-nized, highly structured reaction to an event that is relevant to the needs, goals, or survival of the organism. Furthermore, an emotion contains at least four interrelated but differentiable components, each of which is crucial in understanding its evolutionary origins and adaptive signifi-cance: (1) a prototypical form of expression (typically facial), (2) a pattern of consistent autonomic changes, (3) a distinct subjective feeling state, and (4) a characteristic form of adaptive behavior. For instance, the emo-tion of fear is characterized by a distinctive facial expression in which the eyebrows are raised and drawn together, the eyes are opened widely, the lower lip is tensed, and the lips are stretched back (Ekman & Friesen, 1975; Izard, 1971). At the same time, fear also is associated with marked autonomic changes, including rapid increases in heart rate and sweating (Ekman, Levenson, & Friesen, 1983). In addition, this emotion involves a characteristic experiential state in which the individual reports feeling scared, nervous, and apprehensive (Izard, 1977, 1991; Watson & Clark, 1992a). Finally, fear is a reaction to situations of perceived risk or danger and motivates various behaviors (especially fleeing and freezing) that are designed to eliminate that danger (e.g., Izard, 1991).

A substantial body of evidence has documented the distinctiveness and specificity of these fundamental emotions. For instance, numerous studies have demonstrated that the prototypical facial expressions of several emotions are both distinct from one another and universal across a wide range of cultures (Ekman, 1982, 1994; Ekman et al., 1987; Izard, 1971, 1994). Similarly, Ekman and his associates have identified specific autonomic substrates for various emotions (Ekman et al., 1983; Levenson, Ekman, & Friesen, 1990). Finally, studies of self-rated affect (i.e., in which people rate the extent to which they are experiencing various feeling states) have identified specific content factors that correspond to most of the discrete emotions postulated in the various models (e.g., Izard, 1972; McNair, Lorr, & Droppleman, 1971; Watson & Clark, 1992a, 1994b). Having said this, however, I also should acknowledge that other researchers have challenged this evidence and, indeed, the whole notion of "basic" emotions (for dissenting views, see Averill, 1994; Ortony & Turner, 1990; Russell, 1994; Turner & Ortony, 1992).

Defining "Moods"

What, then, is a mood, and how exactly does it differ from an emotion? Moods are transient episodes of feeling or affect. As such, moods are highly similar to the subjective, experiential component of emotions. Thus, at one level, one could argue that mood research simply restricts itself to studying the phenomenological aspect of emotions while ignoring their other components. This conclusion is mistaken, however, because it overlooks some important differences between these concepts. One key difference involves the typical duration of the affective episode. Emotions generally are intense, high-activation states. Because of their intensity— and because they typically are associated with massive expenditures of energy—they tend to be extremely brief, lasting perhaps only a few seconds (e.g., Izard, 1991). One occasionally observes more prolonged emotional states in certain individuals, but these extended reactions tend to be

dysfunctional and, in fact, frequently are manifestations of psychopathology (see Clark & Watson, 1994).

In contrast, moods typically are much longer in duration. For example, whereas the full emotion of anger may last for only a few seconds or
minutes, an annoyed or irritable mood may last for several hours, or even
for a few days.

Second, emotions usually are viewed as *response* systems that are activated by certain eliciting stimuli: Fear is a response to threat or danger,
anger is a reaction to frustration or insult, disgust is a response to noxious
substances, and so on. Thus, emotions are viewed primarily as reactions
to important events and circumstances: They do not arise randomly and
without good reason. The broader implications of this view have been expressed most forcefully by Izard (1991): "All emotions, as contrasted with
drives, are noncyclical. One does not become interested or disgusted or
ashamed two or three times a day in rhythm with ingestion, digestion,
and metabolic processes" (p. 44).

In sharp contrast, the existing data establish that moods are strongly
influenced not only by external events and experiences but also by various internal processes; furthermore, because of these important endogenous influences, mood states *do* show strong cyclic patterns of variation.
In Chapter 4, for example, I demonstrate that positive mood states display a consistent circadian rhythm, such that we tend to be more enthusiastic, energetic, and alert at certain times of the day.

Third, the concept of mood is much broader and more inclusive than
the subjective component of the emotions. That is, mood refers to *all* transient feeling states, not simply to those feelings that accompany specific,
discrete emotions such as fear, anger, and joy. Thus, mood researchers do
not restrict themselves only to those feelings that clearly represent emotions. There are at least three ways in which the concept of mood is more
inclusive and encompassing than that of experienced emotion. First,
moods include many important and commonly experienced feeling states
that reflect milder, attenuated versions of the classic emotions. For example, the participants in our studies often report feeling annoyed and irritated (subthreshold manifestations of anger), nervous and tense (mild
forms of fear), and cheerful and pleasant (attenuated versions of joy).

I also should acknowledge, however, that one major emotion theo-
rist—Carroll Izard—has adapted his "differential emotions theory" to encompass these milder, subthreshold states. Specifically, he has argued that
emotions do not exist as simple *categories* (i.e., phenomena that either are
completely present or absent); rather, they represent *dimensions* that vary
on a continuum of intensity from very mild to very strong (Izard, 1991).
For example, annoyance, anger, and rage can be characterized as increas-

ingly intense points on a single emotional continuum. Furthermore, Izard has created the Differential Emotions Scale (DES; Izard, Dougherty, Bloxom, & Kotsch, 1974), an instrument that allows researchers to assess emotions as continuous dimensions. Viewed in this way, the gap between moods and emotions narrows considerably.

Nevertheless, the gap persists even if one adopts Izard's approach. A second conceptual difference concerns the inclusion versus exclusion of deactivated, low-energy states such as fatigue (e.g., feeling tired or drowsy) and serenity (e.g., feeling calm and relaxed). Given that fatigue and serenity reflect low levels of activation and arousal—and that emotions are conceptualized as intense, high-activation episodes—they have not been classified as emotions and have been excluded from the major models discussed earlier. If anything, these deactivated states typically have been viewed as reflecting the general *absence* of strong feeling or emotion (for a discussion, see Zevon & Tellegen, 1982). Nevertheless, fatigue and serenity are important feelings that are commonly experienced in everyday life. Accordingly, they clearly are encompassed within the definition of mood and are of general relevance to its study; in fact, we will see in subsequent chapters that these deactivated, low-energy states have been widely studied by mood researchers and play a significant role in contemporary mood theory.

The third—and more general—point is that it is impossible to capture the nuances of everyday affective experience without including a number of states that do not clearly represent one of the classically defined discrete emotions. For instance, nonspecific negative mood terms such as "upset" and "distressed" do not clearly or unambiguously correspond to any single emotion. But this fact does not render them uninteresting or unimportant. On the contrary, their very generality (note that one can be upset or distressed for a great many reasons and in countless situations) makes them extremely applicable to everyday experience.

Similarly, only two positive emotions—joy/happiness and interest/excitement—are included in most models. The assessment of positive affective states would be severely impoverished if it were restricted only to clear markers of these basic emotions. To assess positive feelings adequately, it is necessary to include several terms (e.g., "lively," "energetic," "active," "alert," and "attentive") that do not clearly represent either of these emotions.

This brings me to a crucial issue in the study of mood. Several writers have criticized mood researchers for including "nonemotion terms" (e.g., "sleepy," "drowsy," "calm," and "alert") in their assessments. This criticism frequently has been leveled against investigators seeking to identify the basic, underlying dimensions of affect (e.g., Clore, Ortony, & Foss, 1987; Lazarus, 1991a, 1991b; Morgan & Heise, 1988; Ortony, Clore, &

Collins, 1988; Ortony, Clore, & Foss, 1987). This criticism, of course, assumes that mood research should be restricted to clear referents of emotion; otherwise, it makes no sense to criticize the inclusion of terms that do not clearly represent emotions. Put another way, these critics assume that the ultimate goal of mood researchers is to assess the experiential component of the emotions. It should be clear from the preceding discussion, however, that mood researchers do not have this as their ultimate goal; consequently, they do not view this restriction as either necessary or desirable. It makes perfect sense to include nonemotion terms in mood studies; indeed, it would be a serious mistake to omit them.

Moods and Emotions in Everyday Life

My primary purpose in writing this book is to provide an integrative account of recent research into the moods and feelings that color our everyday lives. Before leaving the topic of emotion, I need to consider one further issue that strikes at the very heart of this book, namely, Why focus on moods rather than emotions?

There are three reasons why I believe the concept of mood is more useful in understanding the vicissitudes of everyday life. The first of these already was noted in the previous section: Mood is a more encompassing concept that includes *all* subjective feeling states, not simply those that clearly correspond to one of the classic emotions. Emotion researchers necessarily restrict themselves to a subset of the total range of transient feeling states. For many scientific purposes, this restriction is not too onerous. However, if one is primarily interested in understanding feelings per se, the concept of mood clearly provides a more complete and satisfactory conceptual scheme.

Second, full-blown manifestations of emotions—especially the negative emotions—are relatively infrequent in daily life. Before considering some relevant data, I ask the reader to do a simple self-study. Assuming approximately 7 to 8 hours of sleep per night, the average person experiences roughly 1,000 minutes of waking consciousness each day. Try to visualize your feelings and activities over the course of a fairly typical day, and then estimate how many of those 1,000 waking minutes you spend in a classic state of fear (as opposed to mild feelings of nervousness or worry) as it was described earlier. If you are like me—and many others who have performed this same self-study—your best guess is that you typically experience no more than 1 or 2 minutes of real fear over the course of a day. If so, then far less than 1% of your waking life is spent in a classic state of fear.

Next, repeat this process using several other emotions, such as anger (again, the full emotion of anger, not simply feeling annoyed or irritable), sadness, disgust, surprise, and joy; again, rate how many minutes each day you typically experience each emotion. Now sum these estimates to yield an overall "emotion minutes" score for the typical day. Of course, these ratings are only rough guesses, so that the exact number should not be taken very seriously. The important point, however, is that the overall score probably represents a small fraction (most likely, less than 10%) of the total number of 1,000 waking minutes. In other words, this self-study most likely suggests the bulk of an everyday life is spent in nonemotional states.

This self-assessment obviously is highly subjective, but it can be corroborated using more objective evidence. Here are data from two large within-subject studies of current, momentary mood; all the participants were undergraduate students at Southern Methodist University. Both of these studies originally were designed to examine diurnal variation in mood (they are discussed in much greater detail in subsequent chapters); accordingly, the students' moods were assessed at various times of the day, including immediately after rising and shortly before retiring. In the first study, the students rated their current mood once a day for several weeks; at each assessment, they rated themselves on the 60 mood terms comprising the Positive and Negative Affect Schedule—Expanded Form (PANAS-X; Watson & Clark, 1994b). In the second study, the students' moods were assessed approximately seven times a day for 1 week; they rated themselves on the 20 terms comprising the original Positive and Negative Affect Schedule (PANAS; Watson, Clark, & Tellegen, 1988). Note that the 20 PANAS mood descriptors are a subset of those included in the PANAS-X.

To be included in the current analyses, a student had to complete a minimum of 35 momentary mood assessments. Overall, the data in Study 1 are based on a total of 10,169 momentary mood assessments from 226 students ($M = 45.0$ observations per person); those in Study 2 are based on a total of 8,191 assessments from 188 individuals ($M = 43.6$ observations per person). At each assessment, the students rated the extent to which they were currently experiencing the various mood terms on a 5-point scale (1 = very slightly or not a all, 2 = a little, 3 = moderately, 4 = very much, 5 = extremely).

Table 1.1 presents overall reported frequencies—computed across all individuals—for nine affect terms in the first study. The terms that were selected clearly correspond to basic emotions that have been included in one or more of the major contemporary theories: Six of them describe negative, unpleasant feeling states ("afraid," "sad," "angry," "disgusted," "guilty," "scornful"), whereas three represent positive, pleasant states ("joyful," "interested," "excited"). For each term, the table indicates the percentage of the time that the students reported very little (defined as a

TABLE 1.1. The Intensity of Reported Emotions (Shown as a Percent of All Observations) in Momentary Mood Data: Results from the First Sample

Emotion term	Rated intensity		
	Very slightly or not at all	A little/ moderately	Very much/ extremely
Negative emotion terms			
Afraid	73.8%	22.6%	3.6%
Sad	66.5%	28.7%	4.9%
Angry	74.8%	20.0%	5.2%
Disgusted	67.1%	27.5%	5.4%
Guilty	77.2%	19.0%	3.8%
Scornful	74.7%	21.0%	4.3%
M	72.4%	23.1%	4.5%
Positive emotion terms			
Joyful	33.4%	47.9%	18.7%
Interested	30.5%	54.5%	15.0%
Excited	38.4%	43.3%	18.3%
M	34.1%	49.5%	17.3%

Note. These figures are based on a total of 10,169 momentary observations.

rating of "1"), mild or moderate levels (i.e., ratings of "2" or "3"), or more intense levels (i.e., ratings of "4" or "5") of that affect.

Of course, we have no definitive way of estimating the actual occurrence of full-blown emotions from simple self-ratings of this sort; a definitive assessment would require collecting physiological and/or expressive data as well. Nevertheless, let us assume for the sake of argument that self-ratings of "4" (very much) and "5" (extremely) reflect significant episodes of emotion; note that this is an extremely liberal criterion that likely *overestimates* the actual occurrence of classic, full-blown emotions such as fear and anger.

What can be gleaned from these data? First, it is evident that the positive emotions are experienced much more frequently—at both moderate and more intense levels—than are the negative emotions. Moreover, this pattern clearly is quite robust in that all the positive terms were reported with greater regularity than any of the negative terms. I explore the implications of this finding in the following section.

Second, although the positive emotions are experienced reasonably frequently, reports of the various negative emotions are relatively rare. Note that the reported frequency of intense affect was quite low for all six negative emotions, ranging from 3.6% (for fear) to 5.4% (for disgust); overall, the mean value across the six negative terms was only 4.5%. These results converge quite nicely with those of the self-study: Again, we see that the negative emotions comprise only a small fraction of everyday affective experience.

Third, the students frequently experienced mild or moderate levels of affect; in addition, they reported these intermediate states much more often than the intense affect that more closely corresponds to a classic episode of emotion. It also is noteworthy that this pattern held for all nine terms, including both the negative and positive emotions. These results indicate that the bulk of everyday experience consists of feelings of mild to moderate intensity that fall beneath the threshold of the classic emotions (see also Diener, Fugita, & Sandvik, 1994). In other words, researchers focusing only on full-blown manifestations of the classic emotions will miss the rich mixture of less intense feelings that comprise most of daily affective experience.

Table 1.2 presents corresponding data for four of these same terms— two negative ("afraid" and "guilty") and two positive ("interested" and "excited")—that also were included in the second study. It can be seen that these results closely replicate those of the first study. That is, we again see that (1) positive emotions were reported much more frequently than negative emotions, (2) full-intensity negative emotions were reported only rarely, and (3) for all terms, mild to moderate levels of affect

TABLE 1.2. The Intensity of Reported Emotions (Shown as a Percent of All Observations) in Momentary Mood Data: Partial Replication in the Second Sample

Emotion term	Rated intensity		
	Very slightly or not at all	A little/ moderately	Very much/ extremely
Negative emotion terms			
Afraid	71.1%	24.2%	4.7%
Guilty	74.6%	21.6%	3.8%
M	72.8%	22.9%	4.2%
Positive emotion terms			
Interested	25.1%	53.6%	21.3%
Excited	29.4%	50.4%	20.3%
M	27.3%	52.0%	20.8%

Note. These figures are based on a total of 8,191 momentary observations.

were experienced much more often than the intense levels corresponding to classic episodes of emotion.

Taken together, the data from these two tables—representing more than 18,000 individual mood observations—demonstrate that the bulk of everyday affective experience consists of mild to moderate-intensity feelings that fall beneath the threshold of classic, full-blown episodes of emotion. Accordingly, models that focus solely on such episodes fail to capture the essential nature of this experience. At one level these results are hardly surprising, even to emotion theorists: After all, because they represent highly intense states, classic episodes of emotion *should be* relatively rare, and they should be experienced much less frequently than milder affective states. Nevertheless, the crucial point here is that research approaches that are based on these infrequent, high-intensity states are poorly suited to the study of ongoing daily experience.

As discussed earlier, this problem can be mitigated somewhat by adopting a dimensional approach to the emotions, thereby encompassing these mild and moderate feeling states as well (Izard, 1991). This, however, brings us to the third reason why emotion theories provide a relatively poor working model for daily affective life, namely, most of daily experience consists of mixed affective states that reflect complex combinations of the basic emotions. In other words, pure emotional states are exceedingly rare in normal daily life. Chapter 2 examines this issue in much greater detail. For now, I will simply illustrate the nature and extent of the problem using data from the first study. For the sake of simplicity, I will restrict this discussion to the six negative terms (each of which represents a different negative emotion) shown in Table 1.1.

Earlier, I presented results for each affect separately, noting that individuals experienced intense levels of each emotion rather infrequently. For the current discussion, however, it is necessary to examine them together. The first step is to calculate the total number of episodes involving at least one of the negative emotions; collapsing across all six terms, this initial analysis yielded a combined total of 1,429 negative emotional episodes, representing 14.1% of the overall number of 10,169 observations (as before, an emotional episode was defined as a rating of either 4 or 5). Further analysis, however, revealed that in roughly half of these cases (N = 696, or 48.7%), the students actually reported intense levels of *two or more* negative emotions. Furthermore, in approximately one-third of the episodes (*N* = 452, or 31.6%), the individual experienced a moderate amount (i.e., a rating of 3) of at least one other negative emotion. Thus, in only 281 instances (representing 19.7% of the emotion episodes, and 2.8% of the total pool of observations) did a person report an intense level of one negative emotion without experiencing at least a moderate amount of another.

In fact, emotion theorists long have conceded this point, acknowledging that mixed states predominate—and pure emotions are rarely encountered—in daily experience (see Izard, 1972, 1977, 1991; Plutchik, 1980). Izard (1972), for instance, states that "most theorists who deal with discrete emotions have suggested that the existence of a pure emotion, such as pure fear or pure guilt, is probably fairly rare in day-to-day living and virtually impossible to obtain in the laboratory or in any other research setting. I share this position" (p. 103). Similarly, Plutchik (1980) concludes that "emotions are rarely if ever experienced in a pure state" (p. 103).

For the reasons I have discussed, mood offers a much better conceptual framework for everyday affective experience than does emotion; indeed, models that emphasize the importance of basic, discrete emotions ultimately are ill-suited to the study of such experience. In saying this, I am not offering a general criticism of classic emotion theory, and I am not suggesting that discrete emotions are unimportant or uninteresting. Let me emphasize two points in this regard. First, although classic episodes of emotion are relatively infrequent, when they do occur they are extremely important and can have profound consequences. Put another way, the very intensity and extremity that make these emotions uncommon also render them extremely powerful when they do occur.

Second, these emotions exert a profound influence on human life and human behavior that extends far beyond their mere occurrence. Consider, for example, the emotion of fear. Over the course of human history, people have expended enormous time and effort to ensure that they experience as little fear as possible. Freud (1930/1961), for instance, argued that the desire for safety and security was a key factor in the development of human civilization. Similarly, in our own society, we obviously place a high priority on achieving security and avoiding danger. Most of us strongly desire to live in safe neighborhoods, to drive safe cars, and to work in safe environments. We seek to avoid harmful substances, dangerous weather conditions, and violent confrontations of any sort. Note, moreover, that fear can be a powerful motivator of avoidance behavior even when real harm is absent, or at least extremely unlikely. For instance, some people will avoid giving a public speech simply because it makes them fearful. Consequently, fear-related considerations can exert a tremendous influence on our life and our behavior, even if we spend very little time actually experiencing the emotion.

THE STREAM OF AFFECT

Although full-blown episodes of emotion are relatively infrequent, our data establish that everyday experience is replete with milder, less intense mood states. In fact, I would argue that waking consciousness is experienced as a continuous *stream of affect* (see also Watson & Clark, 1994a), such that people are always experiencing some type of mood. Of course, we all show profound fluctuations in *what* we are feeling—sometimes we are excited and energetic but other times bored and lethargic; sometimes we are tense and apprehensive yet other times calm and serene. However, while we are awake and conscious, we are always feeling *something* (for related discussions, see Diener et al., 1994; Izard, 1991). Very rarely, a person might report feeling virtually nothing at all: In the mood literature, the terms that seem to come closest to capturing this state of complete nonfeeling are "quiet," "still," and "quiescent" (see Watson & Tellegen, 1985). These terms—and it is noteworthy that there are few like them in the English language—describe a state that is neither clearly good nor bad and that shows no evidence of marked activation or arousal. But such states of nonfeeling are extremely infrequent, and even when they do occur they are exceedingly brief.

Indeed, I would argue that nonfeeling is a highly unsteady state that cannot persist for very long. This is because valence—or what also has been called hedonic tone (e.g., Watson & Clark, 1992a)—is such a fundamental part of our conscious appraisal process that we almost instantaneously perceive our ongoing state to be either pleasant or unpleasant (see Nesse, 1991). This is true even if we are feeling very little. If I am in a quiet, deactivated state in which little is happening—and if I perceive this situation to be satisfactory and acceptable—then I would describe myself as calm and relaxed. On the other hand, if I deem my current situation to be unsatisfactory, then I would experience unpleasant feelings of dullness and boredom.

The existence of this continuous stream of affect can be demonstrated by again examining data from our two large within-subject studies of momentary mood. Recall that in the first of these studies, undergraduate students rated themselves on the 60 mood terms comprising the PANAS-X. Collapsing across all persons and days, the respondents in this study produced only 19 observations (representing 0.2% of the total pool of 10,169 observations) in which they essentially reported feeling *nothing* (i.e., no mood terms received ratings of 2 or greater). Furthermore, in virtually all instances (10,077, or 99.1%), the students rated themselves as experiencing at least a moderate amount of some affect (i.e., at least one term received a rating of 3 or greater).

The second study (in which students rated themselves on the 20 terms comprising the PANAS) yielded extremely similar results. Again, collapsing across all persons and days, our respondents produced only 78 observations (representing 1.0% of the total pool of 8,191 observations) in which they reported feeling nothing whatsoever. Moreover, in more than

90% of the observations (7544, or 92.1%), they reported at least a moderate amount of some affect. Thus, we again see clear evidence of a continuous stream of affect (for very similar findings, see Diener et al., 1994).

Much of this volume is devoted to exploring the nature of this stream of affect. At the outset, however, let me describe two of its very general attributes, which were first identified by my colleague Ed Diener (see Diener et al., 1994). First, consistent with the data reported in Tables 1.1 and 1.2, daily experience primarily consists of relatively mild, low-intensity affective states. It is noteworthy that the data I presented in these tables—and, indeed, most of the relevant data in the mood literature—are based on the responses of college students, who tend to report intense feelings more frequently than older adults (Diener et al., 1994). Consequently, data collected on older subjects would offer even stronger support for the conclusion that most affective states are relatively mild.

Note that this general characteristic of the affective stream is highly adaptive and makes excellent sense from an evolutionary viewpoint. All other things being equal, low-activation states are preferable to high-intensity states because they (1) burn less energy, thereby reducing the amount of food that is needed for survival; and (2) put less of a strain on bodily resources, thereby lessening the threat of physiological exhaustion and illness (for related discussions, see Beck, 1987; Kasper & Rosenthal, 1989; Selye, 1956; Webb, 1979). Of course, circumstances periodically require greater activation and energy expenditure on the part of the organism. In the absence of such circumstances, however, there should be a natural tendency toward less intense, lower-activation affective states. This is a crucial point that is considered in more detail subsequently.

The second general attribute of this affective stream is that it is typically pleasant or positive; Cacioppo and Berntson (1994) labeled this pervasive tendency the "positivity offset." That is, most people experience a pleasant, positive mood most of the time. This basic quality of affective life is readily apparent in Tables 1.1 and 1.2, which indicate that positive emotions are experienced much more frequently—at both moderate and intense levels—than negative emotions. To further demonstrate this point, I created an overall index of current positive feeling for each observation in both of these data sets; this overall score was calculated by summing the student's ratings on the 10 terms comprising the PANAS Positive Affect scale (e.g., "interested," "active," "alert," and "proud"; see Watson, Clark, & Tellegen, 1988). Similarly, I computed an overall measure of current negative feeling by combining the individual's ratings on the 10 terms comprising the PANAS Negative Affect scale (e.g., "scared," "guilty," "irritable," and "distressed"). Finally, I created an index of general hedonic tone for each observation by subtracting the Negative Affect score from the Positive Affect score.

Combining the data from both studies, these analyses indicated that roughly three-quarters of the observations (13,700, or 74.6% of the total) could be characterized as pleasant (i.e., Positive Affect was greater than Negative Affect), whereas only about one-fifth (3,898, or 21.2%) could be classified as unpleasant (i.e., Negative Affect was greater than Positive Affect); in the few remaining cases, people reported equal amounts of Positive and Negative Affect. Diener et al. (1994) reported similar findings, again using very large data sets. Clearly, the bulk of affective life is experienced as pleasant, at least in people without diagnosed psychological disorders. (In a later chapter, I show that this stream of affect has acquired a largely negative tone in individuals suffering from many forms of psychopathology.)

Thus, putting these two general attributes together, we arrive at the more basic conclusion that this stream of affect typically is experienced as mildly to moderately pleasant. In other words, most people report a mildly pleasant, positive mood most of the time.

TRAITS AND TEMPERAMENTS

Affective Traits

Thus far, I have discussed only short-term, transient feelings, which traditionally have been called state mood or state affect in the psychological literature (Cattell & Scheier, 1961; Eysenck, 1983; Spielberger, Gorsuch, Lushene, Vagg, & Jacobs, 1983; Zuckerman & Lubin, 1985). These transient episodes are extremely important; in fact, they constitute the very core of the subject matter of this book. Accordingly, I will devote several chapters to the causes and consequences of state affect.

Clearly, however, any thorough examination of moods and feelings also must consider consistent, long-term individual differences in affective experience—that is, what traditionally has been called trait affect. Affective traits represent stable individual differences in the tendency to experience a corresponding mood state. For instance, individuals who are high in the trait of fearfulness are prone to more frequent and more intense episodes of fear; conversely, those low in this trait experience fear less frequently and intensely. Similarly, individuals who are high in the trait of happiness report more frequent and intense episodes of joy than those who are low in this trait.

I suspect that few readers will object to the notion that some people are more cheerful—or more nervous, or more irritable—than others. But how do we verify this notion scientifically—that is, how do we confirm the existence of these affective traits? Two types of evidence are critically important in establishing the existence of any trait. First, traits must show evidence of temporal stability. That is, individuals must maintain a relatively consistent rank order in their scores over extended time intervals. For example, individuals who report being relatively happy at an initial assessment should still be relatively happy when retested a few months later; conversely, those who initially describe themselves as relatively gloomy should score similarly upon retest. Second, traits must show consistency across different situations or contexts. For instance, individuals who are relatively cheerful and enthusiastic at work also should report similar feelings at home and at social gatherings. Similarly, those who are lively and ebullient with their friends should also be so when they are with family members, coworkers—even when they are alone.

In Chapter 5, I present extensive evidence demonstrating that affect scores exhibit both of these required characteristics, thereby confirming the existence of affective traits. Indeed, these traits exert a very strong influence on everyday affective experience.

Temperaments

Temperament is another concept that figures prominently in subsequent chapters. In many ways, this concept is quite similar to that of trait affect; however, there are two notable differences (Watson & Clark, 1994a). First, positing the existence of an affective trait simply acknowledges that stable individual differences exist and makes no assumption regarding *why* they exist. In other words, the concept of an affective trait has no necessary implications regarding the nature and origins of the trait. Accordingly, these broad and stable differences in affective experience may arise from hereditary influences, environmental factors, or some interaction between the two. In contrast, the concept of temperament implies that these observed individual differences are at least partly heritable and that they are to some extent already present at birth (Buss & Plomin, 1984).

Second, temperaments emerge as broader, more general dispositional constructs that subsume various emotional traits, along with other associated cognitive and behavioral characteristics. This can be illustrated by considering two general dimensions of temperament that figure prominently in later chapters. First, trait differences in negative mood are a centrally defining feature of a very broad temperamental dimension that is usually called Neuroticism or Negative Affectivity (e.g., Clark, Watson, & Mineka, 1994; McCrae & Costa, 1987; Watson & Clark, 1984, 1992b; Watson, Clark, & Harkness, 1994). Accordingly, individuals who are high in Neuroticism are prone to experience a diverse array of negative mood states, including anxiety, depression, hostility, and guilt.

In addition to this marked affective distress, however, high levels of

Neuroticism also are associated with various other cognitive and perceptual characteristics. For instance, high scorers on this disposition tend to be introspective and ruminative; perhaps as a result, they are prone to various types of psychosomatic complaints. They also have a negativistic cognitive/explanatory style; that is, they interpret ambiguous stimuli as reflecting threat or danger and focus differentially on negative aspects of themselves, other people, and the world in general. Consequently, they evaluate themselves unfavorably and tend to be highly dissatisfied. Finally, they experience high levels of stress in their lives and report that they cope poorly with this stress. In contrast, individuals who are low in Neuroticism tend to be content, secure, and self-satisfied and to report relatively low levels of both physical and psychological problems (McCrae & Costa, 1987; Watson & Clark, 1984; Watson et al., 1994).

In parallel fashion, trait differences in positive mood are a core component of the broad temperamental dimension of Extraversion or Positive Affectivity (McCrae & Costa, 1987; Watson & Clark, 1992b, 1997a; Watson et al, 1994). Extraverts tend to report elevated levels of positive mood; they describe themselves as cheerful, enthusiastic, confident, active, and energetic. In contrast, introverts experience generally lower levels of excitement, energy, and cheerfulness.

In addition to this positive affective core, however, Extraversion has broad social/interpersonal implications. That is, extraverts are gregarious, friendly, assertive, and socially facile, whereas introverts tend to be reserved, retiring, and somewhat aloof. Finally, extraversion may be related to other characteristics, such as the tendency to seek intense, highly stimulating experiences (McCrae & Costa, 1987; Watson & Clark, 1997a).

A SCHEMATIC MODEL OF AFFECTIVE EXPERIENCE

A major and long-standing theoretical issue in psychology—which has been of particular concern to personality researchers (see Kenrick & Funder, 1988)—is the relative importance of persons versus situations in human experience. Some readers may be curious about how this general issue applies specifically to the study of mood, wondering whether person-based factors (e.g., affective traits and temperaments) or situational and environmental factors (e.g., life events and the weather) are more important in understanding the vicissitudes of mood.

It generally is counterproductive to phrase this issue in a simplistic either–or manner, and it certainly makes little sense when it is applied specifically to the study of moods and feelings. This is because it is manifestly evident that trait/temperamental and situational/environmental factors both are extremely important in affective experience. On the one hand, we all experience major mood fluctuations in response to various situational and environmental factors: Giving a speech or going to the dentist may make us extremely apprehensive, whereas winning a contest or receiving praise may make us feel elated. On the other hand, it also is quite clear that the people we encounter in our lives differ markedly in their characteristic affective experience: Some tend to be happy, others more gloomy; some tend to be irascible, others friendly and unflappable.

Accordingly, trait/temperamental and situational/environmental factors both must figure prominently in any comprehensive model of affective experience. A few years ago, Clark and I (Watson & Clark, 1994c) proposed a schematic model that attempts to classify—in a broad and general manner—the incredibly diverse array of forces that can influence our moods and feelings. This conceptual scheme classifies the potentially important factors into four broad types. The first class of factors consists of the *affective traits and temperaments* that I have just discussed. These personological factors provide a long-term baseline or set point that is characteristic for each individual but differs markedly across different individuals (in fact, these characteristic baselines approximate a classic normal curve). Consider, for example, feelings of happiness, energy, and enthusiasm. At one extreme, relatively few individuals characteristically approach life with unrelenting exuberance, elation, and vigor; at the other, only a small group typically reports chronic feelings of unhappiness, disinterest, and gloom. Most of us, of course, fall somewhere between these two extremes, typically experiencing more moderate levels of cheerfulness, energy, and enthusiasm. These trait and temperamental factors are examined in Chapters 5 through 7.

Of course, each individual's mood varies considerably around his or her baseline. The three remaining classes of factors are responsible for these enormous fluctuations. The second class consists of various *exogenous factors*, that is, short-term situational or environmental variables that produce significant, transient fluctuations in mood. This class can be further divided into at least three quasi-distinct subgroups: (1) events and activities (e.g., giving a speech, exercising, and going to a party), (2) ingestion of substances (e.g., food and alcoholic beverages), and (3) physical aspects of the environment (e.g., temperature, humidity, noise level, and degree of crowding). These transient exogenous factors are the focus of Chapter 3. Note that because these factors themselves occur irregularly (e.g., most people do not go parties or get the same amount of exercise every day), they give rise to irregular mood fluctuations that are unevenly distributed over time.

In contrast, *endogenous and sociocultural rhythms* are associated with a natural, recurring cyclicity in experienced affect. Mood researchers have been particularly interested in four rhythmic patterns: (1) endogenous circadian or diurnal rhythms that produce systematic mood changes over the course of the day, (2) patterned variation across the days of the week, (3) the influence of the monthly menstrual cycle in women, and (4) systematic mood fluctuations across the seasons of the year (e.g., seasonal affective disorder). These rhythmic cycles are examined in Chapter 4, and we will see that they play an especially important role in positive mood variation.

Finally, recent evidence indicates that there are important individual differences in *characteristic variability.* That is, some individuals consistently display more variable moods than others. In popular terminology, some people simply are "moodier" than others. For example, although most individuals report relatively moderate fluctuations in their feelings of joy, energy, and enthusiasm, those suffering from a bipolar disorder (American Psychiatric Association, 1994) experience more dramatic changes: During a manic or hypomanic episode they may be euphoric, exuberant, hyperactive, and filled with a grandiose sense of optimism; when they are depressed, however, they are likely to be anhedonic, disinterested, listless, and filled with a pervasive sense of hopelessness and despair. These individual differences in characteristic variability have extremely important implications for our understanding of mood (see especially Depue, Krauss, & Spoont, 1987); they are discussed in Chapter 6.

Taken together, these four classes of factors provide a useful heuristic scheme for understanding the vicissitudes of mood. As I have noted, each of them is examined extensively in the chapters that follow.

BASIC THEORETICAL ASSUMPTIONS

Over the years, I have identified several basic theoretical principles that are central to my thinking about mood, and that increasingly have shaped and guided my research on this subject. As I have ventured deeper into this topic, I have become more and more convinced that these tenets are essential to any complete and satisfactory approach to the study of mood. Most of these principles are widely accepted among mood researchers, and some of them already have been formally acknowledged in the literature (cf. Thayer, 1989). On the other hand, none of them is so obvious or self-evident that it would be universally endorsed by all researchers in this area. Consequently, these principles should not be viewed as fundamental features of all contemporary mood models.

Primacy of Conscious, Subjective Experience

Earlier, I defined a mood as a transient episode of feeling or affect. Moreover, I argued that the concept of mood subsumed all subjective feeling states. It is hardly surprising, therefore, that I would maintain further that the scientific study of mood primarily involves an examination of conscious, subjective experience. In other words, rather than being primarily involved with cognitions, behaviors, facial expressions or physiological responses, mood research essentially is concerned with the experienced feelings of the individual. Thayer (1989) has articulated this principle quite well, stating: "Moods may be judged by behaviors, or they may even be inferred by bodily postures, but first and foremost, mood is part of consciousness. Certainly no conclusions regarding mood could be drawn without some sort of description or self-rating by an individual of how he or she feels" (p. 147).

This point may seem self-evident, but it becomes much less so when we consider its further implications. How exactly can we assess this subjective experience? It cannot be measured directly, because we lack direct access to the feelings of others. Ultimately, the best we can do—and this is a crucial point—is to ask people to *report* their feelings to us. Consequently, self-ratings of experienced affect are the clearest and most proximal measures of mood that are available. Of course, mood researchers make use of other forms of relevant data whenever possible, but we must rely primarily on self-reported affect. Moreover, in cases of apparent disagreement, self-ratings generally must be accorded primacy. Suppose, for instance, a person reports feeling extremely tense and nervous, but an electrocardiogram indicates only mild activation; in this case, the self-ratings ultimately provide our best estimate of the person's current mood state.

This point may be rather controversial, as psychologists—with some justification—long have viewed self-report data with considerable suspicion (for discussions, see Thayer, 1989; Watson & Clark, 1991b). This distrust, in fact, has led to the common practice of "validating" self-ratings by relating them to other types of evidence (e.g., peer reports and physiological responses); furthermore, in cases of apparent disagreement, it often has been concluded that the self-reports are invalid and untrustworthy.

Psychologists have voiced several general concerns regarding the use of self-ratings; four of these seem particularly applicable to mood research. First, people may present a biased view of themselves based on the *social desirability* of the terms they are rating. For instance, many people may be reluctant to admit—either to themselves or to others—that they experience socially disapproved feelings of anger, resentment, and rage. Thus, self-ratings often may be biased in such a way that respondents overreport pleasant, socially acceptable feelings and underreport socially undesirable states. Conversely, in certain settings (e.g., when suing for legal damages following an injury) people may be motivated to overreport negative mood states such as anxiety, depression, and hostility.

Second, participants in mood studies generally want to be cooperative. This may lead respondents to distort their ratings so that they support the perceived hypotheses of the study. For instance, suppose a researcher is interested in examining the effects of exercise on mood and therefore collects self-ratings both before and after a vigorous walk. Some participants might guess that the purpose of the experiment is to demonstrate that exercise leads to *improved mood* and adjust their ratings accordingly. A related idea is that mood ratings might be heavily biased by *expectancy effects*; for example, if people generally believe that exercise makes them feel better, they might adjust their self-ratings to match their preexisting expectations (see Thayer, 1989).

Third, if mood is assessed repeatedly (as frequently is necessary), people may begin to respond quickly and carelessly, even randomly. Suppose, for instance, that students are asked to fill out a mood questionnaire once every hour over the course of a day. For the first few assessments they may be eager to help; indeed, they even might find the task somewhat interesting. After several repetitions, however, they may come to view the ratings as intrusive and annoying, so that their primary motivation is to complete them as quickly (and with as little thought) as possible (Stone, Kessler, & Haythornwaite, 1991).

Finally, people might interpret the anchoring points of mood rating scales idiosyncratically, so that they use numbers in characteristically different ways. For instance, recall the 5-point rating scale described earlier (*very slightly or not at all, a little, moderately, very much, extremely*). Some people might interpret the anchoring term "moderately" quite liberally, so that their self-reports are filled with ratings of 3 or greater. In contrast, other people might use much more stringent standards in applying this anchoring term, so that—even when they are experiencing the same intensity of feeling—their ratings consist primarily of 1s and 2s. Idiosyncratic interpretations of this sort can be expected to produce systematic distortions whenever one attempts to compare the responses of these different types of individuals (Green, Goldman, & Salovey, 1993).

These concerns all are quite legitimate. Fortunately, none of them has emerged as a crippling problem in mood research, in large part because researchers have been aware of them and have worked hard to minimize their influence. For instance, although socially desirable responding can be a major problem in some types of psychological assessment (imagine, for example, that you knew that your responses to a personality questionnaire might determine whether or not you were offered a job), it is much less so in mood research because participants typically (1) are assured of confidentiality, so that their responses will be seen only by the researcher, and (2) are tested under circumstances in which socially undesirable responses do not have any obvious negative consequences (such as criticism or disapproval).

Expectancy and related effects can be more of a problem, but they can be minimized through careful research designs. For example, my colleagues and I have conducted a number of studies in which students initially rate their current mood and then note whether or not they engaged in several activities (exercise, social interaction, eating, etc.) during the previous hour. With repeated assessment, the rating process becomes increasingly automatic, so that the students give less and less thought to the significance of their responses; consequently, expectancy effects are of little concern (see also Thayer, 1989). In fact, we will see subsequently that this type of design frequently produces findings that differ quite markedly from the respondents' preexisting expectations.

To reduce fatigue and boredom, mood researchers space out assessments as widely as possible over time; to return to an earlier example, because responding once an hour over the course of a day would be both intrusive and fatiguing, I have never asked study participants to follow this intensive a schedule. For similar reasons, we are careful to terminate within-subject studies of momentary or daily mood before the sheer repetition of responding becomes overwhelming. Furthermore, most investigators maintain periodic contact with participants in these within-subject studies in order to maintain their personal involvement and enthusiasm (see Thayer, 1989; Zevon & Tellegen, 1982).

Finally, as noted earlier, idiosyncratic interpretations and alternative rating strategies can lead to systematic distortions in between-subject analyses (i.e., those in which the responses of different individuals are compared). However, these problems can be circumvented quite easily by employing a within-subject design in which each respondent serves as his or her own control; consequently, mood researchers have relied heavily on these designs in recent years.

Thus, careful research designs can minimize potential problems that frequently arise with self-report data. I emphasize, however, that mood researchers do not accept self-ratings uncritically. Anyone who has ever worked with such data realizes that they are influenced by both random and systematic measurement errors and are far from perfect. Nevertheless, even with these problems and imperfections, self-ratings provide the clearest and best measures of mood that are available.

Moods Are Components of Broader Biobehavioral Systems

Although mood is primarily concerned with subjective experience, this experience obviously does not exist in complete isolation. Rather, subjective mood states are components of broader, more complex biobehavioral systems. Specifically, beginning with the seminal work of Gray (1981, 1982, 1985), a growing body of evidence has suggested that negative mood experience is part of a larger Behavioral Inhibition System (BIS), whereas positive mood experience is linked to what has variously been called the Behavioral Activation System, Behavioral Engagement System, or Behavioral Facilitation System (see Depue & Iacono, 1989; Depue et al., 1987; Depue, Luciana, Arbisi, Collins, & Leon, 1994; Fowles, 1980, 1987, 1992; Tellegen, 1985).

These biobehavioral systems are discussed in much greater detail in subsequent chapters. For now, I note simply that they contain at least four differentiable aspects or components: the affective (i.e., the subjective mood state), the cognitive, the biological, and the behavioral. As an illustration, let us consider the operation of the Behavioral Facilitation System (BFS; Depue & Iacono, 1989). At one extreme, the BFS is associated with elevated levels of positive mood, such that the individual reports feeling elated, enthusiastic, and energetic (affective component). These feelings likely are accompanied by a heightened sense of self-worth and self-efficacy and by a pervasive confidence and optimism (cognitive component). Furthermore, a person in this state is quick and quite active and is either engaged in—or is actively seeking—interesting and rewarding experiences (behavioral component). Finally, this state appears to be associated with heightened activity of the mesolimbic dopaminergic system (biological component; see Depue et al., 1994). At the other extreme, an individual feels depressed, anhedonic, disinterested, and unenergetic; experiences reduced self-esteem and self-efficacy and is overpowered by a pervasive sense of pessimism and hopelessness; is slow and largely inactive and fails to engage in behaviors that normally are pleasurable and rewarding; and shows reduced dopaminergic activity (see Depue et al., 1987).

The existence of these subcomponents inevitably raises the further issue of *causal primacy*. That is, which component emerges first and causes others to occur? For instance, Lazarus (1982, 1984) argued that cognitions arise first and subsequently produce the experienced affect, whereas Zajonc (1980, 1984) asserted that affects can arise independently and induce cognitive changes. In a related vein, James (1884) posited that biological changes precede the onset of subjective experience (James, 1884), whereas Cannon (1927) argued that the two components arise simultaneously. Finally, some models emphasize that affect motivates behavior, whereas other schemes assume that behavior generates affect (see Watson, Clark, McIntyre, & Hamaker, 1992).

I believe that framing the issue in this manner is unproductive. My own view is that these different components naturally exist *in synchrony* with one another. Furthermore, this natural synchrony is no accident but, rather has evolved through natural selection: Specifically, these biobehavioral systems contain feedback loops that pass information between the various subcomponents and ensure that they remain in concert with one another. Because of these feedback loops, certain affective/cognitive/biobehavioral combinations represent stable states that have a higher probability of initial occurrence and are much more likely to persist over time; other combinations, however, represent improbable, unsteady states that quickly necessitate further changes in the system to restore synchrony across the various components.

For instance, a person who is subjectively nervous and apprehensive, and who also is experiencing marked activation of the sympathetic nervous system, is in a synchronous, stable state; in contrast, someone who experiences feelings of panic and terror but is unaroused physiologically would be in an unstable, desynchronous state. In the latter case, strong pressure would be exerted to induce change on one or both of the components, thereby restoring synchrony. In fact, a key principle of systematic desensitization (Wolpe, 1961)—a widely used treatment for fears and phobias—is that it is impossible for a person to remain subjectively anxious and agitated when he or she is physiologically relaxed. Consequently, patients are trained in deep muscle relaxation, which enables them to respond to the phobic object with reduced levels of fear and anxiety.

A further implication of this argument is that *altering the organism's standing on any one component necessarily produces corresponding changes in all the others.* In other words, inducing a change on any one component produces a desynchronous, unstable state and, therefore, strong pressure for further, corresponding changes on the others. For example, although it is synchronous to be depressed, pessimistic, and inactive, it is incongruous to be depressed, *optimistic,* and inactive; accordingly, altering the individual's cognitive state can be expected to generate comparable changes on the other components. In this regard, it is interesting to note that the mood disorder of depression (a state that essentially represents the low end of the BFS; see Depue et al., 1987) can be successfully treated by changing the individual's internal biological state (e.g., Davidson, Giller, Zisook, & Overall, 1988; Elkin et al., 1989), ongoing cognitions (e.g., Beck, 1976, 1991), or physical activity level (e.g., Bosscher, 1993; Martinsen, 1993). Thus, consistent with the model outlined here, inducing change in any part of this biobehavioral system leads to more general changes across all aspects of the system.

Mood Has Important Directive Properties

Because these components exist in synchrony with one another, they all act as both causes and effects. For example, as I have already suggested, altering an individual's cognitive state should produce comparable affective, biological, and behavioral changes in order to restore synchrony. On the other hand, it is equally true that substantial fluctuations in mood will quickly generate corresponding cognitive, behavioral, and biological effects. Similarly, altering the biological or behavioral substrates should cause systematic changes in the remaining components. Thus, no component in the system possesses an intrinsic causal primacy over any of the others.

Consequently, moods are not simply effects. They also are important causal variables that can motivate and direct behavior, produce systematic changes in thoughts and attitudes, and so on. This is a crucial point, because even with the recent upsurge of interest in affect, psychologists have tended to view moods as effects or dependent variables rather than as active causal agents. For instance, cognitive therapists typically have assigned causal primacy to cognitions over affects. That is, they have argued that irrational beliefs (Ellis, 1962, 1987), dysfunctional attitudes and schema (Beck, 1976, 1991), and maladaptive attributions (Abramson, Seligman, & Teasdale, 1978) give rise to negative affective conditions such as depression and anxiety. In contrast, relatively few therapists have entertained the alternative possibility that negative affective states may serve as underlying causal forces that lead to irrational beliefs, dysfunctional attitudes, and maladaptive attributions (for a discussion of this point, see Thayer, 1989). Similarly, many more studies have examined moods as potential effects of various events and activities (e.g., socializing and exercise) rather than as possible causes of such activities.

One of the primary goals of this book is to counteract this unfortunate and unwarranted bias. Accordingly, throughout this book I present evidence establishing that moods are important causal agents that motivate and direct various types of behavior and a wide range of cognitive processes.

Mood-Regulating Systems Evolved and Have Adaptive Value

The next basic principle—which likely is the least controversial of all those I am presenting here—is that the systems that regulate our experienced mood states (i.e., the BIS and BFS) gradually evolved through a process of natural selection. This, in turn, suggests that these evolved systems facilitated the survival of the individual (or, more precisely, that of his or her genes; see Hamilton, 1964) better than any of the earlier alternatives. Thus, even though these systems can go awry and affective states can become highly dysfunctional (which is the focus of Chapter 8), we can assume with some confidence that moods generally serve important adaptive functions and have significant survival value (Beck, 1987; Clark & Watson, 1994; Thayer, 1989). In fact, much of the mystery that traditionally has enveloped mood can be eliminated by considering the adaptive functions that affects normally serve.

What adaptive functions do our moods serve? To answer this question, we need to consider these two general biobehavioral systems in greater detail. As discussed previously, negative mood states (e.g., feelings of sadness, nervousness, irritability, and guilt) have been linked to the BIS. In behavioral terms, the essential purpose of the BIS is to keep the organism out of trouble—that is, it seeks to inhibit behavior that might lead to pain, punishment, or some other unpleasant consequence. Put another way, the primary function of this system is to help the organism *avoid* various types of aversive stimuli. For instance, fear motivates organisms to escape from situations of potential threat or danger. Similarly, anticipatory feelings of apprehension and worry help individuals to avoid situations that have been previously associated with pain and punishment. In a related vein, feelings of disgust and revulsion help to keep organisms away from noxious or toxic substances (Fowles, 1980, 1987, 1992; Tellegen, 1985).

As noted earlier, positive mood states (e.g., feelings of joy, interest, enthusiasm, energy, and alertness) have been linked to a different biobehavioral system, the BFS. The BFS is an appetitive system of behavioral *approach*: It directs organisms toward situations and experiences that potentially may yield pleasure and reward. Fowles (1987) describes it as "a reward-seeking or approach system that responds to positive incentives by *activating* behavior" (p. 418; emphasis in original). The adaptive function of the BFS differs markedly from that of the BIS, but it is crucial nonetheless: In essence, its role is to ensure that organisms obtain the resources (e.g., food and water, warmth and shelter, the assistance of others, and sexual partners) that are necessary for the survival of both the individual and the species.

Positive and Negative Moods Must Be Assessed Separately

It is commonly believed that moods reflect a single, basic continuum of "good versus bad" feeling. In other words, it is assumed that a person's current mood can be broadly characterized as either good/positive or bad/negative (see Thayer, 1989, for a discussion). Although it is usually not formally expressed in these terms, this naive viewpoint further implies that positive and negative moods are contradictory and are mutually exclusive of one another. For instance, if I am feeling cheerful and enthusiastic, I cannot be feeling sad, enraged, or terrified. Note that this view further implies that one can achieve a rough sketch of ongoing mood by assessing a person's standing on this single dimension of good versus bad feeling.

This commonsense model is not entirely wrong. Specifically, extremely high levels of one type of mood tend to be associated with extremely low levels of the other. For instance, it is rare for individuals who report feeling terrified and panic stricken (or, alternatively, enraged and furious) to also describe themselves as extremely cheerful and enthusiastic. Put another way, extremely high levels of negative mood are largely incompatible with high levels of positive mood, and vice versa (Diener & Iran-Nejad, 1986; Watson, 1988b).

However, I already have shown that such extreme episodes are relatively rare in everyday experience; instead, our daily experience consists primarily of low to moderate intensity states. When applied to such states, the commonsense model is no longer accurate. That is, at these more moderate levels of intensity, positive and negative moods are not contradictory or mutually exclusive; rather, they operate largely independently of one another. For example, someone who is mildly or moderately nervous may be very enthusiastic, quite unenthusiastic, or (more likely) somewhere between these two extremes. Conversely, someone who is moderately cheerful and enthusiastic may be nervous, calm, or at some intermediate point. In other words, knowing someone's current level of negative mood says very little about the intensity of his or her positive mood: It may be high, low, or intermediate. Because of this, it is essential that these two types of affective experience be assessed and analyzed separately.

In the next chapter, I present extensive evidence demonstrating that positive and negative moods do, in fact, vary more or less independently of one another. However, because this finding is counterintuitive, it is important to consider *why* it has emerged so clearly in our mood data. In other words, why do positive and negative moods fluctuate independently of one another?

At one level, the answer to this question already is clear from my earlier discussion of the two biobehavioral systems. Recall that positive and negative moods have been linked to two (very different) systems: Negative mood states are related to the BIS, whereas positive moods are associated with the BFS. Consequently, it should not come as a great surprise that these two types of moods operate at least quasi-independently of one another.

However, we can take this analysis a bit further and suggest two specific reasons—both of them arising from the highly distinctive functions of these two systems—for this quasi-independence. First, as discussed earlier, the BIS is primarily concerned with the avoidance of painful and punishing stimuli, whereas the BFS is primarily related to the procurement of pleasurable and rewarding stimuli. Accordingly, positive and negative moods should be associated with different types of events and experiences. On the one hand, negative moods should be highly sensitive to the imminent possibility of danger, pain, or punishment. For instance, negative mood should be significantly elevated under the threat of shock, or when an individual is about to undergo a painful medical or dental procedure. In contrast, because these situations invoke issues that are much less relevant to the logic and operation of the BFS, they should be more weakly related to fluctuations in positive mood. Conversely, appetitive and rewarding behaviors (e.g., eating and sexual activity) should be more strongly associated with fluctuations in positive mood than in negative mood.

In Chapter 3, I show that these expectations are extensively supported by recent data, and that positive and negative moods are, in fact, associated with different types of events and experiences. These differential affinities are an important cause of the observed independence between these two types of mood states.

The second reason can be derived from a basic principle that was briefly discussed earlier, namely, all other things being equal, low-activation states (which consume less energy and put less of a strain on bodily resources) are preferable to high-activation states. In other words, deactivated, low-intensity states represent the normal, baseline "steady" state of the organism. Of course, circumstances frequently require greater expenditures of energy from the organism, but these high-energy episodes should be engaged in sparingly. In fact, we can specify further that *high-activation states are to be avoided unless they are likely to yield some significant advantage to the organism.*

In light of this principle—and considering the very different functions subsumed by the BIS and BFS—negative and positive moods can be expected to show different patterns over time. On the one hand, negative moods should be essentially *reactive* in character. That is, it is inefficient and maladaptive for individuals to experience strong feelings of fear, anger, or disgust in the absence of some clear precipitating stimulus or event. However, when confronted with some type of threat, the individual should experience a sudden, sharp increase in negative mood to help resolve the crisis; after the emergency has passed, negative mood should quickly return to its basal level. Thus, although the individual must remain vigilant for potential threat or danger, negative moods can be expected to remain at low, baseline levels during the bulk of daily life, with periodic sharp elevations corresponding to these short-term crises. In Chapter 3, I present data confirming this predicted temporal pattern.

Note also that according to this same logic, negative moods should not be subject to any strong endogenous cycles. For instance, there is no compelling reason why one should tend to experience a marked upsurge of fear at a particular time each day, such as 10 A.M. or 3 P.M.; rather, whether or not one is fearful and apprehensive should primarily be a function of ongoing events and circumstances.

However, the BFS operates according to a different logic. Recall that the essential function of this system is to ensure that the organism obtains necessary resources. Although the behaviors subsumed by this system (e.g., eating, socializing and sexual activity) are essential to survival, they lack the reactive, context-bound character of those subsumed by the BIS. For instance, it is critically important that animals be alert and apprehensive in situations of potential threat, and that they respond quickly and decisively when danger is apparent. In other words, it is essential that the various components of the BIS be activated in specific circumstances. In sharp contrast, although it is essential that BFS-related behaviors be performed with some frequency, exactly *when, where, and how* they are emitted is much less crucial for survival. For example, although it also is absolutely necessary that an animal consumes enough food to survive, its precise eating regimen (i.e., exactly when and where and what it eats) need not be rigidly specified in advance.

What, then, determines when these appetitive behaviors will be performed? Because these approach behaviors represent high-activation states, they should tend to be emitted when reward is likely and avoided when it is not. Accordingly, these behaviors (and the positive moods associated with them) should show strong, systematic cyclic trends that vary widely across species but are highly consistent within species. For instance, members of a given species should tend be active, alert, and energetic at those times of the day when food and other resources are easily obtainable and the risk of harm is relatively low; conversely, they should be sluggish, unenergetic and disengaged when resources are less available or the threat of danger is relatively greater. Similarly, it is adaptive to be more active during those times of the year when food is plentiful (i.e., the spring and summer) than when it is scarce (i.e., the winter).

Thus, preprogrammed rhythmic variation should be a basic feature of the BFS in general, and of positive moods in particular. In Chapter 4, I offer support for this theoretical argument by establishing that positive affective states vary as a function of endogenous biological rhythms, such as body temperature and the sleep–wake cycle.

It should no longer be surprising that positive and negative moods vary rather independently of one another. As we have seen, the negative affects are highly reactive and are strongly associated with painful and punishing stimuli. They tend to remain at low, baseline levels until the individual is faced with some sort of threat or crisis, at which point the individual experiences a sudden, sharp upsurge in negative mood; after the crisis has been resolved, these moods quickly return to their basal level. In sharp contrast, positive moods are strongly rhythmic and are related to various types of pleasurable and rewarding stimuli. They show broad and systematic fluctuations that result both from preprogrammed cycles and from ongoing feedback from the environment.

CONCLUSION

This opening chapter introduced the basic themes and concepts of this book. I began by distinguishing "moods" from "emotions" and then discussed why the former provides a better working model for understanding everyday experience than does the latter. Next, I examined evidence indicating that waking consciousness is experienced as a continuous *stream of affect*, which typically consists of a mildly positive mood. I then articulated a basic schematic model of affect that included four general classes of variables (affective traits and temperaments, short-term exogenous factors, endogenous and sociocultural rhythms, and individual differences in characteristic variability). Finally, I discussed five basic theoretical assumptions that have guided my thinking in this area. I explore these themes, concepts, and principles in greater detail throughout the remainder of the book.

2

MEASURING MOOD:
A STRUCTURAL MODEL

This chapter discusses key issues in the measurement of mood. This is a crucial topic with profound implications for the remainder of this book. Affective experience clearly is complex, and the number of potentially interesting feeling states (e.g., joy, excitement, love, affection, amazement, nostalgia, contentment, fatigue, irritation, nervousness, guilt, loneliness, and depression) seems virtually limitless. Out of this vast array of candidates, how can one select a manageable set of mood states to study systematically?

Most people intuitively view affective experience in terms of specific, distinct mood states that roughly correspond to the fundamental emotions posited in the classical theories (e.g., feelings of fear, anger, sadness, and joy). For several decades this commonsense view was adopted by psychological investigators, who conducted thousands of studies on such specific affective states as depression, anxiety, hostility, shame and joy (see, e.g., Lubin, Zuckerman, & Woodward, 1985; Spielberger, 1983).

In recent years, however, mood researchers have become increasingly dissatisfied with this discrete affect approach (although specific affects still are very widely studied); in its place, they have turned to models that emphasize the importance of a few general mood dimensions. This conceptual shift has occurred because of a highly robust finding that was briefly discussed in Chapter 1, namely, that pure, unmixed affective states are relatively rare in everyday life. For instance, it repeatedly has been found that individuals who experience prominent levels of depression also report significant amounts of anxiety and hostility (e.g., Gotlib, 1984; Mineka, Watson, & Clark, 1998). In other words, it is difficult to find individuals who report one type of negative affect without also experiencing one or more of the others. Consequently, one encounters serious conceptual and data-analytic problems if one focuses solely on specific types of affect. General dimensional models circumvent these problems by collapsing closely related affects into broader, nonspecific measures of mood. In essence, this dimensional approach assumes that it is better to assess a few relatively independent dimensions than several strongly correlated (and, hence, semioverlapping and redundant) discrete affects.

Two alternative models of this type—both of them consisting of two broad and nonspecific dimensions—figure prominently in the contemporary mood literature. First, many mood researchers advocate an approach consisting of (1) Pleasantness versus Unpleasantness and (2) Activation, Arousal, or Engagement (e.g., Feldman Barrett & Russell, 1998; Larsen & Diener, 1992; Russell, 1980; Russell & Carroll, 1999). The first of these dimensions, Pleasantness–Unpleasantness, has a certain intuitive appeal, as it orders affective experience along a broad continuum of good versus bad feeling. That is, affective experience is reduced to the simple classification of whether it feels good (i.e., pleasant) or bad (i.e., unpleasant) to the individual. At the pleasant extreme, one feels wonderful—happy, enthusiastic, and content—without any substantial problems or concerns. Conversely, at the unpleasant extreme, one feels absolutely terrible—depressed, irritable, tense, and guilty—without any hint of positivity whatsoever. In contrast, Activation represents the extent to which one is feeling aroused and energized. This concept is based on the idea that most states of strong emotion—whether negative (e.g., fear and anger) or positive (e.g., elation and excitement)—are associated both with increased physiological arousal and with a subjective sense of heightened energy and activation (Izard, 1977, 1991; Thayer, 1989).

According to this model, affective experience can be neatly summarized by assessing an individual's position on these two general dimensions. Put another way, finer differentiations (e.g., whether the individual is feeling anxious or guilty) are viewed as relatively unimportant in this approach. Obviously, adopting this model greatly simplifies mood assessment: Instead of measuring multiple discrete affects, one needs only two broad scales, one for each of the general dimensions. Note, moreover, that this model suggests that mood states can be classified into four basic types: pleasant and activated (e.g., elation), pleasant and unaroused (e.g., relaxation), unpleasant and activated (e.g., irritation), and unpleasant and unaroused (e.g., boredom).

My colleagues and I have proposed an alternative two-dimensional model that also has been quite influential in the mood literature (Tellegen, 1985; Watson & Clark, 1997b; Watson & Tellegen, 1985; Watson, Wiese, Vaidya, & Tellegen, 1999). Rather than Pleasantness–Unpleasantness and Activation, it focuses on the general dimensions of Negative Affect and Positive Affect. The Negative Affect dimension represents the extent to which one is (nonspecifically) experiencing some type of negative mood, such as feelings of nervousness, sadness, irritation, and guilt. In contrast, Positive Affect reflects the extent to which one is experiencing some type of positive mood, such as feelings of joy, energy, enthusiasm, and alertness. This model emphasizes the fundamental distinction between positive and negative affective experience, thereby embodying one of the basic principles articulated in Chapter 1. That is, it essentially posits that one can summarize affective experience by assessing the extent to which one is experiencing positive moods and negative moods. Furthermore, because positive and negative moods are viewed as distinct from one another, one again can classify affective states into four basic types: (1) high positive/low negative (e.g., feeling happy), (2) high positive/high negative (e.g., the mixture of fear and excitement one feels on a roller coaster), (3) low positive/high negative (e.g., feeling depressed), and (4) low positive/low negative (e.g., the relatively disengaged state that many people report while watching television).

Although these rival two-dimensional schemes may appear to be quite different, these differences actually are only superficial. In fact, these two models are equally capable of explaining observed phenomena and are mathematically derivable from one another (see Feldman Barrett & Russell, 1998; Larsen & Diener, 1992; Tellegen, 1985; Watson, 1988b; Watson & Tellegen, 1985). Moreover, findings derived from one scheme easily can be translated into the other. For instance, measures of Positive and Negative Affect can be converted into rough measures of Pleasantness and Activation, respectively, by first subtracting them (i.e., Pleasantness = Positive Affect – Negative Affect) and then adding them (i.e., Activation = Positive Affect + Negative Affect). For reasons discussed in Chapter 1, I believe that the distinction between positive and negative affective experience is essential, and I therefore prefer to conceptualize mood in terms of Positive Affect and Negative Affect. Accordingly, I focus on these dimensions throughout this book.

As I stated earlier, these general dimensional models have become quite prominent in the mood literature. Nevertheless, they remain confusing and mysterious to many people. Certainly, some of the key implications of these models are counterintuitive and contrary to traditional thinking in this area. For instance, the subjective experiences of anger and fear seem radically different from one another: Why, then, ignore the distinction between them and simply consider both to be manifestations of general Negative Affect? Furthermore, how is it possible to experience positive and negative feelings at the same time: Is it possible for one to be both happy and sad simultaneously? Because of these lingering doubts and concerns, I devote much of this chapter to an examination of the limitations of the traditional, discrete–affect approach as well as to a review of the evidence that makes these general dimensions essential in the assessment of mood.

THE PANAS-X

As I stated earlier, psychologists have conducted thousands of studies examining specific, discrete mood states. The vast majority of these studies have examined some type of negative affect, largely because of the central importance of negative moods in psychopathology and physical illness (topics I return to in Chapters 8 and 9). Because of this intense interest in the negative affects, researchers have created several widely used inventories to measure depression (e.g., Beck, Rush, Shaw, & Emery, 1979; Radloff, 1977; Zung, 1965), anxiety (e.g., Beck, Epstein, Brown, & Steer, 1988; Spielberger, Gorsuch, Lushene, Vagg, & Jacobs, 1983; Zung, 1971), and anger/hostility (Cook & Medley, 1954; Spielberger, Jacobs, Russell, & Crane, 1983).

In addition, researchers have created more comprehensive measures that are designed to assess several different affective states in a single questionnaire. Three of these have been especially prominent in the mood literature. First, the Profile of Mood States (POMS; McNair, Lorr, & Droppleman, 1971) consists of six basic scales: Tension–Anxiety, Depression–Dejection, Anger–Hostility, Fatigue, Confusion–Bewilderment, and Vigor. Similarly, the revised Multiple Affect Adjective Check List (MAACL-R; Zuckerman & Lubin, 1985) contains five scales, three of which (Anxiety, Depression, Hostility) clearly measure the same basic affects as similarly labeled scales on the POMS. The two remaining MAACL-R scales—Positive Affect and Sensation Seeking—both contain content included in the POMS Vigor scale. Finally, the DES (Izard, Dougherty, Bloxom, & Kotsch, 1974; Izard, Libero, Putnam, & Haynes, 1993) was designed to assess the fundamental emotions posited in the classical theories. It contains 12 affect scales: Fear, Sadness, Anger, Contempt, Disgust, Hostility Inward, Guilt, Shame, Shyness, Surprise, Interest, and Enjoyment.

Clark and I have developed our own comprehensive mood inventory, the Positive and Negative Affect Schedule—Expanded Form (PANAS-X; Watson & Clark, 1994b). The PANAS-X is an extension of an earlier instrument called the Positive and Negative Affect Schedule, or PANAS (Watson, Clark, & Tellegen, 1988). The original PANAS consisted simply of two 10-item scales that measure the general Positive Affect and Negative Affect dimensions discussed in the previous section. In addition to these two general scales, the PANAS-X contains 11 scales that assess specific types of affect. Table 2.1 presents these scales—together with sample items. It can be seen that these PANAS-X scales measure affects that generally correspond to the fundamental emotions of the classical theories. Moreover, they assess states that are comparable to those contained in the POMS, MAACL-R, and DES.

Most of these scales are quite narrow in content, containing closely related terms that reflect a single core mood state. For instance, Fear contains terms such as "scared," "frightened," and "nervous"; Sadness includes "sad," "blue," and "lonely"; and Fatigue contains "sleepy," "sluggish," and "drowsy." In terms of content, the two broadest scales are: (1) Hostility, which contains descriptors reflecting the emotions of anger (e.g., "irritable" and "angry"), disgust ("disgusted") and contempt

TABLE 2.1. The Specific Affect Scales Contained in the Expanded Form of the Positive and Negative Affect Schedule (PANAS-X)

Scale	Sample items	Internal consistency reliability[a]
Basic negative affects		
Fear (6)	Frightened, scared, nervous	.87
Sadness (5)	Sad, blue, lonely	.87
Guilt (6)	Guilty, ashamed, angry at self	.88
Hostility (6)	Angry, disgusted, scornful	.85
Basic positive affects		
Joviality (8)	Happy, enthusiastic, energetic	.93
Self-Assurance (6)	Proud, confident, daring	.83
Attentiveness (4)	Alert, concentrating, determined	.78
Other affective states		
Shyness (4)	Shy, bashful, timid	.83
Fatigue (4)	Sleepy, sluggish, drowsy	.88
Serenity (3)	Calm, relaxed, at ease	.76
Surprise (3)	Surprised, amazed, astonished	.77

Note. The number of items comprising each scale is shown in parentheses.
[a] Cronbach's coefficient alpha. These are median values computed across 11 samples with a total *N* of 8,194 (adapted from Watson & Clark, 1994b, Table 12).

("scornful"); and (2) Joviality, which includes several items related to the basic emotion of joy (e.g., "happy," "joyful," and "cheerful"), as well as terms reflecting enthusiasm ("excited," "enthusiastic") and energy ("lively," "energetic"). Even these broader scales are relatively homogeneous, however, and their content is easily distinguishable from that contained in the other scales.

These 11 PANAS-X scales were developed through factor analysis, a multivariate technique that allows one to identify clusters of interrelated variables. Once these intercorrelated variables have been identified, they can be combined into reliable and homogeneous scales. Consequently, the PANAS-X scales are homogeneous and highly reliable, despite the fact that they are relatively short. This also is shown in Table 2.1, which displays internal consistency reliabilities (Cronbach's coefficient alpha) for each scale. The values shown are median reliability estimates computed across 11 samples. The individual sample sizes ranged from 107 to 1,657, with a combined total of 8,194 observations. The respondents completed the scales using one of eight different temporal instructions, rating how they felt (1) "right now, that is, at the present moment" (Moment instructions), (2) "today" (Today), (3) "during the past few days" (Past few days), (4) "during the past week" (Past week), (5) "during the past few weeks" (Past few weeks), (6) "during the past month" (Past month), (7) "during the past year" (Past year), and (8) "in general, that is, on the average" (General) (see Watson & Clark, 1994b).

The longer (i.e., five- to eight-item) scales all have excellent reliabilities, with values ranging from .83 (Self-Assurance) to .93 (Joviality). Moreover, two of the four-item scales—Fatigue (.88) and Shyness (.83)—also are highly reliable. The three remaining scales—Attentiveness, Serenity, and Surprise—yield slightly lower reliability estimates. Note, however, that their median reliability values (.76 to .78) reflect average interitem correlations of .45 or greater, indicating that these scales are, in fact, homogeneous; their lower reliability estimates simply reflect the fact that they have relatively few items.

Watson and Clark (1994b) present additional evidence that establishes the reliability and validity of the PANAS-X scales. For instance, they showed that trait (i.e., General) forms of these scales were strongly stable over time and systematically related to measures of personality and emotionality. Furthermore, self-ratings on these scales correlated significantly with corresponding judgments made by well-acquainted peers. Similarly, state versions of the scales had strong and theoretically appropriate correlations with commonly used measures of mood and psychopathology. This reliability and validity evidence is examined in detail throughout the remainder of this book. For the current discussion, the crucial point is that these 11 PANAS-X scales were carefully constructed and have been extensively validated. Moreover, the PANAS-X is similar to other widely used mood inventories, such as the POMS, MAACL-R, and DES. Accordingly, the data I present do not reflect problems unique to the PANAS-X; rather, these results are typical of what one obtains with any of the commonly used mood inventories.

RELATIONS AMONG AFFECTS WITH THE SAME VALENCE

The Negative Affects

The 11 specific PANAS-X scales are reliable, valid, and perfectly reasonable measures. Why, then, not focus simply on them? Why have mood researchers increasingly turned to general dimensional measures of Positive and Negative Affect? To answer these questions, we have to explore the underlying *structure* of mood ratings—that is, we have to examine relations among individual mood terms and scales.

I discuss three basic and robust structural properties of mood ratings. The first of these properties (which we can term the "convergent" property) is that affects with the same valence (i.e., both are pleasant/positive or unpleasant/negative) tend to be substantially positively intercorrelated. For instance, on the basis of this principle, one would expect ratings of nervousness to be significantly positively related to reports of annoyance; in other words, as ratings of nervousness increase in magnitude, so should reports of annoyance. Similarly, ratings of two positive mood states—say, enthusiasm and alertness—also should be significantly positively intercorrelated.

To illustrate this properly, I first examine relations among the various negative affects. Table 2.1 indicates that four PANAS-X scales have been classified as "basic negative affects." This classification reflects the fact that these four types of negative mood are especially strongly interrelated. Table 2.2 presents illustrative correlations among these four PANAS-X scales. Shown are data from two large data sets: (1) 1,657 college students who rated themselves using General, trait instructions, and (2) 1,027 students who rated their current, momentary mood.

Let us consider the General ratings first. All four negative mood scales are strongly interrelated in these data; the correlations range from .53 to .62, with a mean value of .57. These data indicate that these negative affects systematically covary with one another such that individuals who report significant amounts of one type of negative emotion also tend to experience elevated levels of the others. Put another way, highly fearful individuals also typically report substantial levels of sadness, anger, and guilt.

TABLE 2.2. Correlations among the Basic Negative Affect Scales of the PANAS-X

Scale	1	2	3	4
1. Fear	—	.57	.56	.53
2. Sadness	.55	—	.62	.55
3. Guilt	.40	.51	—	.57
4. Hostility	.47	.55	.53	—

Note. Correlations above the diagonal are trait ratings (N = 1,657) in which students rated how they "generally" felt. Correlations below the diagonal are state ratings (N = 1,027) in which students rated how they felt "right now, that is, at the present moment." All correlations are significant at $p < .001$.

One might suspect that this correlational pattern is restricted to long-term, trait ratings of affect. For instance, one might plausibly suggest that it largely results from the responses of highly neurotic individuals who eventually report increased problems of all kinds. At any given point in time, these individuals might experience a specific problem such as depression or anxiety; over the long run, however, they will report higher levels of depression, anxiety, hostility, and guilt (and perhaps many other difficulties as well) than anyone else. However, Table 2.2 demonstrates that this type of explanation cannot explain the data, because one sees an extremely similar pattern in momentary mood ratings. The correlations in the moment ratings range from .40 to .55, with a mean value of .50. In other words, even at a specific moment in time, respondents typically do not report pure mood states but, instead, experience mixed states of non-specific negative affect.

The findings presented in Table 2.2 all are based on a classic between-subject design in which large numbers of individuals each are assessed once. In this design, the responses of each person are compared to those of all the others. Accordingly, these data simply establish that some individuals report more fear, sadness, guilt, and hostility than do others. It might still be argued, however, that these results reflect some sort of response bias or other artifact that can plague between-subject designs (see Green et al., 1993) and, therefore, that they might not capture the structure of mood fluctuations *within* an individual. In other words, when I experience an increased level of sadness, do I also report concomitant increases in the other negative affects? To answer this sort of question, we need to conduct within-subject analyses of each individual respondent.

With the collaboration of Cathey Soutter, I have investigated the structural properties of the PANAS-X in two large within-subject data sets. The first consisted of 226 college students who rated their current, momentary mood repeatedly over a 1- to 2-month period. The students completed one mood assessment a day; the times for these ratings varied from day to day according to a prearranged, randomized schedule. These individuals completed a total of 10,169 observations (*M* = 45.0 per person). The second data set consisted of 254 students who rated themselves over a 1- to 2-month period using Today instructions. Again, the students completed one mood questionnaire a day; all ratings were made in the evening so that they would provide a reasonable estimate of their moods over the course of the day. These individuals completed a total of 11,322 mood observations (*M* = 44.6 per person). All students in both data sets completed a minimum of 35 mood assessments.

I computed correlations among the Fear, Sadness, Guilt, and Hostility scales individually for each person, and then calculated overall mean correlations for each scale pair (e.g., between Fear and Guilt) in each data set. Finally, I computed a grand mean correlation in each data set that represents the average of these six overall scale-pair coefficients. Although these correlations tend to be somewhat lower than those observed in between-subject data, the same basic pattern was consistently found. In the momentary mood data, the average correlations ranged from .38 to .54 (grand mean = .47); in the daily mood data, the correlations ranged from .39 to .52 (grand mean = .44).

I again must emphasize that results of this sort do not reflect psychometric limitations of the PANAS-X. In fact, Watson and Clark (1994b, Table 15) collected both PANAS-X and POMS data from a sample of 563 students who rated themselves using "Past few weeks" instructions. In this sample, the PANAS-X Fear, Sadness, and Hostility scales had a mean intercorrelation of .56; in contrast, the average correlation among the three corresponding POMS scales was .66. In other words, these PANAS-X scales actually differentiated these states better than did corresponding scales from the POMS.

Clearly, reports of the various negative affects are substantially interrelated, regardless of whether they are based on state or trait ratings, or whether they are examined on a within-subject or between-subject basis. This robust finding undoubtedly will be puzzling to many readers. After all, these negative affects seemingly represent different subjective experiences, so that we easily can distinguish feelings of fear from anger, anger from sadness, and so on. Moreover, our own subjective sense is that these negative affects arise from rather different circumstances. That is, we perceive that we experience nervousness and anxiety—not hostility and anger—when we anticipate a public speech or a potentially painful visit to the dentist. Similarly, when we are treated unfairly by another person, we feel anger and annoyance, not guilt or nervousness. These considerations lead us to expect that these negative mood states should be largely independent of one another.

Nevertheless, they clearly are not independent. Our data could possibly reflect the fact that prototypical, emotion-specific experiences (such as giving a speech) occur extremely infrequently in our everyday lives and, therefore, exert little effect on observable data. Another possibility, however, is that everyday events actually produce more complex affective reactions than we initially perceive. For example, going to the dentist may indeed arouse feelings of fear and anxiety, but it might also generate substantial levels of guilt and self-blame (e.g., because of the knowledge that one has failed to take proper care of one's teeth). Similarly, a cruel, insulting remark may arouse both anger (because the remark was made in an insensitive manner) and depression (because it is perceived to be true to some extent), and being treated unjustly by another may generate feelings of both anxiety and depression (because it demonstrates one's helplessness in the face of perceived injustice) in addition to anger and resentment.

Whatever the explanation, this strong covariation among the negative affects is a robust empirical fact that cannot be ignored. In fact, it has extremely important implications for mood research (see Watson & Clark, 1992a). As an example, suppose I have hypothesized that elevated levels of depression lead to poorer immune system functioning and, therefore, to increased symptoms of infectious disease. As an initial test of this model, I conduct a simple correlational study and find that there is a significant positive correlation between depressed mood and reported illness symptoms. Of course, this is only a correlational study, so it cannot be interpreted as indicating that depression causes illness. But at the very least, it seems to show that depressed mood has a potentially important association with illness symptoms.

Or does it? In light of the data we have considered, it is entirely possible that depression per se has little or nothing to do with illness symptoms. As we have seen, people who report being depressed also will report elevated levels of anxiety, hostility, and other negative moods. In other words, depressed individuals are not simply depressed but also tend to be anxious, hostile, and guilty. Consequently, any of these other negative affects—rather than sadness or depression per se—actually might be responsible for the observed elevation in illness symptoms.

Thus, each of these negative affects serves as a potential confounding variable for all of the others. Thus, these negative mood states cannot be studied individually, in isolation from one another; rather, they must be examined together. For instance, if researchers only assess current depressed mood, they have no way of knowing whether any observed relations are due to depression or, alternatively, to one of the other negative affects (e.g., anxiety or hostility). Only by assessing *all* these negative affects can one determine which of them really is responsible for observed relations with other variables.

But there is a further complication that must be considered. It is possible that the observed associations are not due to *any* of these individual negative affects per se. Rather, they may reflect what these variables have *in common*, namely, that they are all negative mood states. In other words, these observed relations may reflect the operation of the general Negative Affect dimension discussed earlier. The situation here is exactly analogous to a classic problem in ability testing. Suppose that I find that students who are good spellers get better grades in school: Does this suggest that spelling ability per se is crucial to academic success? Not necessarily, because one could argue that spelling ability is itself a manifestation of general intelligence, and it is this general ability factor—rather than spelling per se—that is critically important in academic success.

In the current context, this general Negative Affect dimension represents the empirical overlap among these specific negative mood scales—that is, it reflects the portion of each scale that is correlated with the others (just as general intelligence causes diverse ability measures to be positively interrelated). Moreover, because these specific negative mood scales all share this common component of general Negative Affect, they tend to have similar associations with other variables; once this general component has been statistically removed, however, these associations may largely or completely disappear.

Watson and Clark (1992a) present several examples that illustrate this point nicely. For instance, in a large student sample, the four PANAS-X negative affect scales all were significantly correlated with a measure of somatic complaints at each of two assessments (r's ranged from .24 to .46). Once the general Negative Affect component was statistically removed, however, these correlations all essentially dropped to zero. In this instance, the observed relations were almost entirely due to the general Negative Affect dimension, rather than any individual affect per se. Further analyses of the same sample indicated that all four scales also were significantly related to perceived stress at both assessments (r's ranged from .31 to .45). Again, once the influence of general Negative Affect dimension was statistically eliminated, these relations essentially vanished.

These data clearly demonstrate that one needs to have some way of measuring this general Negative Affect dimension. There are many ways that this can be accomplished, but the simplest is to develop a scale that assesses it directly. Accordingly, Watson, Clark and Tellegen (1988) created the 10-item PANAS Negative Affect scale. This scale contains a broad range of content; specifically, it includes terms from the Fear ("afraid," "scared," "nervous," "jittery"), Guilt ("guilty," "ashamed") and Hostility ("irritable," "hostile") scales, as well as two nonspecific descriptors of negative mood ("upset," "distressed").

It is noteworthy that no Sadness terms (e.g., "blue" and "lonely") were included in this Negative Affect scale. This is because these terms tend to have somewhat higher (negative) correlations with positive mood descriptors (a point I consider in more detail shortly); consequently, including these terms would have increased the correlation between this scale and our measure of general Positive Affect (see Watson & Clark, 1997b). Unfortunately, the omission of these terms sometimes has been misinterpreted as indicating that sadness and depression are unrelated (or perhaps only weakly related) to this general Negative Affect dimension. Table 2.2, however, clearly establishes that this is not the case; indeed, self-rated Sadness is strongly related to the other negative affects in both sets of ratings. Furthermore, Sadness correlated .67 (General ratings) and .68 (Moment ratings) with the general Negative Affect scale in these same two data sets, despite the fact that these scales share no common content. Accordingly, the general Negative Affect scale is as relevant to sadness as it is to any other type of negative mood.

The Positive Affects

The convergent property also applies to positive mood states. Table 2.1 indicates that three of the PANAS-X scales—Joviality, Self-Assurance, and Attentiveness—have been classified as "basic positive affects"; this designation reflects the fact that these three scales consistently show very strong correlations with one another. Table 2.3 reports correlations among these scales in the same two between-subject data sets that previously were used to examine relations among the negative affects.

These data strongly support the proposition that same-valenced affects are substantially interrelated. In the General ratings, the correlations among the positive mood scales range from .48 to .59 (mean = .52); the co-

TABLE 2.3. Correlations among the Basic Positive Affect Scales of the PANAS-X

Scale	1	2	3
1. Joviality	—	.59	.50
2. Self-Assurance	.65	—	.48
3. Attentiveness	.54	.50	—

Note. Correlations above the diagonal are trait ratings ($N = 1,657$) in which students rated how they "generally" felt. Correlations below the diagonal are state ratings ($N = 1,027$) in which students rated how they felt "right now, that is, at the present moment." All correlations are significant at $p < .001$.

efficients are even higher in the Moment data, ranging from .50 to .65 (mean = .56). Thus, paralleling the negative mood data, we see consistent evidence that the individual positive affects covary with one another, such that individuals who report significant amounts of one also tend to experience elevated levels of the others. That is, individuals who report being cheerful, enthusiastic, and energetic (high Joviality) also tend to describe themselves as proud, confident, and daring (high Self-Assurance) and as attentive and alert (high Attentiveness).

As with the negative affects, it is important to demonstrate that the same general pattern emerges in within-subject analyses of individual respondents. To examine this issue, I again analyzed the two large within-subject data sets collected by Cathey Soutter and myself. Following my earlier procedure, I initially computed correlations among the three positive mood scales individually for each person, and then computed overall mean correlations for each scale pair (e.g., between Joviality and Attentiveness) in each data set; finally, I calculated a grand mean correlation in each data set that represents the average of the three mean scale-pair correlations.

These correlations actually tended to be somewhat *higher* than those seen in the between-subject data. Specifically, in the momentary mood ratings, the average correlations ranged from .61 to .75 (grand mean = .67), whereas those in the daily mood ratings ranged from .52 to .68 (grand mean = .59). These data are quite striking, as they demonstrate that the positive affects covary quite strongly, even on a within-subject basis and even at a specific moment in time. In other words, as a given individual begins to feel happier, livelier, and more enthusiastic, he or she also begins to experience concomitant increases in confidence, boldness, concentration, and alertness. Conversely, as an individual's level of joy, energy, and enthusiasm declines, one also tends to see corresponding decreases in confidence and attentiveness.

Thus, the various positive affects are strongly intercorrelated in both state and trait ratings and in both within-subject and between-subject analyses. The implications of these data are the same as those discussed earlier in the context of the negative affects: Again, each of these positive affects serves as a potential confounding variable for both of the others. Because of this potential confounding, it is essential that these various positive affects be examined together rather than in isolation; otherwise, one has no way of knowing which of them ultimately is responsible for any observed effects. Moreover, one again faces a further complication, namely, the existence of a general Positive Affect dimension. In this case, the general dimension represents the empirical covariation among the various positive mood scales—that is, it reflects the portion of each scale that is correlated with the others. The problem is that it may be this shared, correlated component—rather than the unique portion that is specific to each individual scale—that is responsible for any observed associations with other variables.

To measure this general dimension, Watson, Clark and Tellegen (1988) created the 10-item PANAS Positive Affect scale. This scale includes terms from the Joviality ("excited," "enthusiastic"), Self-Assurance ("proud," "strong") and Attentiveness ("alert," "attentive," "determined") scales, as well as three nonspecific positive mood descriptors ("active," "interested," "inspired"). Although the content of the scale obviously is quite broad, it contains no descriptors that specifically assess feelings of joy or happiness ("cheerful," "joyful"). Paralleling my earlier discussion of Sadness, these terms were omitted because they tend to have somewhat higher (negative) correlations with negative mood descriptors (an issue discussed in the following section); consequently, including them would have increased the correlation between this scale and our measure of general Negative Affect. Their omission, however, should not be misinterpreted as indicating that feelings of happiness and joy are weakly related to other types of positive mood or to the general Positive Affect dimension itself.

To demonstrate this important point, I created a four-item Happiness scale consisting of the terms "happy," "joyful," "cheerful," and "delighted." Note that this scale shares no terms with the PANAS Positive Affect scale. Nevertheless, it correlated .73 (Moment ratings) and .70 (General ratings) with general Positive Affect in the two between-subject data sets. Clearly, the general Positive Affect scale is as relevant to feelings of joy and happiness as it is to any other type of positive mood (see also Watson & Clark, 1997b).

RELATIONS BETWEEN AFFECTS WITH THE OPPOSITE VALENCE

The Independence of the Positive and Negative Affects

The second general property of mood ratings also may be counterintuitive to many readers. As I discussed in Chapter 1, the commonsense view seems to be that negative and positive mood states are contradictory and incompatible, even mutually exclusive of one another. From this naive perspective, if I am feeling happy, I cannot be depressed, resentful, or apprehensive; conversely, if I am embittered or terrified, I cannot be simultaneously experiencing feelings of joy, enthusiasm, and cheerfulness.

As noted in Chapter 1, there is some evidence to support this commonsense view. Most notably, it is rare for individuals who are experiencing extremely high levels of Negative Affect also to report high levels of Positive Affect, and vice versa (Diener & Iran-Nejad, 1986; Watson, 1988b). Thus, it is truly difficult for one to be simultaneously ecstatic and terrified, or to be concurrently enraged and euphoric. In addition, I will present evidence shortly indicating that feelings of sadness and joy show stronger inverse correlations than do other types of negative and positive affect; not surprisingly, it is rather difficult for one to be happy and unhappy at the same time.

Aside from these important qualifications, however, the naive view is inaccurate. The bulk of the empirical evidence demonstrates that positive and negative mood states are not polar opposites or mutually incompatible but, instead, are only weakly to moderately related to one another; in fact, they tend to fluctuate more or less independently of one another. Thus, the second robust property (which we can label the "discriminant" property) is that oppositely valenced affects (e.g., nervous vs. enthusiastic and irritable vs. delighted) tend to be only weakly negatively correlated with one another. In the previous chapter, I discussed possible reasons for this observed independence of the negative and positive affects; in the current discussion, I will concentrate on demonstrating its existence.

Table 2.4 presents correlations between the basic Negative and Positive Affect scales in the two between-subject data sets. Several aspects of these data warrant comment. First, and most important, these correlations generally are quite low; in fact, only 2 of the 24 coefficients are

TABLE 2.4. Correlations between the Basic Negative and Positive Affect Scales of the PANAS-X

Negative Emotion scale	Correlations with		
	Joviality	Self-Assurance	Attentiveness
Moment ratings			
Fear	−.07	−.07	.00
Sadness	−.34	−.20	−.15
Guilt	−.12	−.09	−.13
Hostility	−.19	.03	−.14
General ratings			
Fear	−.02	−.11	−.05
Sadness	−.30	−.23	−.17
Guilt	−.18	−.19	−.20
Hostility	−.18	.05	−.13

Note. N = 1,027 (Moment ratings) and 1,657 (General ratings). Correlations of −.09 or greater are significant at $p < .01$, two-tailed.

greater than −.25. Thus, we see clear evidence of a basic separation between positive and negative affective experience.

Second, the two sets of ratings yielded extremely similar correlational patterns. Most notably, the mean correlations in the two data sets (−.12 and −14 in the Moment and General ratings, respectively) are virtually identical. In other words, the positive and negative affects are largely independent of one another in both state and trait ratings. This is an important point to which I will return shortly.

Third, among the individual scales, Sadness and Joviality showed the strongest association. In fact, these two scales produced the strongest negative correlation in both the Moment ($r = -.34$) and General ($r = -.30$) ratings. As explained earlier, because of relatively high inverse correlations such as these, descriptors of sadness and happiness/joy (which are included in Joviality) were excluded from the PANAS Negative and Positive Affect scales; including items of this sort would have increased the correlation between the scales, thereby lessening their discriminant validity (see Watson & Clark, 1997b).

Once again, it is important to establish that a similar pattern emerges in within-subject analyses of individual respondents. Accordingly, following the same procedure as before, I computed overall mean scale-pair correlations (e.g., between Joviality and Fear) and grand mean correlations separately for each of the two large within-subject data sets. These within-subject correlations were somewhat higher than those obtained in the between-subject analyses, but they still were sufficiently low to indicate that the positive and negative affect scales remained largely independent. Specifically, the grand mean correlations were −.25 and −.29 in the momentary and daily ratings, respectively. Consequently, the observed independence of the positive and negative affects is not an artifact of between-subject designs: It also emerges quite clearly in within-subject analyses of individual respondents. This is also a crucial point to which I return shortly.

Putting the convergent and discriminant properties together, we can identify a basic structural pattern in which (1) same-valenced affects are strongly positively correlated, but (2) oppositely valenced affects tend to be more weakly related. That is, the various negative affects (e.g., Fear and Hostility) tend to be substantially interrelated, as do different types of positive affect (e.g., Joviality and Self-Assurance); however, the cross-valence correlations (e.g., between Fear and Self-Assurance) generally are rather low. This pattern has clear implications for the measurement of mood. It indicates that the most parsimonious approach is to combine same-valenced terms into two separate scales that reflect negative and positive affective experience. And this is precisely what Watson, Clark, and Tellegen (1988) did when they created the PANAS: They summed 10 negative mood terms into a general Negative Affect scale and 10 positive descriptors into a general Positive Affect scale. Consistent with the data shown in Table 2.4, the correlation between these general Positive and Negative Affect scales is consistently low (I present some relevant evidence shortly). Finally, as I demonstrate throughout the remainder of this book, these two general scales have highly distinctive correlates and tend to be related to different classes of variables. These differential correlates confirm the basic distinction between positive and negative affective experience and demonstrate the desirability of assessing these two types of experience separately.

Challenges to This Independence

Although the evidence I have presented appears to be clear and straightforward, it has not gone unchallenged in the mood literature. Perhaps because this independence between positive and negative affective life seems so counterintuitive, many researchers have approached it skeptically and have questioned it—or at least tried to qualify it—on various grounds. Three of these challenges have been particularly prominent in the mood literature and are discussed here.

First, various researchers have argued that this apparent independence reflects the use of improper or inappropriate *response formats*. By "response format" I mean the rating scale that is used to generate a person's actual responses. For instance, the PANAS-X employs an "extent" format (see Watson, 1988b); that is, people are asked to indicate "to what extent" they have experienced each mood term over a specified time span. As such, this type of format essentially asks respondents to quantify *how much* of each affect they have experienced during the specified time frame (1 = very slightly or not at all, 2 = a little, 3 = moderately, 4 = quite a bit, 5 = extremely). Note that this format does not specify precisely how people are supposed to convert their experiences into numbers; for most respondents the quantification process probably involves some consideration of both the duration (i.e., how long one actually spent in the state) and intensity (i.e., the perceived strength of one's feeling while in that state) of the experience.

Clearly, however, there are many other possible formats that can be—and have been—used to generate mood ratings. Over the years, mood researchers have worried that different formats might yield highly discrepant results and, moreover, that some of these formats might be more valid than others. One particularly relevant concern is that improper response formats may artifactually weaken what actually are strong negative correlations between positive and negative mood terms. The earliest challenge of this sort was offered by Meddis (1972). Meddis was especially critical of a 4-point response format (1 = definitely do not feel, 2 = cannot decide, 3 = feel slightly, 4 = definitely feel) that was widely used in early studies of mood and is still being employed in some contemporary research. According to Meddis, this format is problematic for two reasons. First, it is asymmetric—that is, it contains two categories of endorsement (feel slightly, definitely feel) but only one of rejection (definitely do not feel). Second, it is unclear whether a "cannot decide" response really should be considered intermediate between "definitely do not feel" and "feel slightly." He maintained that these undesirable characteristics might serve to weaken the size of observed negative correlations. Furthermore, he demonstrated that when these problems were corrected, stronger negative correlations were obtained between opposite mood terms.

Meddis's analyses initially caused great concern among mood researchers. However, when Russell (1979) attempted to replicate Meddis's findings, he concluded that this problematic format "contributes at most a modest bias" (p. 350). Moreover, other researchers found that the structural properties of mood ratings actually were highly robust across different response formats (Hendrick & Lilly, 1970; Thayer, 1986). Similarly, Watson and Tellegen (1985) demonstrated that the positive and negative affects remained largely independent of one another even using formats that were not subject to Meddis's criticisms. Consequently, the problems noted by Meddis (1972) cannot explain the observed independence of positive and negative mood terms.

Warr, Barter, and Brownbridge (1983) subsequently offered another influential format-based explanation. Warr et al. (1983) argued that most of the widely used response formats do not require people to make any logical or empirical connection between positive and negative mood states. For instance, over a period of a few weeks many people may have experienced prolonged episodes of both joy and sadness; consequently, on an extent-type format—such as that used with the PANAS-X—these individuals would rate themselves as being high on both of these affects. Obviously, this sort of process would serve to weaken the correlations between positive and negative mood states.

Warr et al. (1983) argued, however, that a fundamentally different type of response format should lead to much stronger correlations between the positive and negative affects. Specifically, the independence between these states should disappear if people were asked to rate *what proportion* of a specified period they had experienced each affect. For example, if during the past the past few weeks a person had felt happy most of the time, he or she could not possibly have felt sad most of the time. According to Warr et al., hedonically opposite mood states (such as joy and sadness) are mutually exclusive in this type of "frequency" format.

Hence, in this rating scheme, any increment in one affect necessarily implies a decrement in its opposite; this, in turn, should lead to very strong negative correlations.

Warr et al. (1983) presented data that provided preliminary support for their assertions. Watson (1988b) subsequently subjected them to a more exhaustive test, collecting mood ratings from two large college student samples: The ratings in one group were based on a 5-point "extent" format, whereas those in the other reflected a 4-point "frequency" format (1 = little or none of the time, 2 = some of the time, 3 = a good part of the time, 4 = most of the time). The responses in both groups were based on "Past few weeks" time instructions, thereby controlling for the rated time frame. The results indicated that the response format did influence the strength of the relation between negative and positive mood states, but the effect generally was rather small. Most notably, the correlation between the PANAS Negative and Positive Affect scales was −.16 and −.28 in the "extent" and "frequency" ratings, respectively. Thus, these scales remained relatively independent of one another, even when a "frequency" format was used. More generally, the data I have reviewed indicate that the structural properties of mood ratings (including the independence of the positive and negative affects) are highly robust across different response formats.

The second major challenge to independence involves the role of the rated time frame. Specifically, it has been argued that negative and positive mood terms are substantially negatively correlated when people rate how they have felt during a relatively brief time period (e.g., at the current moment, today), and that they become independent only as the rated time frame lengthens (e.g., during the past month or year) (for discussions, see Watson, 1988b; Watson & Clark, 1997b). The logic underlying this argument actually is quite similar to that offered by Warr et al. (1983) to explain the influence of different response formats. In both cases, it is assumed one cannot possibly experience two opposite mood states simultaneously; for instance, one cannot be happy and sad at the same time. Because of this, one would expect to see strong negative correlations between negative and positive mood states when the ratings are based on short time intervals. However, as the rated time frame lengthens, it becomes increasingly possible to experience two or more apparently incompatible affects. For example, over the course of a month, it is entirely possible that one has experienced substantial levels of both joy and sadness. Accordingly, the negative correlations between positive and negative states should become weaker as the rated time frame lengthens.

Although this argument seems quite plausible, it is wrong. In actuality, the independence of the positive and negative affects is unaffected by the time frame that is used. I already have presented some data relevant to this issue in Table 2.4. In discussing these results, I noted that the average correlation between the basic Negative and Positive Affect scales of the PANAS-X was –.12 and –.14 in the Moment and General ratings, respectively. In other words, these scales were similarly independent of one another in both short-term "state" ratings and long-term "trait" ratings.

Although these data seem straightforward, it nevertheless might be helpful to examine this issue in more detail. Table 2.5 presents correlations between the general Positive and Negative Affect scales in eight large samples (with a combined total of 14,463 observations), each of which completed the scales using one of eight different temporal instructions (these data originally were reported in Watson & Clark, 1997b, Table 5). All the respondents were students enrolled in psychology courses at Southern Methodist University (SMU), thereby controlling for age and other demographic variables.

The data in Table 2.5 require little comment. One sees no tendency for the correlation between Negative Affect and Positive Affect to decline as the rated time span lengthens. In fact, the two weakest coefficients were obtained in the Moment ($r = –.06$) and Today ($r = –.05$) ratings, whereas the strongest correlation (–.23) was found in the Past year ratings. Clearly, the relation between the positive and negative affects is unaffected by the rated time frame. Moreover, these two types of affect remain largely independent of one another even when people are rating their current, momentary mood.

Echoing my earlier discussion of response formats, the third major challenge again is based on an assertion that the apparent independence of the negative and positive affects is artifactual; in this case, it is argued that the observed data reflect systematic measurement errors such as response sets and rating biases (for discussions, see Bentler, 1969; Feldman

TABLE 2.5. The Correlation between the General Negative Affect and Positive Affect Scales as a Function of the Rated Time Frame

Rated time frame	N	NA–PA correlation
Moment	2,213	–.06
Today	1,664	–.05
Past few days	1,577	–.17
Past week	1,521	–.14
Past few weeks	2,076	–.13
Past month	1,006	–.15
Past year	964	–.23
General	3,622	–.13

Note. NA, Negative Affect; PA, Positive Affect. Adapted from Watson & Clark (1997b, Table 5). Copyright 1997 by Lawrence Erlbaum Associates, Inc. Adapted by permission.

Barrett & Russell, 1998; Green et al., 1993; Russell, 1979, 1980; Tellegen, Watson, & Clark, 1999). Most of the attention in this area has focused on the *acquiescence* response bias. Russell (1979) has defined acquiescence as "an individual-difference variable in the tendency to agree or disagree with an item regardless of its content" (p. 346). The acquiescence bias is potentially relevant to almost any type of assessment instrument, although there is a long-standing controversy as to whether or not it really represents a serious problem in psychological measurement (see Wiggins, 1973).

The concept of acquiescence originally was applied to measures using a "true–false" response format. In this case, it represents a tendency to answer "true" regardless of the content of the item (in contrast, the "nay-saying" bias reflects a tendency to answer "false" irrespective of content). Thus, an extremely acquiescent individual tends to answer "true" even when confronted with contradictory statements; for instance, highly acquiescent respondents might endorse various statements indicating that they are both friendly and hostile, both honest and dishonest, and both popular and unpopular.

However, as noted earlier, the concept of acquiescence can be applied to almost any form of assessment. For example, in the case of adjective checklists (such as MAACL), it reflects a general propensity to "check" items regardless of their particular content. In other words, some people simply are more likely to check items as being self-descriptive—irrespective of the content of these items—than are others. In fact, carefully conducted studies have suggested that the adjective checklist format is particularly susceptible to this type of rating bias, causing psychometricians to recommend that this method be avoided (see Bentler, 1969; Green et al., 1993).

In the case of Likert rating formats (such as the one used with the PANAS-X), the acquiescence bias would be reflected in a general tendency to respond with the same rating to a broad range of content. In other words, highly acquiescent people tend to use the same number when responding to very different—even contradictory—items. Note, however, that although any given acquiescent individual should be highly self-consistent (i.e., he or she should tend to use the same number over and over again), there is no reason to expect consistency across different individuals who exhibit this bias (i.e., various acquiescent individuals may prefer to use different numbers). That is, one acquiescent respondent may tend to assign 5's to all items, whereas another might prefer to use 3's, or even 1's. Accordingly, if everyone in a sample were to respond in a completely acquiescent manner, all items would correlate approximately +1.00 with each other.

Because of this, the acquiescence bias will distort observed correlations by shifting them toward greater positivity: That is, it moves them away from −1.00 and toward +1.00. If two variables have a true positive correlation, then acquiescence will inflate the magnitude of the observed coefficient. For instance, if the "true" correlation between *happy* and *enthusiastic* is +.40, then the presence of this bias might artifactually strengthen the association into an observed correlation of +.60.

However, if two variables have a true negative correlation, then acquiescence will weaken the strength of the observed relation, shifting it away from −1.00 and toward 0. As an example, consider the relation between *happy* and *sad*. Suppose that the true correlation between these states is −1.00, such that the presence of one necessarily implies the absence of the other. Suppose, furthermore, that acquiescence exerts no influence on mood ratings. Table 2.6, which shows ratings of *happy* and *sad* from 12 hypothetical individuals, illustrates this idyllic situation. Because a high score on one variable necessitates a low score on the other—and because the acquiescence bias is completely absent from these data—the observed correlation is, in fact, −1.00.

Suppose, however, that we alter the situation so that two individuals—one preferring 5's and the other tending toward 1's—respond in a perfectly acquiescent manner. In sharp contrast to the other respondents (all of whom score high on one variable and low on the other), one of these respondents receives a very high score on both items, whereas the

TABLE 2.6. Illustrative Data Showing the Effect of Acquiescence Response Bias on the Observed Correlation between Positive and Negative Mood States

Person No.	Bias-free ratings		Acquiescence-biased ratings	
	Happy	Sad	Happy	Sad
1	5	1	5	1
2	5	1	5	1
3	5	1	5[a]	5[a]
4	4	2	4	2
5	4	2	4	2
6	4	2	4	2
7	2	4	2	4
8	2	4	2	4
9	2	4	2	4
10	1	5	1[a]	1[a]
11	1	5	1	5
12	1	5	1	5
Happy–Sad *r*	−1.00		−.47	

[a]Ratings of individuals exhibiting the acquiescence response bias.

other obtains an extremely low score on both. Clearly, ratings of this sort will lower the observed negative correlation substantially: In fact, Table 2.6 shows that the presence of two such individuals is sufficient to reduce the observed correlation to −.47.

Thus, samples containing a relatively large number of highly acquiescent individuals may yield seriously distorted correlations; most important, they may yield data spuriously demonstrating the supposed independence of the positive and negative affects, even though these two types of affect actually are strongly negatively correlated.

Does acquiescence produce spuriously low negative correlations in mood data? To date, the available evidence suggests that acquiescence and other sources of systematic error exert a moderate influence on mood ratings (Diener, Smith, & Fujita, 1995; Tellegen et al., 1999). Nevertheless, distinctive, separable Positive and Negative Affect dimensions can be identified even after controlling for systematic measurement error, including acquiescence. Tellegen, Watson, and Clark (1994), for instance, constructed simple 5-item scales to measure general Positive and Negative Affect. Without correcting for acquiescence, the observed correlation between these scales was −.28. Controlling for acquiescence increased the strength of their interrelation, but the corrected correlation still was only moderate ($r = −.43$). Thus, the positive and negative affects remained relatively independent even after controlling for acquiescence.

The studies conducted by Diener et al. (1995) and Tellegen et al. (1999) are based on between-subject analyses in which structural equation modeling was used to eliminate the influence of systematic measurement error. There is, however, a different way to examine the possible influence of response biases such as acquiescence. As stated earlier, acquiescence is defined as an *individual difference variable*—that is, it is a tendency that some people exhibit but others do not. Accordingly, its influence necessarily is confined to between-subject analyses in which the ratings of one individual are compared with those of another. The problem of acquiescence therefore can be bypassed completely by conducting separate within-subject analyses of individual respondents.

Thus, the strength of the acquiescence bias can be estimated by comparing correlations derived from between-subject versus within-subject analyses (see Watson & Clark, 1997b). I already have presented some data along these lines and they are quite consistent with my earlier conclusion that acquiescence exerts a moderate influence on mood ratings. Specifically, between-subject analyses yielded average correlations between the basic Negative Affect (Fear, Sadness, Guilt, Hostility) and Positive Affect (Joviality, Self-Assurance, Attentiveness) scales of −.12 and −.14 in Moment and General ratings, respectively (see Table 2.4). By comparison, the average within-subject correlations between these scales were −.25

and –.29 in the momentary and daily ratings, respectively. In other words, although the within-subject correlations generally were higher, these scales remained largely independent even in these data.

It also is interesting to examine parallel data for the general Positive and Negative Affect scales. In between-subject analyses, the correlation between these scales ranges from –.05 to –.23 (see Table 2.5). These low values suggest that the positive and negative affects are essentially unrelated.

These correlations can be compared with corresponding values derived from within-subject analyses. I have collected within-subject data from 414 SMU students who rated their current, momentary mood, and from 453 students who rated their daily mood; as before, all participants completed a minimum of 35 mood assessments. Because the between-subject data reported in Table 2.5 also were collected from SMU students, demographic characteristics should not exert any influence on these results.

The average within-subject correlations in these two data sets were –.25 (momentary ratings) and –.33 (daily ratings). These numbers certainly are higher than those observed in the between-subject analyses, but they still reflect only a moderate association. Thus, these results again indicate that acquiescence exerts a moderate influence on mood ratings; they also demonstrate that positive and negative mood states remain largely independent even in within-subject analyses in which the acquiescence bias is bypassed.

In summary, I have discussed several challenges to the observed independence of the positive and negative affects. These challenges have made an important contribution to the mood literature because they have forced mood researchers to investigate possible methodological problems and measurement artifacts. Nevertheless, even when these various problems and artifacts are corrected or controlled, the positive and negative affects remain distinct, separable, and largely independent of one another.

OTHER AFFECTIVE STATES

Thus far, I have discussed two robust structural properties of mood ratings. These properties are highly relevant to 7 of the 11 specific PANAS-X scales. As we have seen, four of the scales are strongly interrelated and jointly define a nonspecific dimension of general Negative Affect; similarly, three scales are substantially intercorrelated and demonstrate the existence of a general Positive Affect dimension. Furthermore, these basic Negative and Positive Affect scales (and, hence, the general dimensions themselves) tend to be relatively independent of one another. Accordingly, the most parsimonious approach is to recognize this basic distinction between positive and negative affective experience and to focus assessment on these two general dimensions.

However, I have not yet discussed the structural characteristics of the four remaining PANAS-X scales—Shyness, Fatigue, Serenity, and Surprise. I must begin by emphasizing that each of these scales is significantly related to the negative and/or positive affects, so that they also can be viewed in terms of the general Negative Affect and Positive Affect dimensions. Accordingly, everyday affective experience can be neatly summarized using these two general dimensions (Tellegen, 1985; Tellegen et al., 1999; Watson, 1988b; Watson & Clark, 1997b; Watson & Tellegen, 1985).

To examine the structural properties of these scales in a relatively concise manner, I will concentrate on their correlations with the general Negative and Positive Affect scales. Keep in mind, however, that these results easily can be understood in terms of the basic negative and positive affects. That is, a scale that correlates strongly with general Negative Affect also will tend to correlate strongly with the Fear, Sadness, Guilt, and Hostility scales individually; moreover, as its correlations with the general dimension increase in magnitude, so will its associations with these specific types of negative affect. Similarly, a scale that is highly related to general Positive Affect also tends to be substantially related to Joviality, Self-Assurance, and Attentiveness. Finally, a scale that correlates significantly with both of the general scales also will be significantly related to all of these specific affects.

With this in mind, Table 2.7 presents correlations between Shyness, Fatigue, Serenity, and Surprise and general Negative and Positive Affect in the two between-subject samples. In addition, Table 2.8 reports corresponding average within-subject correlations in the two within-subject data sets. Consistent with my earlier suggestion, these data demonstrate that these four scales are each moderately to strongly correlated with at least one of the general mood dimensions. Beyond this basic finding, however, what do these results tell us about these PANAS-X scales? First, they indicate that Shyness essentially represents another variety of negative affect. Note that this scale has moderate positive correlations with general Negative Affect in both the between-subject and within-subject analyses. In contrast, its correlations with Positive Affect consistently are quite low.

Why, then, did I exclude Shyness from my earlier discussion of the individual negative affects? The answer is that Shyness contains less of the shared, overlapping variance—which represents the influence of the general Negative Affect dimension—than do scales such as Fear and Sad-

TABLE 2.7. Correlations between General Negative Affect and Positive Affect and the Shyness, Fatigue, Serenity and Surprise Scales (Between-Subject Analyses)

	Correlations with	
Scale	Negative Affect	Positive Affect
Moment ratings		
Shyness	.41	.03
Fatigue	.29	−.32
Serenity	−.45	.22
Surprise	.37	.36
General ratings		
Shyness	.46	−.14
Fatigue	.42	−.27
Serenity	−.29	.32
Surprise	.30	.40

Note. $N = 1,027$ (Moment ratings) and 1,657 (General ratings). Correlations of $|.09|$ or greater are significant at $p < .01$, two-tailed.

TABLE 2.8. Average Within-Subject Correlations between General Negative Affect and Positive Affect and the Shyness, Fatigue, Serenity, and Surprise Scales

	Correlations with	
Scale	Negative Affect	Positive Affect
Momentary data		
Shyness	.30	−.15
Fatigue	.26	−.62
Serenity	−.43	.21
Surprise	.12	.35
Daily data		
Shyness	.30	−.12
Fatigue	.30	−.41
Serenity	−.48	.37
Surprise	.08	.32

Note. The momentary data are based on the responses of 226 students and 10,169 total observations. The daily data are based on the responses of 254 students and 11,322 total observations.

ness. For example, as noted earlier, Sadness—which, similar to Shyness, shares no terms with the general Negative Affect scale—correlated .68 (Moment ratings) and .67 (General ratings) with general Negative Affect in the two between-subject analyses, compared with corresponding values of .41 and .46, respectively, for Shyness. Similarly, Sadness had average within-subject correlations of .56 and .57 with general Negative Affect in the momentary and daily data, respectively, compared with corresponding values of .30 and .30, respectively, for Shyness. Thus, although Shyness contains a component of nonspecific Negative Affect, it clearly has much less of it than scales such as Sadness and Fear.

The data for the three remaining scales are more complex in that each is related to both of the general dimensions; moreover, the results for these scales are inconsistent across the various analyses. For instance, Surprise has moderately positive correlations with both Negative and Positive Affect in the between-subject analyses, suggesting that it essentially represents a state of high activation or arousal. In the within-subject data, however, although it still is moderately correlated with general Positive Affect, it is largely unrelated to Negative Affect.

The findings for Fatigue are even more inconsistent. The earliest studies indicated that fatigue-related terms (e.g., "sluggish," "sleepy," and "exhausted") were strongly negatively correlated with positive mood states and more weakly (positively) related to various types of negative affect (see Larsen & Diener, 1992; Watson & Tellegen, 1985); subsequent data, however, have provided inconsistent support for this notion (Burke, Brief, George, Roberson, & Webster, 1989; Mayer & Gaschke, 1988; Meyer & Shack, 1989; Watson & Clark, 1997b). The current data indicate that this early conclusion was indeed accurate, but only when applied to within-subject analyses of momentary mood. Note that Fatigue had a strong mean correlation with Positive Affect ($r = -.62$)—and a relatively modest relation with Negative Affect ($r = .26$)—in the momentary mood ratings. In other words, at the momentary, within-subject level, Fatigue essentially represents the *absence* of positive affective experience. That is, if I currently am feeling tired and sluggish, I likely will not report substantial levels of energy, enthusiasm, and alertness. In contrast, Fatigue varies much more independently of negative feelings such as fear and anger. As we will see in Chapter 4, these within-subject correlations reflect, in large part, the influence of a strong circadian rhythm that produces marked fluctuations in Fatigue and the various positive affects (but not the negative affects).

In the other three analyses, however, Fatigue has similarly moderate correlations with both of the general scales. Specifically, its correlations with Positive Affect range from −.27 to −.41, whereas those with Negative

Affect vary from .29 to .42. Fatigue's structural properties clearly fluctuate across different types of analyses.

Similar considerations apply to Serenity. In this case, the early evidence indicated that serenity-related terms (e.g., "relaxed," "placid," and "at rest") were strongly negatively correlated with negative mood states and more weakly (positively) related to various types of positive affect (Larsen & Diener, 1992; Watson & Tellegen, 1985); again, however, subsequent data have not consistently supported this notion (Burke et al., 1989; Meyer & Shack, 1989; Watson & Clark, 1997b). The current results also provide only inconsistent support. The most supportive evidence comes from the two analyses of momentary mood: Note that Serenity has moderately strong negative correlations with general Negative Affect in both the between-subject and within-subject analyses; moreover, in both cases its correlations with Positive Affect are much lower. Similarly, it also shows a moderately strong association with Negative Affect in the within-subject analysis of daily mood; in this instance, however, it also has a moderately strong relation with Positive Affect. Finally, Serenity has similar relations with both of the general scales in the between-subject analysis of the General ratings. As with Fatigue, it appears that Serenity's structural properties vary across different types of analyses.

Generally speaking, the results for these scales are less clear and consistent than those for the basic positive and negative affects. Nevertheless, these scales all consistently show significant (at times, strong) associations with at least one of the general dimensions. This again demonstrates that affective experience can be parsimoniously summarized using the general dimensions of Positive and Negative Affect.

THE HIERARCHICAL STRUCTURE OF AFFECT

Is it really possible to reduce the rich complexities of affective life to these two global dimensions? Can one assess mood simply by using these two general scales? The answer to both questions clearly is "no," and no mood researcher has ever seriously suggested otherwise. This brings me to the third robust property of mood data (which we can term the "hierarchical" property). My colleagues and I have presented extensive evidence indicating that mood ratings are hierarchically arranged such that they must be viewed at two fundamentally different levels: a higher-order level that consists of the general Negative and Positive Affect dimensions, and a lower-order level that consists of specific types of affect (see Watson & Clark, 1992a, 1992b, 1997b; Watson & Tellegen, 1985; for an expanded three-level hierarchical scheme, see Tellegen et al., 1999). In this hierarchical model, the upper level reflects the overall *valence* of the affects—that is, whether they represent negative or positive mood states. As we have seen, negative states jointly comprise the higher-order Negative Affect dimension, whereas positive states jointly define general Positive Affect. In contrast, the lower level of the hierarchy reflects the specific *content* of mood descriptors—that is, the distinctive qualities of each specific type of affect.

I already have demonstrated the existence of these general dimensions by showing strong and systematic interrelations among specific types of affect. What sort of evidence indicates that there is a lower-order level to mood structure as well? In essence, the existence of a hierarchical structure can be established by demonstrating that different manifestations of the same basic affect are more strongly related than are measures of different affects. For example, a given measure of fear should correlate more highly with another measure of fear than it does with measures of sadness or hostility. Note, however, that these cross-affect correlations (e.g., between fear and hostility) nevertheless may be substantial, thereby reflecting the influence of the higher-order dimension.

My colleagues and I have presented evidence of this sort in a number of studies (see Watson & Clark, 1991b, 1992a; Watson & Tellegen, 1985). Watson and Clark (1992a), for instance, reported four studies demonstrating the hierarchical arrangement of the negative affects. In their Study 1, various measures of sadness/depression were shown to correlate more highly with one another than with scales assessing fear/anxiety and anger/hostility. Similarly, Studies 2 and 3 demonstrated that a given Time 1 measure (e.g., Time 1 Guilt) correlated more strongly with its Time 2 counterpart (e.g., Time 2 Guilt) than with a Time 2 measure of another negative affect (e.g., Time 2 Sadness). Finally, Study 4 indicated that trait self-ratings (e.g., self-reported Sadness) correlated more highly with their peer-rated counterpart (e.g., peer-rated Sadness) than with comparable judgments of the other negative affects (e.g., peer-rated Hostility). Berenbaum, Fujita, and Pfennig (1995) subsequently replicated these findings in another series of four studies.

As with the other general properties of mood ratings, the existence of this hierarchical structure has important implications for mood assessment and research. Most notably, it clearly is necessary to examine both levels of the hierarchy in any complete investigation of mood. Consider, for instance, feelings of anxiety and anger. In many important respects, these feeling states are similar and must be understood together. That is, both of them are negative mood states and both, therefore, contain a strong component of nonspecific Negative Affect. Furthermore, as we have seen, scales assessing these two affects are substantially intercorrelated and represent important potential confounds for one another. On the other hand, these two types of affect are not completely interchangeable; each has its own unique properties as well. After all, the correlation between them does not approach +1.00, even if it is corrected for measurement error. Thus, there will be some situations in which an individual experiences substantial anxiety but not anger, and vice versa. Moreover, in certain cases these two affects actually may correlate quite differently with other variables. For instance, I demonstrate in Chapter 6 that the PANAS-X Fear and Hostility scales show somewhat different associations with general dimensions of personality (see also Watson & Clark, 1992b). In other words, negative affects such as anxiety and anger are strongly correlated and intimately interconnected, but they nevertheless remain at least partly distinct from each other.

Throughout the rest of this book, I have adopted a general approach that serves the scientific goal of parsimony but also is sensitive to this observed hierarchical arrangement of affective experience. In the interest of parsimony, I believe that the best approach is to begin with an examination of phenomena at the higher-order level. For instance, in discussing possible relations between mood and weather (see Chapter 3), I begin by reporting correlations between various weather indices and the general Negative Affect and Positive Affect scales. At this higher-order level, we will see that a great many phenomena are related either to the negative affects or to the positive affects, but not to both.

Whenever possible, however, I then go beyond this general level and examine each of the specific affects to see whether these lower-order analyses help to clarify our understanding of mood-related phenomena. In some cases I show that different types of negative or positive affect display similar patterns, which indicates that the phenomena under consideration are more meaningfully viewed at the higher-order level. For example, I show in Chapter 4 that the various positive affects all display extremely similar cycles of fluctuation over the course of the day. Accordingly, it appears that the circadian cycle influences positive mood in a very broad and nonspecific manner. In other cases, however, the individual affects exhibit somewhat different patterns, indicating that it may be more useful to conceptualize these phenomena at the lower-order level. For instance, I also demonstrate in Chapter 4 that the various positive affects show different patterns of fluctuation across the days the week.

CONCLUSION

I have established the existence of three highly robust properties of mood ratings. First, affects with the same valence tend to be substantially positively intercorrelated (the convergent property). Second, affects with the opposite valence tend to be relatively independent of one another (the discriminant property). Because of these two properties, mood can be conceptualized in terms of two general dimensions: Negative Affect and Positive Affect. Finally, affective experience is hierarchically arranged such that these general dimensions can be decomposed into substantially intercorrelated—but nevertheless distinct—types of affect (the hierarchical property). With these structural properties in mind, we are now ready to examine recent research on mood.

3

SITUATIONAL
AND ENVIRONMENTAL
INFLUENCES ON MOOD

Our mood is influenced by an incredible variety of factors, including ongoing events and experiences, the environmental milieu in which we find ourselves, our current physical state—and much, much more. This chapter discusses many of these variables. Specifically, it examines the influence of short-term *exogenous* factors on mood. By "exogenous," I mean situational factors, current life events, and environmental variables that are external to the experiencing organism (in Chapter 4, I consider internal *endogenous* processes). The relevant literature is huge and cannot possibly be summarized in a single chapter. Consequently, I only highlight some of the most important findings that have emerged in the recent mood literature, making particular use of the extensive within-subject data my colleagues and I have collected.

Before reviewing the evidence, I must emphasize two general points that will help readers to organize and interpret the findings that follow. First, the research literature suggests that people actually are rather poor at identifying the specific factors that influence their mood. Put another way, recent evidence has established some important disjunctions between our beliefs and our actual affective experience. In this chapter, we see some outstanding examples of such disjunctions.

Second, in the two preceding chapters I strongly emphasized the basic distinction between positive and negative mood states. Nowhere is this distinction more apparent than in the study of situational and environmental factors. Positive and negative mood states clearly are influenced by different classes of variables. Generally speaking, negative mood increases in response to various types of unpleasant events and aversive stimuli, whereas positive mood is relatively unaffected by such variables; conversely, positive mood states are much more responsive to pleasant events and pleasurable, rewarding stimuli (e.g., Goldstein & Strube, 1994; Headey, Holmstrom, & Wearing, 1984; Stone, 1981; Warr et al., 1983; Zautra & Reich, 1983).

This fundamental asymmetry still may be puzzling to many readers. It therefore may be helpful to conduct a simple self-study. Begin by imagining yourself in a relatively neutral, low-activation state. Next, think of some events or experiences that likely would make you upset or distressed (i.e., a state of elevated negative mood), at least for a few minutes. In my own case, some of the first things that come to mind are (1) having car trouble when I am in a hurry to get somewhere, (2) being criticized for something that really wasn't my fault, and (3) hearing some bad news about a family member. Now think of some events or experiences that would make you happy, cheerful, or excited (i.e., a state of elevated positive mood), at least briefly. My own introspection yielded such experiences as (1) having a very stimulating conversation with someone, (2) playing football with my children on a brisk fall day, and (3) listening to some engaging music. Of course, different people generate different lists, but I suspect that most people will produce two sets of events—one related to negative mood change and the other to positive mood change— that differ quite markedly in their character and quality. In other words, the events that make us feel bad are quite different from those that make us feel good.

Note, moreover, that the *absence* of one type of event has implications that differ markedly from the *presence* of the other. For instance, although I may become upset when I experience car trouble, I don't necessarily feel happy, cheerful, and enthusiastic when my car is working perfectly. In other words, the performance of my car has a much greater capacity to induce negative mood change than positive mood change. Conversely, I very much enjoy those times in which I am able to engage in an activity such as football with my children. Nevertheless, I rarely become upset or distressed because I currently am not engaging in such activities. Thus, this type of interpersonal, physical activity has a much greater capacity to induce positive mood change than negative mood change.

Goldstein and Strube (1994) conducted a study that illustrates this point nicely. They assessed mood in college students (1) at the beginning of a class session and (2) after receiving feedback regarding their performance on the first course examination. Students who received failure feedback (i.e., they learned that they had performed below the class average) showed a significant increase on the PANAS Negative Affect scale but no corresponding decrease on Positive Affect. Conversely, those who received success feedback (i.e., they performed above the class average) displayed a significant elevation on Positive Affect but no corresponding decline in Negative Affect. These results were later replicated at the time of the second course examination. Thus, hearing bad news (in this case, feedback indicating poor performance) apparently has stronger and more immediate implications for negative mood change, whereas receiving good news (e.g., feedback indicating success) has greater implications for positive mood change.

The asymmetry between positive and negative mood is further reflected in their markedly different distributions over time. Zevon and Tellegen (1982), for example, plotted the distribution of nearly 2,000 Negative and Positive Affect scores derived from the daily mood ratings of 21 students. They found that the Negative Affect scores were positively skewed and leptokurtic (i.e., more "peaked" than a normal distribution); that is, most of the scores were packed within a relatively narrow range slightly below the mean. However, they also observed a relatively large number of extremely elevated scores that appeared to represent "emergency reactions" to current crises. In contrast, Positive Affect scores showed a roughly normal distribution, displaying substantial variability across a much broader range. My colleagues and I later identified the same basic distributional patterns in more than 1,500 daily mood ratings derived from the responses of 18 Japanese college students (Watson, Clark, & Tellegen, 1984).

To further illustrate this point, I examined the responses of students who completed a minimum of 35 PANAS assessments in our studies of momentary or daily mood. This yielded a total of 18,362 momentary mood observations from 414 students and 20,240 daily mood observations from 454 students. I then standardized the PANAS Negative Affect and Positive Affect scale scores on a person-by-person basis, such that each student now had an overall mean of 0 and a standard deviation of 1 on both scales, which put all of the scores on the same metric so that they could be collapsed across individuals.

Figures 3.1 and 3.2 display the resulting distributions for the momentary and daily ratings, respectively. In each figure, the ordinate represents the proportion of all scores falling within each designated interval, whereas the abscissa indicates the midpoint of that interval (for instance, –1.2 is the midpoint for the scores falling between –1.05 and –1.35, and 0 is the midpoint for the scores falling between –0.15 and +0.15). Repli-

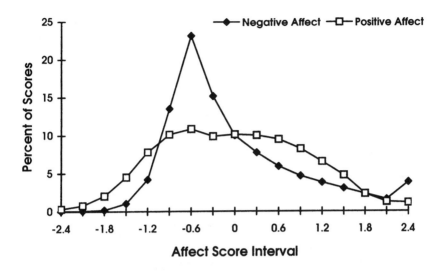

FIGURE 3.1. Overall distribution of Negative and Positive Affect scores (momentary mood data).

cating the findings of earlier studies, ratings on Negative Affect are positively skewed, with most of the scores falling below the mean. Moreover, the bulk of the scores are tightly packed within a relatively narrow range. Nevertheless, one also sees a relatively large number of extremely high scores, which correspond to episodes of marked distress. Thus, it appears that an individual's negative mood level remains low and relatively stable until a crisis occurs, at which point the person is roused into action by a sharp increase in Negative Affect. After the emergency has passed, Negative Affect quickly returns to its low, baseline level. In other words, this distinctive distribution reflects the inherently reactive, crisis-driven character of the negative affects.

Clearly, a different logic underlies positive mood fluctuation. Positive Affect scores are roughly symmetrical around 0 and show substantial variability across a broad range. In fact, they are slightly platykurtic, which means that their distribution is slightly "flatter" (i.e., shows less of a peak at the mean) than that of a classic normal curve. As we will see, positive moods do not show the same close association with ongoing crises and, therefore, do not exhibit the sudden, sharp elevations that are characteristic of the negative affects. As Clark and Watson (1988) put it, "Positive Affect ebbs and flows with the daily tide of events, whereas

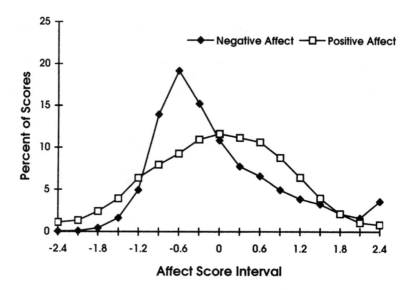

FIGURE 3.2. Overall distribution of Negative and Positive Affect scores (daily mood data).

Negative Affect crashes upon us in times of trouble only to disappear just as quickly when the storm is over" (p. 305).

STRESSFUL EVENTS AND AVERSIVE STIMULI

Relations with General Negative and Positive Affect

An enormous literature has examined the short-term effects of stressful and aversive stimuli on mood. The large majority of the relevant studies have focused on the negative affects, especially anxiety. These studies clearly establish that anxious mood increases significantly in response to various kinds of stressors. For instance, anxiety is substantially elevated in situations involving pain or the threat of physical harm; thus, marked increases in anxiety have been identified in individuals undergoing surgery (Auerbach, 1973b; Martinez-Urrutia, 1975), awaiting a painful dental treatment (Lamb, 1976; McNair et al., 1971), or anticipating shock (Hodges & Spielberger, 1966; Scarpetti, 1973). Similarly, people report increased feelings of anxiety while watching a gruesome or disgusting film (Kendall, 1978; Kendall, Finch, Auerbach, Hooke, & Mikulka, 1976).

Anxiety also increases in situations involving evaluation or scrutiny by others, such as being interviewed (Johnson, 1968), taking an examination (Kendall et al., 1976; Zuckerman, Lubin, & Rinck, 1983), and giving a public speech (Lamb, 1972). Interestingly, people also display vicarious anxiety while observing others in socially embarrassing situations (Kendall, Finch, & Montgomery, 1978). Finally, anxiety increases markedly in response to failure, criticism, or other negative feedback (Auerbach, 1973b; Kendall, 1978; Watson & Clark, 1984).

Not surprisingly, several studies have demonstrated strong correlations between state anxiety and measures of general negative mood, such as the PANAS Negative Affect scale (e.g., Watson & Clark, 1984; Watson, Clark, & Tellegen, 1988). Thus, we can anticipate that various types of stressors (examinations, criticism, shock, etc.) will be associated with marked increases in general Negative Affect. I should add, however, that some anxiety scales also show weaker negative correlations with measures of positive mood, such as the PANAS Positive Affect scale (Watson & Clark, 1984; Watson, Clark, & Tellegen, 1988). Consequently, these older studies of state anxiety do not rule out the possibility that stressful events also lead to significant decrements in positive mood.

Our own data have extended this earlier literature by demonstrating that the effects of stress are almost entirely confined to Negative Affect (see Watson, 1988a; Watson & Pennebaker, 1989). That is, stressful events are strongly associated with transient elevations in negative mood but are more weakly and inconsistently related to changes in positive mood. Some of the clearest and most compelling evidence of this point comes from our extensive within-subject studies of momentary and daily mood. Table 3.1 presents relevant data from three samples. In two of these samples, students rated their momentary mood (one on the original 20-item PANAS, the other on the expanded 60-item PANAS-X); in the third, they rated their daily mood. In addition to reporting on their mood, students also rated their current or daily level of stress on a 1–5 scale (1 = very slightly or not at all, 2 = a little, 3 = moderately, 4 = quite a bit, 5 = extremely). All respondents completed a minimum of 35 mood/stress assessments; overall, these three samples represent a combined total of 16,635 observations derived from 382 students.

Table 3.1 reports the average within-subject correlations between rated stress and the general Negative and Positive Affect scales in each sample. These data establish a strong link between perceived stress and experienced Negative Affect, with mean correlations ranging from .44 to .56 across the three samples. In contrast, the average within-subject correlations with Positive Affect are substantially weaker, ranging from only −.07 to −.18. Similar findings have been obtained using between-subject designs: Current stress levels are substantially correlated with individual

TABLE 3.1. Average Within-Subject Correlations between Perceived Stress and General Negative and Positive Affect

			Correlation with	
Time frame/sample	No. of participants	Total No. of observations	Negative Affect	Positive Affect
Momentary data				
Sample 1	187	8,038	**.56**	−.07
Sample 2	115	5,043	**.50**	−**.18**
Daily data				
Sample 1	80	3,554	**.44**	−**.11**

Note. Correlations of |.10| or greater are shown in **boldface.**

differences in Negative Affect but are unrelated to Positive Affect (Watson, 1988a; Watson & Pennebaker, 1989).

These correlational findings perhaps may be a bit too abstract for some readers. In everyday terms, just how strong are these effects? To explore this point, I conducted additional analyses on the combined momentary mood samples. I began by dichotomizing each person's ratings into "low stress" (i.e., a rating of 1, 2, or 3) and "high stress" (i.e., a rating of 4 or 5) responses. For each person, I then computed separate mean Negative and Positive Affect scores for the low- and high-stress conditions; these analyses were restricted to the 218 students who produced at least 10 ratings of each type. Finally, I calculated overall mean Negative and Positive Affect scores for the low and high stress conditions across all 218 individuals. These analyses revealed that the mean Negative Affect score during moments of high stress (18.5) was nearly 5 points higher than the corresponding average during times of low stress (13.7); in contrast, the mean Positive Affect score during times of high stress (23.8) was only slightly lower than the corresponding average during moments of low stress (25.5).

One possible objection to these data is that the stress ratings were not anchored to any specific life event; rather, the respondents simply estimated their overall level of stress in a vague and subjective manner. In fact, it could be argued that the students essentially treated the stress rating as another negative mood term. In other words, when people reported that they were currently under stress, this simply may have been another way of saying that they were feeling distressed and upset (for a related discussion, see Watson, 1988a). Even if one accepts this criticism, however, these data still have important implications, in that they establish a specific affinity between stress and Negative Affect. That is, for whatever reason, stress appraisals are largely unrelated to variations in positive mood. Apparently, one can continue to feel cheerful and enthusiastic (i.e., high Positive Affect), even in the face of perceived stress and strain.

Nevertheless, it still is highly desirable to circumvent this problem entirely by measuring stress more objectively. My colleagues and I therefore examined mood fluctuations as a function of a stressful examination (McIntyre, Watson, & Cunningham, 1990). In this study, college students completed the PANAS Negative and Positive Affect scales (1) in a relaxed baseline setting and (2) immediately prior to a course examination. Consistent with the other results I have discussed, this stressor had no effect on Positive Affect but was associated with a marked elevation in Negative Affect (which increased from an average score of 17.3 at baseline to a mean score of 25.3 before the examination). Curt McIntyre and I (1991) replicated these findings in a second study in which mood was assessed both before and after course examinations (these data are discussed in more detail shortly). These findings clearly demonstrate that stressful events primarily result in elevated levels of negative mood.

Relations with Specific Types of Mood

I have not yet addressed the key issue of *specificity*. That is, are stressful events associated with nonspecific increases in negative mood, or do they instead show specific affinities with a particular type of affect? For instance, does watching a gruesome film lead only to increased levels of fear and anxiety, or is it nonspecifically associated with elevations in hostility, sadness, and guilt as well? Similarly, does receiving failure feedback lead to feelings of depression, anxiety, or both?

Unfortunately, most of the relevant studies have assessed only a single type of negative mood (e.g., anxiety), thereby precluding any analyses of specificity. Furthermore, of the studies that actually assessed multiple types of negative affect, most used scales that clearly lacked discriminant validity (i.e., are very highly intercorrelated), such as the original scales of the MAACL (Zuckerman & Lubin, 1965). These studies tended to find little or no evidence of specificity, but this is hardly surprising in light of the high scale intercorrelations. For instance, Polivy (1981) reported two studies that examined the effects of shock threat on anxious, depressed, and hostile mood. She found that the threat of a painful shock produced significant increases in depression and hostility in addition to the expected elevation in anxiety, thereby suggesting that the effects of shock are largely nonspecific. However, her measures of anxious, depressed, and hostile mood had intercorrelations ranging from .61 to .82 across the two studies. It is virtually impossible to establish the existence of specific effects when mood scales are this highly interrelated!

Tests of specificity require scales with better discriminant validity, such as those included in the revised MAACL (Zuckerman & Lubin, 1985) and the PANAS-X (see Watson & Clark, 1997b). Some relevant data are available using such scales, and they provide some limited evidence of specificity. Generally speaking, specificity appears to be quite poor when people are asked to rate their current stress levels—that is, when the assessed variable is *perceived stress* rather than the occurrence of a stressful event per se. Clark and I demonstrated this point quite clearly (Watson & Clark, 1992a, Study 2). College students completed general, trait versions of the PANAS-X basic Negative Affect scales (Fear, Sadness, Guilt, Hostility) at two assessments separated by a 2-month time interval. At each assessment, the students also completed a 55-item adaptation of the Revised Hassles Scale (DeLongis, Folkman, & Lazarus, 1988). On this scale, the students rated the extent to which each of the items (e.g., "your work load," "your friends," "the weather") bothered or upset them during the past month. Responses to the 55 items were then summed to yield a Total Hassles score at each assessment.

The four Negative Affect scales showed virtually identical associations with Total Hassles at the Time 1 assessment (r's ranged from .31 to .37). In other words, current life stress was nonspecifically related to various types of negative affect. Moreover, when the influence of the general Negative Affect dimension was eliminated, these relations completely vanished (the partial r's now ranged from only .03 to –.01). The same pattern emerged at the second assessment. Again, the four Negative Affect scales all correlated similarly with Total Hassles (r's ranged from .35 to .45), and these relations essentially vanished if the nonspecific effect of general Negative Affect was removed (the partial r's ranged from only .13 to –.11). Clearly, when assessed in this manner, perceived stress is nonspecifically related to general Negative Affect.

These data are based on trait versions of the PANAS-X scales and so might not generalize to short-term fluctuations in mood. Moreover, it might be argued that within-subject designs might yield better evidence of specificity. However, our subsequent within-subject analyses of short-term mood fluctuations have yielded essentially the same results. Table 3.2 reports further analyses of the second momentary mood sample (previously discussed in connection with Table 3.1), in which students rated themselves on the complete PANAS-X. This table presents average within-subject correlations between ratings of perceived stress and the 11 specific PANAS-X mood scales. These data again demonstrate that the four basic Negative Affect scales all have similar associations with perceived stress. Taken together, these findings indicate that ongoing stress is

TABLE 3.2. Average Within-Subject Correlations between Perceived Stress and Specific Types of Affect (Momentary Mood Ratings)

Scale	Mean within-subject correlation
Basic negative affects	
Fear	.39
Hostility	.38
Guilt	.36
Sadness	.28
Basic positive affects	
Joviality	−.31
Self-Assurance	−.21
Attentiveness	−.02
Other affective states	
Shyness	.11
Fatigue	.18
Serenity	−.32
Surprise	−.04

Note. These correlations are based on 5,043 observations from 115 students. Correlations of |.10| or greater are shown in **boldface**.

associated with nonspecific increases in negative mood, such that stressed individuals report elevated levels of nervous, fear, sadness, guilt, shame, anger and irritability.

One aspect of these results deserves some further comment. Note that the data in Table 3.2 suggest that the various positive affects have rather different associations with current stress. On the one hand, Joviality (i.e., feelings of cheerfulness, joy, enthusiasm, and energy) had a mean coefficient of −.31, which is comparable in magnitude to the correlations for the various negative affects. In contrast, the average correlation (−.21) for Self-Assurance (i.e., feelings of confidence and daring) was somewhat lower, and that for Attentiveness (−.02) was essentially 0. These data therefore establish that current stress appraisals are related to at least some types of positive mood.

I explored this issue further by examining the average within-subject correlations for each individual positive mood term. Consistent with the scale-level findings, terms reflecting joy and enthusiasm ("happy," "cheerful," "joyful," "delighted," "enthusiastic," and "excited") showed the strongest stress-related effects. Conversely, the terms showing the weakest stress effects all were markers of Attentiveness ("alert," "attentive," "determined," and "concentrating"). These findings suggest that although ongoing stress does not produce a strong general decrement in positive affective experience, it is associated with decreased feelings of cheerfulness, joy and enthusiasm.

However, the most noteworthy aspect of Table 3.2 is that it again demonstrates a nonspecific relation between stress appraisals and negative mood. Are there, in fact, any data to suggest that more specific affinities exist? Evidence of specificity can be obtained when one examines the effects of stressful events per se rather than subjective stress appraisals. Zuckerman et al. (1983), for instance, found that anxious mood was significantly elevated immediately before a course examination but feelings of depression and hostility were not.

Curt McIntyre and I obtained particularly striking evidence of specificity in our studies of examination stress (McIntyre & Watson, 1991). We conducted two tests of this issue. In the first, 44 college students rated their current, momentary mood (1) shortly before their first course examination, (2) immediately following the examination, and (3) from 1 to 2 hours postexamination. The students completed the PANAS-X Fear, Sadness, Guilt, and Hostility scales at each assessment, thereby allowing us to determine whether the examination had specific or nonspecific mood effects.

Mean scores on these four PANAS-X scales at each assessment are displayed in Figure 3.3, and they show impressive evidence of specificity. Repeated measures analyses of variance (ANOVAs) revealed significant

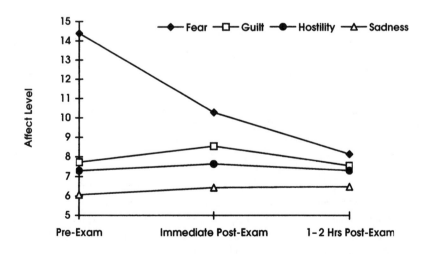

FIGURE 3.3. Effects of examination stress on the basic negative affects (Exam 1).

effects for Fear and Guilt but not for Sadness or Hostility. Furthermore, an inspection of Figure 3.4 indicates that only Fear scores were substantially elevated *before* the examination; in contrast, ratings of Guilt increased slightly immediately *after* the test. Thus, the anticipatory effects of the stressful event were specifically confined to feelings of nervousness and fear.

We subsequently attempted to replicate these findings at the time of the second course examination. The procedure was the same as before, using 40 of the 44 original students. These analyses again revealed impressive evidence of specificity (see Figure 3.4 for the mean scale scores at each assessment). Repeated measures ANOVAs revealed a significant effect for Fear but not for any of the other scales. Thus, replicating our earlier results, this stressor produced a significant elevation in nervousness and anxiety without influencing any other types of negative mood.

These data demonstrate that specific stress-related effects can be established under certain conditions. It appears that two methodological features are crucial in establishing specificity. First, considerable evidence now indicates that subjective perceptions of stress are nonspecifically related to general Negative Affect, whereas analyses of particular stressful events seem much more likely to yield evidence of specific effects. The implications are clear: In the future, mood researchers interested in establishing specific effects should use the latter approach to assessing stress rather than the former.

Second, it is essential to use mood measures that show a reasonable

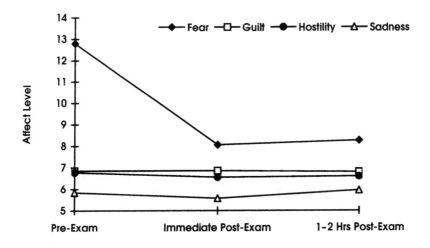

FIGURE 3.4. Effects of examination stress on the basic negative affects (Exam 2).

level of discriminant validity. This does *not* mean that one needs to use negative mood scales that are entirely uncorrelated with one another, because such scales do not exist. Furthermore, mounting evidence suggests that the various negative affects are truly interrelated; consequently, it is difficult to imagine how one could construct valid measures of fear, sadness, hostility, and guilt that were entirely independent of one another (see Watson & Clark, 1992a). Thus, some level of overlap is both desirable and inevitable. Nevertheless, some mood measures clearly show better discriminant validity than others; it is much easier to establish specific effects when better, more precise measures are used.

SOCIAL ACTIVITY

Relations with General Positive and Negative Affect

In contrast to stressful events, social interaction has a much stronger association with positive mood than with negative mood. This important finding initially emerged from between-subject studies showing that individual differences in Positive Affect—but not Negative Affect—are broadly and consistently related to various indexes of social behavior, including frequency of contact and satisfaction with friends and relatives, making new acquaintances, and involvement in social organizations (e.g., Beiser, 1974; Bradburn, 1969; Phillips, 1967; Watson, 1988a; Watson & Clark, 1997a).

My colleagues and I subsequently established that this same basic pattern emerges in within-subject analyses as well. In addition to rating their current affect, the students in our two momentary mood samples indicated whether or not they had interacted socially within the past hour. Table 3.3 reports the average within-subject correlations between this dichotomous social interaction index and general Negative and Positive Affect across the combined samples; these mean values represent a total of 18,359 observations from 414 respondents. Replicating the data from the between-subject studies, social interaction had a mean correlation of .24 with Positive Affect but only –.08 with Negative Affect. In other words, recent social activity was associated with a significant, short-term elevation in positive mood but was largely unrelated to negative mood.

When compared to the strong within-subject correlations between perceived stress and Negative Affect, this mean coefficient of .24 might seem weak and unimpressive. However, in evaluating the magnitude and importance of these effects, two considerations should be kept in mind. First, in these samples we assessed social activity simply as the occurrence versus nonoccurrence of an interaction within the past hour. Many mood effects are quite evanescent (e.g., Thayer, 1989); consequently,

TABLE 3.3. Average Within-Subject Correlations between Social Interaction and Momentary Mood

Scale	Mean within-subject correlation
General affect scales	
Negative Affect	−.08
Positive Affect	**.24**
Basic negative affects	
Fear	−.05
Hostility	**−.12**
Guilt	−.05
Sadness	−.05
Basic positive affects	
Joviality	**.29**
Self-Assurance	**.26**
Attentiveness	**.21**
Other affective states	
Shyness	−.05
Fatigue	**−.20**
Serenity	.09
Surprise	**.14**

Note. The correlations for the general affect scales are based on 18,359 observations from 414 students; all other correlations are based on 10,168 observations from 226 students. Correlations of |.10| or greater are shown in **boldface.**

much of the actual affective response may have dissipated by the time of the rating, especially if the interaction occurred relatively close to the maximum time limit of one hour. Furthermore, because of practical limitations, we could not measure the extent, intensity, or nature of the reported interaction; as we will see, all these variables can influence the magnitude and character of the mood response. Finally, we made no attempt to capture the overall *valence* of the social activity. That is, although many of these interactions presumably were quite pleasant and stimulating, others undoubtedly were relatively mundane and uninspiring, and still others (e.g., fights and arguments) were actively unpleasant (Berry & Hansen, 1996; Rook, 1984). Put another way, these data demonstrate that a typical episode of social activity—without any consideration of the nature, extent, duration, or valence of the interaction—has a distinctly positive quality. Viewed in this light, it seems remarkable that we were able to find any significant mood effects at all.

Second, as long as the pattern is systematic, even relatively small effects can exert a powerful influence on mood over time. At a given moment in time, a person's mood may be influenced by countless variables (e.g., current stressors, level of social interaction, recent physical activity, consumption of food or other substances, current health status, the time of day, and the day of the week). Because of this, the impact of any one factor—such as the occurrence versus nonoccurrence of socializing—is likely to be relatively weak when mood is assessed on a single occasion. Over time, however, as these variables recur again and again, these small momentary influences are gradually transformed into much more substantial effects (see Thayer, 1989). For instance, one's mood on any given Monday or Friday depends on a host of variables: A particular Monday can be quite enjoyable if it happens to be a holiday, whereas a given Friday can be extremely onerous if one is ill. Nevertheless, over the long haul, people do report substantially better moods on Fridays than on Mondays (a topic considered in Chapter 4).

To illustrate this point—and to demonstrate the real-world magnitude of this social interaction effect—I computed separate mean affect scores for each individual across (1) those occasions in which they reported socializing versus (2) those in which they reported no recent social activity. These analyses were restricted to the 339 students who reported at least 10 observations of each type. I then calculated overall mean Negative and Positive Affect scores for the socializing and nonsocializing occasions across all individuals.

These results clearly demonstrated that recent social activity has a substantial effect on positive—but not negative—mood. The mean Positive Affect score during times of recent social activity (25.8) was 4 points higher than the corresponding average during times with no such activity (21.8). In contrast, the mean Negative Affect scores differed by slightly less than 1 point (15.1 vs. 16.0 for the social and nonsocial occasions, respectively).

The data I have examined thus far are based on momentary mood ratings, and it is important to note that similar findings have emerged in studies of daily mood. My colleagues and I initially conducted two studies that also used simple measures of social activity. First, Clark and I examined daily mood variation in 18 Japanese college students over a 3-month period (a total of 1,612 observations; see Clark & Watson, 1988). The students also kept a brief diary in which they recorded important events and concerns for each day; a dichotomous index of social activity was constructed by noting whether or not they spontaneously reported some type of interpersonal event in their diary record for that day. We obtained an average within-subject correlation of .25 between this index of social activity and daily Positive Affect; the corresponding value for Negative Affect was only −.05.

In the second study, I collected daily mood and activity questionnaires from 80 U.S. college students over a 6- to 7-week period (a total of 3,554 observations; see Watson, 1988a). On each day, the students indicated the number of hours (to the nearest half hour) that they had spent with friends. Consistent with our other data, reported social activity had a significantly higher mean within-subject correlation with Positive Affect (.14) than with Negative Affect (−.07).

Although these data are interesting, it clearly is desirable to measure social activity more thoroughly. Accordingly, my colleagues and I constructed a 21-item survey of daily social activity, which we included in a study of 127 college students who were assessed over a 1- to 2-month period (a total of 5,424 observations; see Watson et al., 1992, Study 2). The survey items were selected to sample broad classes of social activity; the assessed items included romantic activity or dating, going out for a meal, exercise or playing sports, going to a movie or play, having a serious discussion, watching television, running errands, helping someone, and religious activities. The students rated the amount of time (not at all, 1–15 min, 15–30 min, 30–60 min, more than 1 hr) they had spent in each of these activities during the day. An index of Overall Social Activity was then constructed by summing the responses to the individual items.

As shown in Table 3.4, Overall Social Activity had a significantly higher average within-subject correlation with Positive Affect (.26) than with Negative Affect (−.05). Thus, this differentiated, multi-item survey of

TABLE 3.4. Average Within-Subject Correlations between Daily Mood and Various Types of Social Activity

Affect scale	Overall social activity	Social activity subscales		
		Active participation	Social entertainment	Social responsibilities
General affect scales				
Negative Affect	−.05	−.03	−.03	.02
Positive Affect	**.26**	**.23**	**.12**	.05
Basic positive affects				
Joviality	**.31**	**.29**	**.15**	.03
Self-Assurance	**.26**	**.24**	**.12**	.03
Attentiveness	**.16**	**.10**	.06	.09

Note. Correlations with the general affect scales are based on the responses of 127 students and 5,424 total observations; all other correlations are based on the responses of 96 students and 4,117 observations. Correlations of |.10| or greater are shown in **boldface**. These data are adapted from Watson et al. (1992, Study 2).

interpersonal activity yielded results that were virtually identical to those obtained using simple measures of socializing.

Watson et al. (1992, Study 1) obtained similar results in analyses of weekly mood. In this study, 85 college students completed a mood and social activity questionnaire once a week for 13 weeks; they all completed a minimum of seven weekly assessments (a total of 1,037 observations). Weekly social activity was measured using a 15-item survey that was quite similar to the 21-item questionnaire described previously; the one major difference was that the students indicated how frequently they had engaged in each of these activities during the past week on a 4-point scale (not at all, once, twice, three or more times). Across the 13 weeks, Overall Social Activity again had a significantly stronger mean correlation with Positive Affect (.30) than with Negative Affect (–.18).

We also have obtained similar findings in two more controlled studies (McIntyre, Watson, Clark, & Cross, 1991). In the first study, students rated their current mood on the PANAS three times during a 2-hour class: (1) at the beginning of the class, (2) 1 hour into the class, and (3) after a period of social interaction. During this social interaction, the students were required to get acquainted with a classmate that they had not previously met. This brief social interaction produced a significant, marked elevation in Positive Affect (which increased nearly 6 points) but had no effect on Negative Affect. The procedure for the second study was identical except that the social activity consisted of having lunch with the same classmate with whom they had gotten acquainted earlier. Again, the social episode produced a significant elevation in Positive Affect (which increased more than 4 points) but had no effect on Negative Affect.

Note that these data have important *causal* implications. Because all the previously reviewed evidence had been collected from naturalistic correlational designs, it was causally ambiguous and could be interpreted in various ways. One obvious possibility is that social interaction leads to increased positive affect. In other words, most interpersonal activity is pleasurable and rewarding and, therefore, produces transient feelings of joy and enthusiasm. Another possibility, however, is that causality actually flows in the opposite direction, and elevated Positive Affect increases the likelihood of socializing. That is, feelings of joy and enthusiasm may be associated with an enhanced desire for affiliation and an increased preference for interpersonal contact (see Watson & Clark, 1997a; Watson et al., 1992).

These two possibilities are not necessarily mutually exclusive. In fact, the available data suggest that both are true to some extent. On the one hand, considerable evidence indicates that elevated Positive Affect does lead to an increased desire for social and prosocial activities and to actual increases in social and prosocial behavior (e.g., Cunningham, 1988a,

1988b; Shaffer & Smith, 1985; Strickland, Hale, & Anderson, 1975). On the other hand, the students in the McIntyre et al. (1991) studies were required to engage in social interactions at designated times, regardless of their current level of Positive Affect. Accordingly, these data strongly suggest that social activity produces transient elevations in positive mood.

Relations with Specific Types of Mood

Again, it is important to assess the specificity versus generality of this observed relation between social activity and positive mood. Table 3.3 reports average within-subject correlations between the dichotomous index of social interaction (i.e., whether or not the person socialized within the past hour) and the 11 specific PANAS-X scales in the second momentary mood sample; these data are based on a total of 10,168 observations from 226 individuals. The most notable finding is that socializing had similar, moderate correlations (ranging from .21 to .29) with the three basic positive affect scales. Thus, social interaction tends to be broadly associated with increased positive mood.

Furthermore, consistent with the results observed at the general dimensional level, all four basic negative affects had substantially lower associations with socializing. In fact, only Hostility had an average coefficient greater than −.05. Interestingly, Shyness also was essentially unrelated to interpersonal activity, again demonstrating its consistent links with negative—but not positive—mood.

We obtained similar results in our intensive, within-subject analysis of daily mood and social activity (Watson et al., 1992, Study 2). As discussed earlier, students completed a 21-item survey of daily interpersonal interaction that was summed into an index of Overall Social Activity. In addition to the general affect scales, 96 of these students completed the basic Positive Affect scales of the PANAS-X each day over a 1- to 2-month period (a total of 4,117 observations). As can be seen in Table 3.4, Joviality and Self-Assurance both showed moderately strong associations with daily social activity that were essentially the same as those observed in the momentary mood data. Attentiveness again had the lowest association with socializing, so we can tentatively conclude that feelings of alertness and concentration are more weakly related to interpersonal activity than are other types of positive mood. Nevertheless, the overall pattern again suggests that interpersonal activity is broadly related to positive affective experience.

One final aspect of this study deserves mention. We constructed a three-item Sociability scale that consisted of the terms "friendly," "sociable," and "warmhearted"; the students also completed this measure on a daily basis. Analyses of this scale yielded two interesting results. First, despite the frankly interpersonal nature of its component items, this scale (mean $r = .29$) was no more highly related to Overall Social Activity than were Joviality and Self-Assurance. Second, Sociability was moderately to strongly correlated with the various positive affects, with average within-subject correlations ranging from .45 (with Attentiveness) to .73 (with Joviality). (In fact, this strong correlation with Sociability played a crucial role in the naming of the Joviality scale. Note that the term "joviality"—in addition to reflecting jollity and good-humor—conveys a strong sense of conviviality, of enjoying the company of others.) Thus, these data establish a strong and pervasive link between affiliative feelings and positive mood (see also Watson & Clark, 1997a).

Analyses of Different Types of Social Activity

I have not yet considered how different types of social events are related to mood. This clearly is a crucial issue, as some types of interpersonal activities obviously are more pleasurable and rewarding than others. Clark and I conducted the first systematic analysis of this issue in our daily mood study of Japanese college students (Clark & Watson, 1988). We again found a broad association between positive mood and socializing such that most types of social events were significantly related to elevations in Positive Affect. Finer-grained analyses, however, revealed that physically active, informal, and Epicurean events (e.g., skiing, hiking, parties, and eating and drinking with others) were associated with extremely high levels of positive mood, whereas relatively formal and sedentary interpersonal activities (e.g., club meetings and lessons) were entirely unrelated to mood. Finally, and not surprisingly, one class of social events (arguments with others) was extremely unpleasant to the students and was associated with a highly dysphoric mood (i.e., very high Negative Affect and very low Positive Affect).

My colleagues and I further examined this issue by factor analyzing our 21-item survey of daily social activity (Watson et al., 1992, Study 2). We identified three interpretable factors and created subscales to measure each of them: Social Entertainment (e.g., going to a movie or play, going to a concert, and playing cards or other games), Active Participation (e.g., going to or giving a party, going out for a drink, and romantic activity or dating), and Social Responsibilities (e.g., having a serious discussion, helping someone, running errands or chores, and studying). Table 3.4 reports average within-subject correlations between these subscales and various PANAS-X scores. On the basis of our earlier findings (Clark & Watson, 1988), one would expect Active Participation to have the strongest association with positive mood. This expectation was clearly confirmed. Active Participation had moderately strong mean correlations with general Positive Affect, Joviality, and Self-Assurance that are substantially higher than the corresponding values for the other two subscales. Social Entertainment had significantly lower associations with these mood scales, but all three of these mean correlations still differed significantly from 0. Finally, Social Responsibilities displayed relatively weak associations with mood; in fact, only its mean correlation with Attentiveness differed significantly from 0.

However, we obtained somewhat different results in our analyses of weekly mood and social activity (Watson et al., 1992, Study 1). Using modified versions of the social activity subscales that were derived from a 15-item survey, we found that Social Responsibilities and Active Participation both had relatively strong associations with general Positive Affect and much weaker relations with Negative Affect. In contrast, Social Entertainment had both the strongest average correlation with Negative Affect and the weakest mean coefficient with Positive Affect.

These discrepant findings make it difficult to draw general conclusions. However, one finding did emerge consistently across all three studies, namely, physically active and engaging social events (e.g., hiking, partying, and eating or drinking with others) are associated with marked elevations in positive affective experience; moreover, they are especially strongly related to feelings of joy, excitement and energy (Joviality) and confidence and daring (Self-Assurance).

These differential relations lend further credence to the idea that socializing is causally responsible for elevations in positive mood. As noted earlier, considerable evidence suggests that positive mood states produce an enhanced desire for social interaction. However, if this were the sole basis for the observed correlations between socializing and positive mood, then Positive Affect should be more or less equally related to all types of social events. This clearly is not the case: Although some types of events are associated with strong elevations in Positive Affect, others are completely unrelated to mood. Moreover, the events showing the strongest mood effects (e.g., skiing, partying, and dating) intuitively seem much more pleasurable and rewarding than those displaying the weakest effects (e.g., lessons and studying). Consequently, it seems reasonable to conclude that certain types of social activity lead to increased levels of Positive Affect.

Conceptual Implications

In Chapter 1, I suggested that negative moods should be essentially *reactive* in character. That is, negative moods should remain at relatively low, baseline levels during the bulk of everyday life—in the absence of some precipitating event or stimulus, it is maladaptive for an individual to experience strong feelings of fear, anger, or any other type of negative mood. However, when confronted with a threat or crisis, the individual should experience a sudden, sharp increase in negative mood that is designed to help resolve the crisis by (1) signaling that a threat is imminent and (2) mobilizing resources for quick and decisive action. After the crisis has passed, negative mood should return quickly to its basal level.

The reviewed data strongly support this basic model. We have seen, for instance, that negative moods do remain at low, baseline levels throughout most of everyday life, but they show sharp, periodic "emergency reactions" that represent responses to current crises (see Figures 3.1 and 3.2). What are these crises? For the most part, they are the stresses and strains of everyday life—painful medical and dental treatments, being interviewed, taking an important examination, giving a public speech, being criticized or insulted, confronting an uncooperative car, and so on. Negative moods display marked, transient reactions to stressful events of this sort and then quickly return to baseline.

On the other hand, social interactions rarely represent threats or crises, so it is not surprising that Negative Affect is largely unrelated to various indicators of socializing. In this regard, it is interesting to note that one type of social event—having an argument with another—is psychologically threatening and is also associated with a marked elevation in negative mood (Clark & Watson, 1988; see also Rook, 1984). These data further demonstrate the crisis-driven quality of negative affective experience.

In contrast, positive moods are not designed to help the individual cope with threat and crisis. Rather, their basic function is to ensure that organisms obtain the resources that are necessary for the survival of both the individual and the species. Note that they may do so in various ways. For instance, feelings of energy, enthusiasm, and alertness help to activate behavior by providing the physical and cognitive resources necessary for sustained performance. Moreover, heightened feelings of confidence and daring lead to an increased expectancy that behavior will be rewarded with a successful outcome. Finally, the successful attainment of these resources is accompanied by transient feelings of joy and well-being that help to maintain the behavior and ensure that it will recur in the future.

Because many—perhaps most—stressful events lack clear and immediate implications for resource acquisition and maintenance, it is not surprising that positive moods do not strongly or consistently vary as a function of ongoing stresses and strains. Note, however, that certain types of stressors (e.g., the loss of a loved one through death, separation, or rejection, or being demoted or fired) may be associated with a significant loss of resources. Following the logic of the model outlined here, such stressors may be associated with a marked decrement in Positive Affect in addition to the more typically observed elevation in Negative Affect. I return to this idea in Chapter 8 in discussing recent theorizing and evidence regarding depression.

Clearly, however, humans are highly social organisms that depend heavily on others in numerous ways (e.g., physical care and comfort, psychological support, and affectional and sexual needs) so that interpersonal activity plays an extremely important role in resource acquisition and maintenance. Consequently, it is unsurprising that there should be broad and pervasive links between social activity and positive mood. Moreover, the fact that positive mood appears to be both a cause and an effect of social interaction (see also Watson et al., 1992) is entirely consistent with the model I have outlined. On the one hand, elevated levels of positive mood serve to energize the individual, motivating him or her to seek pleasurable and rewarding stimuli through various behaviors, including social activity; on the other hand, positive feelings represent affective rewards that help to maintain these behaviors and ensure that they will be repeated in the future.

EXERCISE AND PHYSICAL ACTIVITY

General Evidence of Mood Effects

As we have seen, social interactions involving strenuous physical activity (e.g., hiking and skiing) are associated with especially strong elevations in positive mood (Clark & Watson, 1988). These data suggest that physical activity per se may have important mood effects. This suggestion is confirmed by an extensive research literature indicating that exercise and intense physical activity have a significant—and generally beneficial—effect on mood (for reviews, see Byrne & Byrne, 1993; Simons, McGowan, Epstein, Kupfer, & Robertson, 1985; Thayer, 1989).

Much of the evidence comes from between-subject designs comparing the mood reports of regular exercisers versus nonexercisers (e.g., joggers vs. non-joggers). Although the results vary somewhat from study to study, regular exercisers generally experience higher levels of positive mood and often report reduced levels of negative mood as well (e.g., Aganoff & Boyle, 1994; Hayden & Allen, 1984). It is noteworthy moreover, that these beneficial mood effects have been observed across many different forms of exercise. Thus, significant mood improvement has been demonstrated for runners (e.g., Morgan, O'Connor, Sparling, & Pate, 1987), body builders (Fuchs & Zaichkowsky, 1983), wrestlers (Nagle, Morgan, Hellickson, Serfass, & Alexander, 1975), and rowers (Morgan & Johnson, 1978).

One obvious limitation of these studies is that they use naturally occurring groups of exercisers and nonexercisers. It is entirely possible that these differences in mood actually are the cause—rather than the effect—of exercise. That is, higher levels of current well-being (i.e., higher positive mood and/or lower negative affect) may increase one's willingness to engage in regular, strenuous physical activity.

Within-subject designs eliminate this problem, however, by using each respondent as his or her own control; these designs also have been used extensively to study the effects of exercise. One common approach is to examine the effects of an intensive exercise training program (e.g., aerobics and weightlifting) on people whose pretraining lifestyle was rather sedentary. Studies of this sort have demonstrated consistently that a regular exercise regimen produces a significantly improved mood in individuals who are initially dysphoric, such as depressives or the highly anxious. Results with nondysphoric, normal-range individuals have been more mixed, however: Some studies have reported significant exercise-related effects, but others have not (e.g., Harris, 1987; Long, 1984, 1985; Norvell & Belles, 1993; Simons et al., 1985).

Another common approach is to examine mood both before and immediately following exercise. The large majority of studies have found that mood is significantly improved (i.e., increased positive mood and/or decreased negative mood) following various types of intense physical activity (e.g., Berger, Owen, & Man, 1993; Lichtman & Poser, 1983). Moreover, the beneficial effects of exercise have been shown to last up to 2 to 3 hours postexercise (Raglin & Morgan, 1987; Thayer, 1987a, 1989). However, a few studies have failed to find consistent mood effects (Sime, 1977; Wood, 1977).

Relations with General Positive and Negative Affect

The bulk of the evidence indicates that exercise has significant effects on mood, especially in individuals who are initially dysphoric. In addition, the data tentatively suggest that exercise may exert stronger and more consistent effects on positive mood than on negative mood; however, no definitive conclusions can be drawn from these studies, most of which used measures that did not clearly distinguish between these two types of affect.

How does exercise, in fact, influence positive and negative mood? My colleagues and I have conducted a number of analyses to answer this question. Table 3.5 presents average within-subject correlations between exercise and the general Negative and Positive Affect scales in four samples. In two of the samples, students rated their current, momentary mood; in the others, they rated their mood over the course of the entire

TABLE 3.5. Average Within-Subject Correlations between Exercise and General Negative and Positive Affect

Time frame/ sample	No. of subjects	Total No. of observations	Correlation with	
			Negative Affect	Positive Affect
Momentary data				
Sample 1	132	5,768	−.05	**.14**
Sample 2	194	8,740	−.07	**.19**
Daily data				
Sample 1	79	3,501	−.04	**.13**
Sample 2	156	7,287	−.09	**.16**

Note. Correlations of | .10 | or greater are shown in **boldface**.

day. Students in the two momentary mood samples indicated whether or not they had exercised during the past hour. Similarly, in the first daily mood sample, the students simply checked whether or not they had exercised at some point during the day; thus, in all these studies, we simply assessed the occurrence versus nonoccurrence of exercise. In the second daily mood sample, however, students were asked to indicate *how many minutes* they had spent exercising that day. Overall, these four samples represent a total of 25,296 observations from 561 individuals.

The results are remarkably consistent across the four samples. The average within-subject correlations between exercise and Positive Affect ranged from .13 to .19, indicating that students tended to report slightly higher levels of positive mood during times of intense physical activity. In contrast, the mean correlations with Negative Affect were consistently lower, ranging only from −.04 to −.09. In fact, in all four samples, the mean correlation with Positive Affect was significantly stronger than the corresponding value for Negative Affect. Thus, we see consistent evidence that exercise is more strongly related to positive mood than to negative mood.

On the other hand, these mean correlations clearly are lower than those seen previously in connection with stress and socializing. Because of this, one may be tempted to conclude that exercise is only weakly related to mood. For various reasons, however, the actual, everyday effect of exercise may be much more substantial than these average correlations suggest. Note, for example, that mood was not assessed immediately after exercise; rather, the ratings tended to be completed somewhat later, especially in the daily mood samples. Although the beneficial effects of exercise may persist for a few hours (Thayer, 1989), much of the actual affective response may have dissipated by the time the mood rating was completed. Moreover, the correlations in the momentary mood samples likely were attenuated due to the low frequency of recent exercising (which, in turn, reduces variability). In the first momentary mood sample, students reported exercising in only 7.8% of the assessments; this translates into an average of only 3.4 exercise observations (out of a total of 43.7) per person. Similarly, in the second momentary mood sample, exercise was reported in only 11.5% of the assessments; this represents an average of only 5.2 exercise observations (out of a total of 45.1) per person. These factors clearly limit the magnitude of the correlations that can be expected.

These considerations notwithstanding, exercise does have a substantial influence on mood when these variables are aggregated over time. To demonstrate this point, I again computed overall mean affect scores in the combined momentary mood samples. In this case, I computed separate mean scores for each student as a function of whether or not they reported exercising within the past hour. Paralleling the earlier analyses for stress and socializing, these analyses were restricted to the 112 students who reported at least 5 observations of each type (this relaxed criterion was necessitated by the infrequent reporting of exercise). Finally, I computed overall mean Negative and Positive Affect scores for the exercising and nonexercising occasions across all of the students.

These analyses demonstrated that exercise has a substantial effect on positive mood and is more weakly related to negative mood. Specifically, mean Positive Affect following exercise (28.9) was 3.5 points higher than the corresponding average across the nonexercising occasions (25.4). In contrast, the Negative Affect means differed by only 1.5 points (15.3 vs. 16.8 for the exercising and nonexercising assessments, respectively).

My colleagues and I also have conducted several studies that were specifically designed to examine the association between mood and exercise. These studies again have demonstrated that strenuous physical activity is strongly and consistently associated with elevations in positive mood but is less clearly or systematically related to negative mood. For instance, we asked students to rate their current, momentary mood on the PANAS scales at baseline and again after 20 minutes of exercise (brisk walking, jogging, swimming, aerobics, or bicycling; see McIntyre et al., 1990). This strenuous physical activity produced a significant elevation in Positive Affect (which increased from 31.4 at baseline to 38.3 after exercise) but had no effect on Negative Affect.

Schneider (1986) investigated the impact of a 6-week exercise regimen on mood and depressive symptoms. The participants were dysphoric students who scored in the mildly to moderately depressed range on the Beck Depression Inventory (BDI; Beck, Ward, Mendelson, Mock, & Erbaugh, 1961) at an initial assessment. Mood ratings on the PANAS were obtained both pre- and posttraining. Regardless of the level of exercise (mild, moderate, or strenuous), the students reported both significantly higher Positive Affect (a mean increase of 7.5 points) and lower Negative Affect (a mean decrease of 5.7 points) following the exercise program.

This study had another noteworthy aspect. Not surprisingly (in view of their relatively high BDI scores), the students' initial mood ratings differed significantly from normative values. Specifically, they initially reported unusually high levels of Negative Affect and atypically low levels of Positive Affect. (These findings are consistent with an affective model of depression that I describe in Chapter 8.) After the exercise regimen, their mean Negative Affect levels still were significantly higher than the established norms; Positive Affect, however, increased to essentially normal levels.

Clark, Ingersoll, Soutter, Hook, and Watson (1989) conducted an intensive, longitudinal analysis of exercise and mood among 55 students enrolled in physical conditioning classes. Mood levels were assessed on the PANAS immediately before and after exercise on 6 class days over the course of the semester, with 2-week intervals between each assessment. At the beginning of the semester (Week 1), an initial measure of aerobic fitness was obtained. On Weeks 3, 7, and 11, the students ran or walked for 30 minutes; a target distance was set and periodically updated by the instructors, based on the individual's fitness level. At the other three assessments (Weeks 5, 9, and 13), exercise consisted of a 1.5-mile fitness test; note that the students' time on these tests contributed to their class grade, so that these runs should constitute mild stressors that are comparable to other types of course examinations.

As expected, the students showed improved aerobic fitness over the course of the semester. In addition, repeated measures ANOVAs indicated that exercise was associated with significant improvements on both Positive and Negative Affect. That is, students reported significantly higher levels of positive mood—and lower levels of negative mood—following exercise. Moreover, the effect on Positive Affect (an overall mean increase of 2.2 points from pre- to postexercise) tended to be greater than that on Negative Affect (a mean decline of 0.8 points), but this difference was only marginally significant. Finally, as expected, Negative Affect— but not Positive Affect—was significantly higher on the fitness test days.

Robert Thayer and his colleagues also conducted several important studies of mood and exercise (for a review, see Thayer, 1989). These studies all employed the Activation–Deactivation Adjective Check List (ADACL; Thayer, 1978a, 1986), which contains four subscales. Two of these subscales—Energetic Arousal and Tense Arousal—essentially represent alternative measures of Positive Affect and Negative Affect, respectively. That is, Energetic Arousal consists of various high-activation positive mood terms ("active," "energetic," "lively," "vigorous"), where-as Tense Arousal consists of descriptors reflecting tension and anxiety ("jittery," "tense," "fearful," "clutched up"). Accordingly, research using these scales is easily integrated into a discussion of Positive and Negative Affect. It also should be noted that the two remaining ADACL sub-scales—Deactivation–Sleep ("sleepy," "tired," "drowsy" vs. "wide awake," "wakeful") and General Deactivation ("placid," "calm," "still," "quiet," "at rest")—correspond closely to the Fatigue and Serenity scales, respectively, of the PANAS-X.

Using the ADACL, Thayer and his colleagues have reported seven studies examining the mood-related effects of a brisk 5- to 10-minute walk (Thayer, 1978b, 1987a, 1987b, Studies 1 and 2; Thayer & Cheatle, 1976; Thayer, Peters, Takahashi, & Birkhead-Flight, 1993, Studies 1 and 2). In all seven analyses, walking produced a marked elevation in Positive Affect. Moreover, Thayer (1987a) demonstrated that this enhanced positive mood persisted for up to 2 hours. In contrast, Negative Affect showed a significant decline in only three of these studies (Thayer, 1987a; Thayer & Cheatle, 1976; Thayer et al., 1993, Study 2). Saklofske, Blomme, and Kelly (1992) also used the ADACL to assess the effects of two different walking conditions (independent vs. monitored). They found that Positive Affect was significantly elevated following both of the walking conditions, whereas Negative Affect decreased only after the independent walk.

These ADACL data closely replicate the findings we have obtained using the PANAS. Moderate and strenuous exercise consistently produce significant elevations in Positive Affect. Although Negative Affect does show some significant exercise-related effects, it is less strongly and systematically related to vigorous physical activity.

Relations with Specific Types of Mood

Virtually no studies have investigated whether physical activity is differentially associated with specific types of affect. It is true that many early studies in this area reported rather broad and nonspecific effects (e.g., exercise sometimes was found to be associated with various types of negative mood, such as depression and anxiety), but this simply may reflect the use of mood measures lacking good discriminant validity.

In fact, the best available data come from our own within-subject analyses of momentary and daily mood. Table 3.6 presents average within-subject correlations for one momentary (194 students, 8,740 observations) and one daily (156 students, 7,287 observations) sample. As discussed earlier (in connection with the Table 3.5 data), the students in this momentary mood sample simply indicated whether or not they had exer-

TABLE 3.6. Average Within-Subject Correlations between Exercise and Specific Types of Affect

Scale	Momentary data	Daily data
Basic negative affects		
Fear	−.04	−.08
Hostility	−.07	−.06
Guilt	−.05	−.06
Sadness	−.06	−.07
Basic positive affects		
Joviality	**.17**	**.14**
Self-Assurance	**.18**	**.14**
Attentiveness	**.14**	**.11**
Other affective states		
Shyness	−.05	−.03
Fatigue	**−.14**	**−.11**
Serenity	−.01	.08
Surprise	.06	.03

Note. The correlations for the momentary data are based on 8,740 observations from 194 subjects; the correlations for the daily data are based on 7,287 observations from 156 subjects. Correlations of |.10| or greater are shown in **boldface.**

cised within the past hour. In contrast, those in the daily mood sample indicated how many minutes they had spent exercising over the course of the day.

Two aspects of these data are noteworthy. First, consistent with the findings shown in Table 3.5, we again see that the momentary and daily mood samples produced extremely similar results. Second, these data show virtually no evidence of specificity. Table 3.5 indicated that general Negative Affect was weakly related to exercise; Table 3.6 extends this finding by demonstrating that various types of negative affect (e.g., Fear, Sadness, and Guilt) all have more or less equally weak associations with physical activity. Similarly, Table 3.5 showed that general Positive Affect was more moderately related to exercise; Table 3.6 demonstrates that all three basic Positive Affect scales (Joviality, Self-Assurance, and Attentiveness) have similar, moderate relations with physical activity. Note, moreover, that Fatigue (which tends to be inversely related to positive mood in within-subject data; see Chapter 2) also has correlations of roughly the same magnitude.

Clearly, these findings require replication in studies that are specifically designed to assess the mood-related effects of exercise. Nevertheless, they tentatively suggest that the effects of exercise are largely non-specific. In other words, it appears that physical activity is broadly associated with elevated levels of positive mood (e.g., enthusiasm, cheerfulness, confidence, and alertness), as well as decreases in sluggishness and lethargy.

Further Implications of the Findings

The exercise data further illustrate the distinctive properties of positive and negative mood states. In this regard, other evidence indicates that elevated levels of negative mood are associated with a pronounced tendency toward rumination and self-focused attention (see Ingram, 1990; Pyszczynski & Greenberg, 1987; Watson & Clark, 1984). Heightened levels of rumination and self-awareness have been related to both depression (e.g., Lyubomirsky & Nolen-Hoeksema, 1993; Pyszczynski & Greenberg, 1987) and anxiety (e.g., Hope & Heimberg, 1985; Hope, Heimberg, Zollo, Nyman, & O'Brien, 1987). Accordingly, high levels of negative mood are associated with a general tendency to turn *inward* and to focus attentional and cognitive resources on oneself. Moreover, other studies suggest that when distressed individuals do turn their attention outward toward the environment, they do so with uncertainty and apprehension, scanning the environment for signs of impending trouble (see Tellegen, 1985; Watson & Pennebaker, 1989).

Putting these considerations together, it appears that negative mood is broadly associated with a sense of separateness and estrangement from one's environment; in a state of high distress, a person perceives and experiences the world as threatening and problematic (Watson et al., 1994). Note also that this distress state contains a highly salient cognitive component in which the individual is introspective, ruminative, apprehensive, and unsettled. In fact, hard and intensive *thinking* is more likely to lead to Negative Affect than to Positive Affect, especially if that thinking is directed inward (Ingram, 1990; Pyszczynski & Greenberg, 1987; Taylor & Brown, 1988).

In contrast, positive mood appears to be related to a much more expansive orientation in which the person approaches and actively engages the environment (Cunningham, 1988a, 1988b; Tellegen et al., 1988; Watson et al., 1992). Cunningham (1988a), for instance, has argued that "positive mood is associated with a social, expansive, approach motivation" (p. 283). Similarly, Tellegen et al. (1988) maintain that individuals experiencing high levels of Positive Affect are prepared to experience "active, pleasurable, and efficacious transactions with their environment" (p. 1033). Thus, in contrast to negative mood, positive mood is associated with a tendency to turn *outward* and to view the environment as a source of pleasure and reward.

Furthermore, this expansive orientation actually is associated with various types of pleasurable and rewarding activities. As we have seen, positive mood both (1) motivates the individual to engage in such activities and (2) serves as an affective reward for these behaviors. In other words, Positive Affect is both a cause and effect of rewarding activities. Thus far, we have seen two broad classes of behavior that illustrate this point: socializing and intense physical activity. On the basis of these findings, we can further suggest that Positive Affect is more related to action than to thought, and that it is easier to induce a state of high Positive Affect through *doing* than through *thinking* (see also Watson & Clark, 1994c). In fact, Csikszentmihalyi (1991) argues that episodes of intense positive mood (which he terms "flow states") are characterized by a merging of action and awareness in which the "person's attention is completely absorbed by the activity. There is no excess psychic energy left over to process any information but what the activity offers" (p. 53). Because of this, individuals in this state "stop being aware of themselves as separate from the actions they are performing" (p. 53).

WEATHER AND THE PHYSICAL ENVIRONMENT

Earlier Studies of Mood and Weather

Physical aspects of the environment also must be considered in any thorough discussion of external influences on mood. In this section, I consider relations between mood and various aspects of the weather. My subjective impression—which is based, in part, on having given several public lectures and academic colloquia on this topic—is that virtually everyone believes that his or her mood is significantly affected by the weather. It is rather surprising, therefore, to find that few studies actually have examined this issue. Moreover, the few available studies are problematic because of small sample sizes, questionable mood measures, and other methodological problems (Sanders & Brizzolara, 1982; Howarth & Hoffman, 1984). Furthermore, the results that have emerged from these studies have tended to be weak, complex, and inconclusive.

One of the earliest published studies was conducted by Goldstein (1972), who assessed seven New York City college students over 11 consecutive Tuesdays and Thursdays in late October. Mood was rated on scales representing the basic semantic differential dimensions of evaluation, activity, and potency; the assessed weather variables included temperature, humidity, barometric pressure, wind speed, and clearness (vs. cloudiness). Results indicated that the students evaluated their mood more positively on days characterized by lower humidity and higher barometric pressure. Similarly, higher activity ratings were associated with lower humidity and higher barometric pressure and with lower wind speed as well. Finally, higher ratings of potency were related to lower temperatures and increased barometric pressure.

Sanders and Brizzolara (1982) examined 30 students enrolled in a 5-week summer course at Towson State University in Baltimore, Maryland. Mood was assessed each day using a short form of the Mood Adjective Checklist (MACL; Nowlis, 1965). The only significant finding was that positive mood (i.e., feelings of elation, vigor, and affiliation) was inversely related to humidity. The other assessed weather variables (temperature and barometric pressure) showed no significant effects; moreover, negative mood was entirely unrelated to weather.

Howarth and Hoffman (1984) studied 24 university students in Edmonton, Alberta, over a 11-day period in November and December. They analyzed 10 different mood scores (e.g., anxiety, depression, aggression, and optimism) and 7 weather variables (e.g., sunshine, temperature, humidity, and barometric pressure). Although these authors reported several significant relations, it is noteworthy that the strongest correlation was only −.15, indicating that levels of concentration declined slightly as humidity increased. Overall, these data suggest that weather has an extremely weak effect on mood.

Charry and Hawkinshire (1981) examined the effects of atmospheric electricity on mood. Current mood was measured twice (on Nowlis's MACL) in a carefully controlled laboratory setting in which temperature and humidity were kept constant. The first assessment occurred under normal atmospheric conditions; at the second assessment, however, the laboratory room contained an excess of small positive ions (a prominent feature of hot, dry winds such as the Santa Ana in California, the Chinook in the Pacific Northwest, the Sirocco in Italy, and the Sharav in Israel). Interestingly, positive mood decreased significantly in the ionized room; negative mood, however, was completely unaffected by the atmospheric manipulation.

Finally, several small-scale studies provide some suggestive evidence that sunshine is associated with a significantly better mood. For instance, Cunningham (1979) reported that level of sunshine correlated .60 with an increasingly good mood among waitresses at a Chicago-area restaurant; unfortunately, however, this correlation was based on only 13 observations. Stronger evidence comes from two studies conducted at the University of Illinois in the early spring. In the first study, Schwarz and Clore (1983) telephoned 84 students on either a sunny or a rainy weekday; students contacted on a sunny day felt significantly happier than those assessed on a rainy day. In the second study, Parrott and Sabini (1990) assessed 65 students on sunny and cloudy days as they entered the university library; again, students assessed on a sunny day reported feeling significantly better than did those contacted on a cloudy day. Sinclair, Mark and Clore (1994) reported similar findings in a sample of 122 students at the University of Alberta.

Intensive Analyses of Sunshine and Rain

It is impossible to draw any firm conclusions from data that are so sparse and inconsistent. This motivated my colleagues and me to conduct much more extensive analyses of the relation between mood and weather. I should begin by noting that I expected to find strong and systematic effects in this area—in no small part because I, too, believe that my mood is strongly influenced by the weather.

For three reasons, I expected to find especially strong associations between Positive Affect and sunshine. First, earlier studies had provided at least suggestive evidence of this relation (e.g., Cunningham, 1979; Schwarz & Clore, 1983). Second, other research (to be discussed in Chapter 4) suggested that positive mood shows a significant seasonal trend, such that it tends to be the highest in the spring and early summer and lowest in the late fall and winter (Bradburn, 1969; Smith, 1979). One obvious explanation is that this seasonal trend reflects systematic changes in the weather, such as the length of the day and the relative frequency of sunshine. Indeed, related research on seasonal affective disorder suggests that positive mood might be substantially influenced by naturally occurring variations in the duration and intensity of light (Kasper & Rosenthal, 1989). Third, as we have seen, Positive Affect is highly responsive to fluctuations in physical and social activity. I therefore expected that certain weather conditions (such as rain or other precipitation) would be associated with reduced opportunities for physical and interpersonal activity, and hence, with decrements in Positive Affect.

My optimistic expectations quickly were quashed. Our initial investigation of this issue was conducted in Kyoto, Japan, between February and June 1980 (Clark & Watson, 1988). In this study, we assessed daily mood in 18 college students over a 3-month period (a total of 1,613 observations). We then correlated these ratings on a person-by-person basis with daily weather summaries for the Kyoto area. We performed extensive analyses on these data using both continuous and dichotomous weather indexes, and lagging the weather variables up to two days in either direction. To our great surprise, these analyses all demonstrated that mood was unrelated to variations in the weather.

These initial findings were quite discouraging. Note, however, that this study was based on a small sample of students. Moreover, because it was conducted in Japan, our null findings might have resulted from translation problems or other difficulties that frequently are encountered in cross-cultural research. I therefore resolved to investigate this issue on a much grander scale in the United States.

Since then, I have collected extensive mood and weather data from eight samples of students at SMU in Dallas, Texas. All the students completed a minimum of 30 daily assessments in which they rated the extent to which they had experienced each mood term over the course of the day. The ratings were all completed in the evening (anytime after 5 P.M.) so that they would provide a reasonable estimate of the person's mood over the course of the entire day. At each assessment, the students also noted the current date, so that their ratings later could be linked with the actual weather conditions for that day. After the completion of the rating period, daily weather data were obtained from official U.S. government records as compiled by the Environmental Data Service of the National Oceanic and Atmospheric Administration.

Table 3.7 provides basic information regarding each of the samples. Five samples were assessed during the fall academic semester (depending on the sample, this could be anytime between late August and early December), whereas the other three were measured during the spring term (anytime between the middle of January and early May). Overall, these data sets represent more than 20,000 observations from 478 students. I should note that these same data sets have been used in previously reported analyses of daily mood; in these earlier analyses, however, they were combined into larger samples (e.g., Table 3.5). In this case, they

TABLE 3.7. Basic Characteristics of the Data Sets Used in the Within-Subject Analyses of Daily Mood and Weather

Sample	Time of assessment	No. of students	Total No. of observations
1	Fall 1985	80	3,523
2	Fall 1989	33	1,360
3	Spring 1990	97	4,152
4	Fall 1990	94	4,125
5	Fall 1991	55	2,200
6	Spring 1992	21	849
7	Fall 1992	48	2,290
8	Spring 1993	50	2,319
Overall		478	20,818

will be analyzed separately to determine whether relations between mood and weather vary across different times of the year.

The Dallas–Fort Worth metropolitan area has a continental climate that is characterized by substantial changes in temperature across seasons; compared to cities that are further north, it has relatively mild winters and extremely hot summers (Ruffner & Blair, 1977). It also tends to be sunnier than many northern cities. It must be emphasized, however, that all these students were subjected to widely varying weather conditions; most notably, they all experienced days characterized by brilliant sunshine as well as extended periods in which the sun was completely absent. Moreover, the average level of sunshine varied enormously across these data sets, ranging from a minimum of only 45% of possible sunshine (Sample 5) to a maximum of 70% of possible sunshine (Sample 2).

Our analyses of these data indicate that mood is not strongly or consistently related to *any* of the assessed weather variables, including temperature, barometric pressure, and level of sunshine. I focus this discussion on (1) the total minutes of sunshine for that day and (2) the measurable precipitation in inches (this being Dallas, Texas, the only measurable precipitation fell as rain). These variables are especially interesting for several reasons. First, as noted earlier, some suggestive evidence indicates that these variables have significant effects, particularly on positive mood. Second, it is reasonable to predict that they will exert simple, linear effects on mood. For instance, it is reasonable to hypothesize that people will be happier on sunny days than on cloudy, rainy days. In contrast, variables such as temperature and humidity might relate differently to mood at different times of the year and in varying conditions. For example, warmer temperatures might be associated with a better mood in the winter but a worse mood in the summer.

Third, these variables have a particularly powerful hold on popular consciousness. There is a strong and pervasive belief in our culture that sunshine improves our mood and, conversely, that cloudiness and rain worsen it. This belief is reflected in countless sayings and songs, such as "keep on the sunny side of life," "into every life some rain must fall," and "you are my sunshine." Indeed, we even use the term "sunny mood" to characterize someone who is cheerful and optimistic, whereas a "dark mood" is used to describe someone who is dismal and sad.

With this in mind, Table 3.8 reports the average within-subject correlations between these weather variables and general Negative and Positive Affect in each of the eight samples. Contrary to both my initial expectation and the prevailing cultural view, sunshine and rain both are completely unrelated to mood. Note that the overall mean correlations with Negative Affect were .00 and –.01 for sunshine and precipitation, respectively; similarly, the average correlations with Positive Affect were

TABLE 3.8. Average Within-Subject Correlations between Weather and General Negative and Positive Affect

	Negative Affect		Positive Affect	
Sample	Minutes of sunshine	Inches of rain	Minutes of sunshine	Inches of rain
1	.04	−.02	.00	.01
2	−.01	−.03	−.05	.04
3	.00	−.03	.04	−.02
4	.02	−.04	.05	−.02
5	.00	.04	.02	−.01
6	.05	−.02	.04	.01
7	.00	−.02	.04	−.04
8	−.04	.00	.07	.00
Overall	.00	−.01	.03	−.01

only .03 and −.01, respectively. Moreover, none of the individual samples showed any evidence of a strong association between mood and these variables.

The students in Samples 4 through 8 completed the full PANAS-X, which allows us to examine whether specific types of mood show somewhat stronger weather-related effects. Table 3.9 reports average within-

TABLE 3.9. Average Within-Subject Correlations (Pooled across Samples 4 through 8) between Weather and Specific Types of Affect

Affect scale	Minutes of sunshine	Inches of rain
Basic negative affects		
Fear	.00	.00
Hostility	.00	.01
Guilt	.00	.00
Sadness	.02	−.01
Basic positive affects		
Joviality	.05	−.01
Self-Assurance	.04	.00
Attentiveness	.02	−.01
Other affective states		
Shyness	.05	−.01
Fatigue	.03	−.01
Serenity	.05	−.01
Surprise	.01	−.01

subject correlations (pooled across these five samples) between the weather variables and the 11 lower-order PANAS-X scales. These analyses lead to exactly the same conclusion: Again, we simply see no evidence that mood is substantially influenced by sunshine or rain.

It is possible that mood is influenced only by more extreme weather conditions. I conducted two additional series of analyses to examine this issue. In both series, I initially standardized all of the scale scores for each person, such that every student had a mean of 0 and a standard deviation of 1 on every mood measure. This procedure eliminates between-subject variance, allowing one to pool observations across individuals. Note that it also yields an overall mean score of 0 on each mood variable. Consequently, negative mean values indicate that the scores were lower than the overall average, whereas positive values indicate that the scores were above average.

The first series of analyses compared mood on entirely sunless (i.e., 0% of possible sunshine) versus completely sunny (i.e., 100% of possible sunshine) days. Table 3.10 presents the mean affect scores for each set of

TABLE 3.10. Standardized Mean Affect Scores on Completely Sunless (0% Sunshine) versus Sunny (100% Sunshine) Days

Affect scale	Sunless days	Sunny days
General affect scales		
Negative Affect	−.019	.025
Positive Affect	−.053	.012[a]
Basic negative affects		
Fear	.138	.054
Hostility	−.088	.074[a]
Guilt	−.042	.062
Sadness	−.132	.068[a]
Basic positive affects		
Joviality	−.056	.004
Self-Assurance	−.034	.035
Attentiveness	.082	.011
Other affective states		
Shyness	−.091	.053[a]
Fatigue	−.091	.029[a]
Serenity	−.136	.007[a]
Surprise	−.101	.064[a]

Note. For Negative Affect and Positive Affect, $N = 1,530$ (sunless days) and 2,217 (sunny days). For all other scales, $N = 451$ (sunless days) and 1,087 (sunny days).
[a]means differ significantly at $p < .05$, two-tailed.

days. Significant mean differences were found for 7 of the 13 scales, but it is the direction of these differences that is most noteworthy. That is, the completely sunny days were associated with higher scores on all 13 mood scales. Thus, the students experienced greater levels of Serenity and general Positive Affect, but they also reported corresponding elevations in Sadness, Hostility, Fatigue, Shyness, and Surprise. These findings suggest that sunshine may act primarily on the *intensity* of experienced affect, such that people report stronger levels of both positive and negative mood with increased sunlight.

The second series of analyses examined mood on dark, rainy days, which were defined as days in which (1) it rained 1 inch or more and (2) there was no more than 10% of possible sunshine. Mood on these days was tested to determine whether it differed significantly from 0—which, as noted earlier, represents the overall mean value for each mood scale. As can be seen in Table 3.11, these analyses yielded no significant effects whatsoever. In other words, the students reported normal, average mood levels on these dark and rainy days.

TABLE 3.11. Standardized Mean Affect Scores on Dark and Rainy Days (1 Inch or More of Rain, 0–10% Sunshine)

Affect scale	M
General affect scales	
Negative Affect	−.039
Positive Affect	−.013
Basic negative affects	
Fear	−.017
Hostility	.104
Guilt	.089
Sadness	.024
Basic positive affects	
Joviality	.024
Self-Assurance	.044
Attentiveness	.021
Other affective states	
Shyness	.000
Fatigue	.005
Serenity	−.001
Surprise	−.042

Note. For Negative Affect and Positive Affect, $N = 393$. For all other scales, $N = 167$. None of these means differs significantly from 0 at $p < .05$, two-tailed.

Thus far, all of the results I have presented were derived from within-subject analyses. In a final series of analyses, I examined whether a between-subject design might yield stronger evidence of mood-related effects. In each sample, I computed mean affect scores—collapsed across all students who were assessed on that day—for each day in the daily rating period. For instance, in Sample 1, I computed mean Positive and Negative Affect scores for September 30, October 1, and so on; these average daily scores were then correlated with the weather variables for that day. To ensure that an adequate number of mood ratings had been collected, I eliminated any days on which there were fewer than 15 observations. Moreover, to control for any spurious person-related effects (resulting from the fact that not every student completed a rating on every usable day), I again standardized the data on a within-subject basis. Table 3.12 displays the number of days—and the average number of observations per day—in each data set used in these between-subject analyses. Across the eight samples there were a total of 394 usable days.

Table 3.13 reports the resulting between-subject correlations between the weather variables and general Negative and Positive Affect. Replicating the within-subject findings, Negative Affect again was unrelated to both sunshine and rain. None of the individual sample correlations is significant, and the overall mean coefficients are only .03 (sunshine) and −.08 (rain). The results for Positive Affect are slightly better (e.g., four of the eight samples yielded correlations of .20 or greater with sunshine), but they still are rather unimpressive, with weighted mean correlations of only .13 (sunshine) and −.03 (rain). Overall, therefore, we must again conclude that mood is essentially unaffected by variations in sunshine and rain.

TABLE 3.12. Basic Characteristics of the Data Sets Used in the Between-Subject Analyses of Daily Mood and Weather

Sample	Number of days	Mean No. of observations per day
1	61	56.4
2	44	30.4
3	46	89.2
4	61	64.0
5	42	51.1
6	42	20.1
7	49	46.6
8	49	47.2
Overall	394	51.7

TABLE 3.13. Between-Subject Correlations between Weather and General Negative and Positive Affect

	Negative Affect		Positive Affect	
Sample	Minutes of sunshine	Inches of rain	Minutes of sunshine	Inches of rain
1	.20	−.10	.00	.08
2	−.07	−.14	−.18	.10
3	−.03	−.18	.22	−.13
4	.14	−.18	.20	−.11
5	−.05	.16	.10	−.03
6	.18	−.05	.13	.03
7	−.04	−.08	.21	−.16
8	−.16	.01	.31*	.00
Weighted M	.03	−.08	.13	−.03

$*p < .05$, two-tailed.

Implications of the Weather Data

Contrary to the prevailing cultural view, these data indicate that people do not report a better mood on bright and sunny days (or, conversely, a worse mood on dark and rainy days). I must emphasize that it would be premature to conclude that variables such as sunshine and rain are completely unrelated to mood. It is possible, for instance, that significant mood effects can be identified only when more extreme weather phenomena are examined. For example, it may be that a single day of rain—perhaps even 2 or 3—has little effect on mood but that more prolonged periods of precipitation produce states of sadness and depression. Moreover, my colleagues and I have studied weather-related effects in only two locations: Kyoto, Japan, and Dallas, Texas. Before any firm conclusions can be drawn, it is important to obtain data from additional sites reflecting different weather patterns. Finally, I only examined simple linear main effects in these analyses, and it is possible that mood effects actually emerge through complex interactions among several weather-related variables, such as sunshine, temperature, humidity, wind speed, and barometric pressure. Consequently, future researchers will need to consider more complex models of the relation between mood and weather.

Nevertheless, even if future studies do succeed in identifying significant relations between sunshine, rain, and mood, we still would be confronted with a clear disjunction between people's beliefs and perceptions on the one hand and the reality of their affective reactions on the other. Most people—including most of the students in our studies—believe that they are much happier on sunny days than on cloudy, rainy days; our data, however, demonstrate that this simply is not the case.

Why do people greatly overestimate the mood-related effects of sunshine and rain? It appears that this phenomenon is another example of an *illusory correlation* (e.g., Chapman, 1967; Chapman & Chapman, 1969; Johnson & Mullen, 1994; Stroessner, Hamilton, & Mackie, 1992). That is, when a given association already is *believed* to exist, people tend to notice and recall instances that are consistent with this relation—and to ignore those cases that disconfirm it. In other words, illusory correlations represent instances of biased perception and recall in which individuals selectively attend to occurrences that confirm their preexisting beliefs and prejudices.

In this case, it appears that people selectively notice and remember those times in which (1) they were unhappy and the sky was dark and gloomy, or (2) they were happy and the day was sunny. However, they tend to ignore days that disconfirm their preexisting expectations—for instance, sunny days on which they felt depressed and irritable. The actual process may proceed in the following manner. When a person is feeling down and depressed, it is natural to try to figure out why. If he or she then looks outside and sees that it is dark and rainy, it is easy to conclude that this pervasive gloominess is the underlying cause of the bad mood. Note that this perception also serves to reinforce the person's preexisting belief that cloudy, rainy days are depressing. In contrast, if the person glances outside and sees that the day is bright and sunny, he or she would immediately conclude that the weather cannot possibly be an appropriate explanation; this appraisal—which would be made almost instantaneously—then would be quickly followed by a resumption of the search for the "true" underlying cause of the dysphoria. Put another way, because we do not believe that sunshine causes dysphoria, we are prone to ignore those instances in which sunshine and dysphoria co-occur.

Although this explanation can account for the persistence of mistaken beliefs about the weather, it inevitably leads to another crucial question: How did these erroneous beliefs arise in the first place? In other words, if we really do not feel any better on sunny days, how did we ever come to believe that we did? No research exists to answer this question definitively, but let me suggest two possibilities. First, it may be that the weather actually exerted a stronger influence on mood in the past. Except for those who work outside (e.g., farmers and construction workers), most individuals in modern, industrialized societies have little day-to-day contact with naturally occurring environmental conditions such as the weather. In fact, given a certain level of affluence, we are capable of spending virtually all of our lives in climate-controlled homes, cars, offices, shops, and theaters, spending little time outside at all. Thus, it is possible that we have become so estranged from nature that weather has ceased to influence us significantly. Weather beliefs simply may be archaic vestiges of an earlier way of life that has now largely vanished.

Second, these weather beliefs may be *overgeneralizations*. That is, some individuals actually might be very sensitive to variations in sunshine versus cloudiness. After all, some of the respondents in our within-subject analyses did show significant correlations in the expected direction, reliably reporting that they felt better on sunny days than on dark and rainy days. In a related vein, it is noteworthy that a small minority of individuals show extreme mood fluctuations across the seasons of the year (Kasper & Rosenthal, 1989). Over the course of centuries, the atypical experiences of these individuals may have been encoded into the folk wisdom of our culture and gradually come to be applied to everyone.

Whatever their source, these erroneous beliefs about the weather strikingly suggest that people may not understand their moods as well as they think they do. In the next chapter, I present further evidence indicating that people lack good insight into the factors that influence their mood.

CONCLUSION

To summarize, three important conclusions can be drawn from the enormous body of evidence I have reviewed. First, positive and negative mood states serve very different functions and, therefore, are related to different classes of variables. Specifically, negative mood states are much more responsive to ongoing stress and current life crises; in contrast, positive mood states are more strongly and consistently associated with social interaction and physical activity. On the basis of these and other data, I speculated that positive mood is more related to action than to thought, and that it is easier to induce a state of elevated Positive Affect through *doing* than through *thinking*. Conversely, hard and intensive *thinking* is more likely to lead to Negative Affect than to Positive Affect, especially if that thinking is directed inward toward oneself.

Second, we saw little evidence of specificity in these relations; rather, most of the observed associations were quite consistent across the individual negative and positive affects. Our analyses of examination-related stress provided the most notable exception to this generalization; here, we found that the anticipatory effects of stressful examinations were specifically confined to feelings of nervousness and fear. Generally speaking, however, the bulk of the data suggest that relations with external variables are better understood at the general, higher-order level.

Third, we have seen striking evidence that people may not be particularly adept at discerning the factors that influence their mood. Specifically, although most people believe that they feel much better on sunny days than on cloudy, rainy days, the extensive data I have collected suggest that mood is almost entirely unrelated to sunshine and rain. It therefore appears that people are subject to self-perpetuating beliefs and biases that do not conform well with actual affective experience. I return to this theme in Chapter 4, which examines cyclic fluctuations in mood.

4

THE RHYTHMS
OF EVERYDAY EXPERIENCE:
PATTERNED CYCLICITY
IN MOOD

Variables such as exercise, stress, and socializing tend to occur irregularly over time. For example, for more than 20 years I have tried to maintain a schedule of running at least three times a week. However, because my work and family responsibilities are constantly changing, it has been impossible for me to maintain a consistent schedule from week to week. That is, I might exercise on Monday, Thursday, and Saturday one week but on Tuesday, Friday, and Sunday the next. Variables such as exercise therefore give rise to mood fluctuations that also are unevenly distributed over time. To return to my earlier example, if exercise is associated with short-term elevations in Positive Affect, then I would expect to see transient increases in my positive mood on Monday, Thursday, and Saturday of the first week but on Tuesday, Friday, and Sunday of the second. Consequently, if my positive mood level were plotted over time, its course would appear to be random and irregular.

In contrast, this chapter focuses on processes that produce recurring, systematic patterns in mood over time. These cycles can be classified into those arising from (1) lifestyle, (2) sociocultural, and (3) endogenous factors. The first type—rhythms related to current lifestyle—will produce patterns that are consistent and systematic within a given individual but essentially random across different people. For instance, my life might fall into a stable and predictable pattern such that each Thursday is an extraordinarily busy and stressful day crammed with work and family responsibilities. In light of this stable pattern, one might expect to see a consistent elevation in my negative mood every Thursday. If plotted over time, this pattern would be regular and systematic.

However, because different individuals lead different lives and follow different schedules, there is no reason to suspect that most people would show a similar trend across the days of the week. For some people, Monday might be the most stressful day, whereas for others it might be Wednesday or Saturday. Of course, many people would be less predictable and fail to show a consistent pattern at all. Consequently, if we assessed the mood of a large group of individuals, averaged their responses, and then plotted them over time, these differing lifestyles would tend to cancel each other out and produce essentially random temporal patterns. Because of this, although lifestyle variables may lead to recurring patterns in particular individuals, they do not produce consistent patterns across individuals and need not concern us further.

The second type—rhythms produced by sociocultural factors—give rise to patterns that are reasonably consistent across different individuals within the same culture but might differ dramatically across different cultures and historical periods. For instance, contemporary Americans might report an unusually good mood on the fourth Thursday of November each year, presumably because our society has designated this day as the holiday of Thanksgiving. However, there is no reason to suspect that individuals in other times or in different cultures would report a similar mood on this particular day.

The most obvious example of a sociocultural rhythm concerns the days of the week (although there is some evidence that the 7-day week is itself a product of an endogenous "circaseptum" rhythm; see Larsen & Kasimatis, 1990). Weekly schedules differ enormously across individuals. Nevertheless, the dominant pattern in U.S. society long has been for adults to maintain a weekly schedule of working Monday through Friday, with Saturdays and Sundays off. Students traditionally have followed a similar pattern, attending classes on Monday through Friday, again with Saturdays and Sundays off. In light of this prevailing pattern, if we assessed the mood of a large group of individuals, averaged their responses, and then plotted them over time, we might expect to see highly systematic fluctuations across the days of the week; for example, we might predict that both adults and students generally would report a better mood on Saturdays and Sundays than during the rest of the week.

Clearly, however, this consistent weekly pattern ultimately depends on the sociocultural context in which it occurs; if this context is somehow altered, we would expect corresponding changes in the pattern of mood fluctuation. For instance, if the 4-day workweek (stretching, say, from Monday through Thursday) gradually evolved to be the dominant societal pattern, we would expect corresponding changes in the weekly pattern of mood variation such that adults now would report a better mood on Fridays as well. Consequently, similar to other sociocultural rhythms, there is no reason to expect weekly variation to be highly consistent across different cultures and historical periods.

Sociocultural rhythms may produce systematic patterns in either positive or negative mood. For example, it is reasonable to hypothesize that stressful events occur more frequently on workdays than during the weekend. If so, negative mood levels might be significantly elevated during the "workweek" of Monday through Friday. On the other hand, it also is plausible to predict that positive mood would be elevated during the weekend because of increased opportunities for socializing and physical activity. Consequently, there is no a priori reason to assume that sociocultural rhythms necessarily produce stronger effects on one type of mood versus the other.

The situation is far different when we consider the third type of cycles, namely, those due to endogenous biological factors. These endogenous rhythms reflect the operation of internal "clocks" or oscillators that control the patterning of a large number of bodily functions (e.g., body temperature and the sleep–wake cycle) and also lead to systematic fluctuations in mood over time (see Clark, Watson, & Leeka, 1989; Thayer, 1978b, 1989). Because they reflect adaptive biological processes that have developed over the course of human evolution, these endogenous rhythms should produce cyclical patterns that are reasonably consistent across individuals, cultures, and historical periods.

Furthermore, as noted in Chapter 1, these endogenous rhythms can be expected to have much stronger effects on positive mood than on negative mood. This asymmetry results from two basic considerations. First, as discussed earlier, there is a natural tendency toward lower-activation states in affective life. All other things being equal, low-intensity states are preferable to high-activation states because they (1) burn less energy, thereby reducing the amount of food that is necessary for survival; and (2) put less strain on bodily resources, thereby lessening the danger of physiological exhaustion (Beck, 1987; Kasper & Rosenthal, 1989; Selye, 1956; Webb, 1979). Consequently, it is evolutionarily adaptive to experience high-activation states (e.g., fear, anger, and exuberance) only when there is a good reason to do so. Put another way, in the absence of some reason that justifies an increased expenditure of energy, animals (including humans) should be preprogrammed by evolution to remain in less intense, lower-activation states.

The second consideration involves the different functions served by negative and positive mood states. As noted in Chapter 1, negative mood states primarily keep the organism out of trouble. Thus, the negative mood system is designed to be highly reactive in character. That is, negative mood should be elevated in response to threat or danger but remain at relatively low levels in the absence of danger. For instance, it is highly adaptive for individuals to experience a sudden, sharp increase in fear when they are being chased by a bear or threatened with a gun.

Note, moreover, that because environmental threats tend not to occur at regularly scheduled times (e.g., rampaging bears do not plan their attacks for precisely 2 P.M.), there is no compelling reason why an individual should consistently experience a sudden upsurge of fear or anger at a particular hour of the day, such as 2 P.M. In light of the earlier principle that energy should be expended judiciously, we therefore would expect endogenous rhythms to have little systematic influence on negative mood states.

In contrast, the essential function of the positive mood system is to ensure that the organism obtains the resources that are necessary both for its own survival and for that of its species. The approach and appetitive behaviors mediated by this system (eating, drinking, socializing, sexual activity, etc.) are extremely important for survival, but they lack the temporally and spatially bound quality of the activities subsumed under the negative mood system. For example, unless the fear response is emitted at a particular place and time (e.g., in response to a rampaging bear), it is of little use to the organism. However, the situation is quite different for the approach behaviors mediated by the positive system. To be sure, these behaviors must be performed with a certain frequency, but it rarely is essential that they be emitted at a particular time or place. For instance, although it is necessary that an animal eats periodically, its survival rarely depends on eating a certain amount at a specific time. Consequently, the positive mood system possesses considerable flexibility regarding exactly where and when these approach behaviors are performed.

When are these approach behaviors likely to be performed? Consistent with the principle outlined earlier, these high-activation behaviors should tend to be emitted when reward is likely and avoided when it is not. To a considerable extent, this means that the positive mood system also has a strongly reactive component and is highly responsive to current environmental conditions. For instance, if an animal receives clear indications that food or other resources are readily available (e.g., a hungry predator catches the scent of its prey), it is likely to initiate approach behaviors.

However, the relative availability of resources—and the relative risk of harm—often can be predicted in advance as a function of time. For instance, foraging is much more likely to be rewarded when food is relatively available (as in the spring and summer) than when it is extremely scarce (as in the dead of winter). Similarly, for animals with poor night vision, foraging will be rewarded more often during the daylight hours than after dark. Because the probability of risk and reward often can be specified in advance, it is plausible to propose that the positive mood system is subject to preprogrammed endogenous cycles that will vary widely across species but are highly consistent within a given species. The function of these endogenous biological rhythms is to increase the probability that species members will be active, alert, and energetic at those times that food and other required resources are easily obtainable and the risk of harm is relatively low. Conversely, animals should be preprogrammed to be sluggish, unenergetic, and inactive when resources tend to be scarce or when the threat of danger is high.

As the previous examples suggest, two cycles that conform to this model especially well are (1) diurnal or "circadian" variation over the course of the day and (2) seasonal variation over the course of the year. In the former case, the diurnal rhythm of a given species should be programmed to maximize the likelihood that approach behaviors will be performed during those hours of the day or night when required resources (food, potential mates, etc.) are plentiful and the risk of harm is relatively low. In humans, the times of peak energy and activity (and, hence, the highest levels of Positive Affect) would be expected to occur during the daylight hours, with relative lassitude and lethargy (i.e., low Positive Affect) after dark.

This conceptual analysis of diurnal mood variation converges nicely with a prominent theory regarding the function and evolutionary origins of sleep. The "energy conservation hypothesis" is based on the finding that sleep is associated with a lower metabolic rate. Accordingly, as animals sleep more, they burn fewer calories and require less food to survive (Allison & van Twyver, 1970; Berger & Phillips, 1995; Walker, Garber, Berger, & Heller, 1979; Webb, 1979). Moreover, proponents of this model further argue that periods of sleep/inactivity and wakefulness/activity do not alternate randomly; rather, consistent with the argument I have developed here, sleep is most likely to occur when approach behaviors are risky and unlikely to result in reward. Consequently, sleep (especially slow-wave sleep) can be viewed as the extreme low end of the positive mood continuum (i.e., it represents the lowest possible levels of alertness and activity).

Similar considerations apply to seasonal variation. Again, animals should be relatively sluggish and inactive during the winter (when resources are scarce) and more active, alert, and energetic during the spring and summer (when resources are more plentiful). Many animal species do, in fact, show substantial variations in specific behaviors (such as reproduction) and in general activity level across the seasons of the year (e.g., Dark & Zucker, 1985; Kasper & Rosenthal, 1989; Tamarkin, Baird, & Almeida, 1985). Seasonal variation is seen most dramatically in hibernation, which involves a marked reduction in body temperature and the metabolic rate, thereby serving as an extremely powerful mechanism for energy conservation (Walker et al., 1979). In this regard, it is interesting to note that hibernation is now considered to be an extension of slow-wave sleep (e.g., Mrosovsky, 1988; Walker et al., 1979).

Hibernation per se is a phenomenon that is confined to small mammals such as hamsters and ground squirrels, which normally cannot survive long without eating; larger mammals can survive much longer without eating and hence have no need for this mode of adaptation (Mrosovsky, 1988). Accordingly, there is no reason to believe that hibernation ever evolved in humans. Nevertheless, many researchers have noted the striking parallels between hibernation and seasonal affective disorder, an illness that is characterized by a severe, atypical depression during the late fall and winter. This depression often is followed by a hypomanic episode in the spring or summer (see Kasper & Rosenthal, 1989; Mrosovsky, 1988). In fact, these clear parallels led Kasper and Rosenthal (1989) to suggest that this fall/winter depression originally developed as a highly efficient means of energy conservation during a time of scarce food supplies.

To summarize, cyclical patterns in mood can arise from either environmental (lifestyle or sociocultural rhythms) or biological (endogenous rhythms) sources. Whereas the former type is equally likely to produce systematic fluctuations in either positive or negative mood, the latter can be expected to exert a much stronger influence on positive states. In the remainder of this chapter, I consider evidence related to mood fluctuations over (1) the course of the day, (2) the days of the week, (3) the monthly menstrual cycle in women, and (4) the seasons of the year.

DIURNAL VARIATION IN MOOD

Earlier Studies of Diurnal Variation

Consistent with expectation, an extensive body of evidence indicates that positive mood states show a replicable diurnal rhythm. In general, Positive Affect tends to be initially low in the morning and rises to a maximum sometime during the day; it then declines during the evening. It is noteworthy, however, that the acrophase—or time of peak affect—has varied widely across studies, in large part because individuals reach their maximum Positive Affect at different times of the day (see Clark et al., 1989; Thayer, 1989). In contrast, most studies have found no systematic diurnal rhythm for negative mood states (Clements, Hafer, & Vermillion, 1976; Froberg, 1977; Froberg, Karlsson, Levi, & Lidberg, 1972, 1975; Monk, Leng, Folkard, & Weitzman, 1983; Taub & Berger, 1974; Thayer, 1987b; Thayer, Takahashi, & Pauli, 1988).

Four studies have reported results that are somewhat inconsistent with this basic pattern. First, Thayer (1978b) and Caminada and de Bruijn (1992) found a significant diurnal pattern on a measure of general Negative Affect; in both instances, however, this effect was substantially smaller than that observed for Positive Affect. Christie and Venables (1973) found positive mood to be lower in the evening than in the morning; however, the participants in this study were assessed only twice a day for 2 days (Monday and Friday), so the reliability of these findings is questionable. Finally, Curtis, Fogel, McEvoy, and Zarate (1966) obtained a typical pattern of positive mood variation (i.e., low in the morning and evening with a peak during the day), but only for women; they also reported a significant diurnal effect for negative mood in one of three groups. Again, however, the participants in this study were assessed only at six points in a single day; thus the reliability of these findings is unclear.

Although these data generally are clear and consistent, three limitations of this research must be noted. First, many studies assessed mood over only 1 or 2 days (Christie & Venables, 1973; Clements et al., 1976; Curtis et al., 1966; Monk et al., 1983; Taub & Berger, 1974; Thayer, 1978b), or at only a few points over the course of the day (Christie & Venables, 1973; Taub & Berger, 1974). Second, much of this research is based on small samples. Especially when time-sampling procedures have been adequate, N's of 20 or fewer are common (e.g., Thayer, 1987b; Thayer et al., 1988). Finally, many earlier studies have used individual mood terms, or else scales of uncertain reliability and validity (e.g., Froberg, 1977; Froberg et al., 1972, 1975; Monk et al., 1983).

Diurnal Variation in General Positive and Negative Affect

These limitations prompted my colleagues and I to conduct three intensive investigations in which (1) large numbers of students, (2) were assessed roughly 40 to 50 times, (3) on mood scales with established reliability and validity. The first of these studies was reported in Clark et al. (1989). In this study, 196 students at SMU rated their current, momentary levels of general Negative and Positive Affect several times a day for a week. Each day, students completed the first mood form within 30 minutes of rising. They then were assessed on a specified 3-hour schedule—6 A.M., 9 A.M., noon, 3 P.M., and so on—until they went to bed, at which time they completed a final mood form. If the rating at rising or retiring was within 30 minutes of one of the scheduled assessments, the students were not required to complete another mood form for that period. Finally, to increase compliance with this rather exacting regimen, the students were required to turn in their mood ratings each day.

In this analysis (and in all subsequent analyses reported in this chapter), we standardized the mood ratings on a within-subject basis such that each individual had a mean of 0 and a standard deviation of 1 on both Positive and Negative Affect. This procedure removes all between-subject variance, allowing us to collapse the data across individuals. Next, we computed overall average scores on both Positive and Negative Affect for each period across all days and individuals. The resulting means for the six most heavily sampled time periods (9 A.M., noon, 3 P.M., 6 P.M., 9 P.M., midnight) are plotted in Figure 4.1. Note that these average scores are based on a total of 7,395 observations ($M = 37.7$ per person), and that each data point is based on more than 1,000 individual assessments.

These data strikingly corroborate the basic pattern that was reported in the earlier studies. Except for a slight elevation at 9 A.M., the curve for

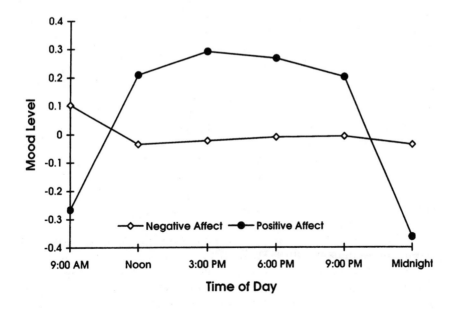

FIGURE 4.1. Diurnal variation in general Positive Affect and Negative Affect (Sample 1).

Negative Affect is essentially flat, showing no systematic diurnal trend whatsoever. In fact, Negative Affect shows little variation at all, ranging from a low of only −.04 (at midnight) to a high of only .10 (at 9 A.M.). In sharp contrast, Positive Affect shows a strong and systematic circadian rhythm. Mean Positive Affect scores were quite low at 9 A.M., but then rose sharply at noon; they remained quite high until 9 P.M., after which they declined dramatically to reach another low at midnight. Note also that Positive Affect scores varied enormously, ranging from a trough of −.36 (at midnight) to a peak of .29 (at 3 P.M.). Thus, we see a clear general pattern in which Positive Affect is quite low at the ends of the day and reaches its acrophase at some point during the middle of the day.

I replicated these findings in a second study that used a somewhat different design (see Watson et al., 1999). In this study, 226 SMU students rated their current, momentary mood on the complete PANAS-X once per day for 45 days; to ensure compliance, they were required to return their ratings twice a week. Each day, they made their ratings during one of five different periods: rising (within 1 hour of getting up in the morning), morning (any time before noon), afternoon (between noon and 6 P.M.), evening (any time after 6 P.M.), and retiring (within 1 hour of going to bed at night). These five periods alternated on a prearranged, random schedule.

I computed overall average Positive and Negative Affect scores for several different periods across all days and individuals. Because of the design of this study, I was able to examine a wider range of hours; specifically, mean scores were computed separately for seven periods: 6 to 9 A.M., 9 A.M. to noon, noon to 3 P.M., 3 P.M. to 6 P.M., 6 P.M. to 9 P.M., 9 P.M. to midnight, and midnight to 3 A.M. These scores are plotted in Figure 4.2. They are based on a total of 9,957 observations (M = 44.1 per person); as in Figure 4.1, each data point reflects more than 1,000 individual assessments.

Although the form of the curves differs somewhat, these data clearly produced the same general pattern found in the first study. Again, we see that Negative Affect shows little systematic diurnal effect; moreover, as in Figure 4.1, it shows little variation at all, ranging from a low of only −.10 (between 9 A.M. and noon) to a peak of only .11 (between 9 P.M. and midnight). In sharp contrast, Positive Affect again exhibited a substantial, systematic circadian rhythm. Mean Positive Affect scores were extremely low during the early morning but then rose steadily until noon; they remained at relatively high levels until 9 P.M., after which they showed a steady decline before reaching another trough at 3 A.M. Again, unlike Negative Affect, Positive Affect scores fluctuated dramatically, ranging from a minimum of −.42 (between midnight and 3 A.M.) to a maximum of .41 (between 6 P.M. and 9 P.M.).

Positive Affect scores do not vary simply with the hours of the day

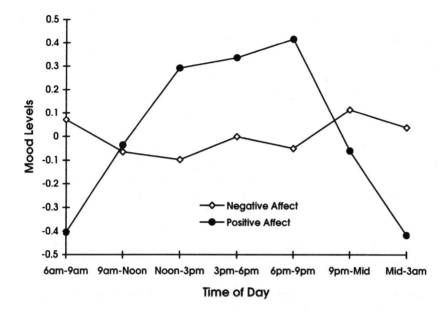

FIGURE 4.2. Diurnal variation in general Positive Affect and Negative Affect (Sample 2).

but also fluctuate as a function of the individual's location on the sleep–wake cycle. Clark et al. (1989) showed that mean Positive Affect scores tended to be particularly low if the individual had recently risen or was preparing to retire. Moreover, this effect persisted regardless of the time of day. For instance, the elevated Positive Affect levels normally seen at noon and 3 P.M. were not evident if the student had recently risen. Similarly, the high Positive Affect customarily observed at 9 P.M. was absent if the student was preparing to retire. Incidentally, these data illustrate one important advantage of assessing diurnal variation in college students, namely, that they follow such chaotic and widely varying sleep–wake schedules. In this study alone, for example, rising times ranged from 5 A.M. to 3:30 P.M., whereas retiring times varied from approximately 8:30 P.M. to 6:30 A.M.

On the basis of these results, Clark et al. (1989) suggested that Positive Affect scores appeared, in part, to be "a function of the proximity of sleep" (p. 225). I tested this idea further in a subset of 104 students from the second diurnal study who noted their exact rising time (as well as the time at which they completed their mood ratings) at each assessment. I computed mean Positive and Negative Affect scores as a function of the time elapsed since rising (i.e., from 0 to 1 hour, from 1 to 2 hours, and at hourly intervals thereafter) across all days and students; these averages are plotted in Figure 4.3. The data shown in the figure are based on a total of 4,494 observations (M = 43.2 observations per person); each of the plotted data points reflects more than 150 individual assessments.

In interpreting these data, it is important to note that rising times again varied enormously across students and days, ranging in this sample from 1 A.M. to approximately 1 P.M. Furthermore, in several of our daily mood studies, we have asked students to record how many hours (to the nearest half hour) they slept the previous night. On the basis of more than 4,500 daily mood observations, we have found that SMU students, on average, sleep slightly more than 7 hours a night. Put another way, the average waking day for an SMU student is slightly less than 17 hours long.

What do the data shown in Figure 4.3 tell us? First, we again see that Negative Affect shows little systematic variation. In fact, except for a sudden, inexplicable increase at approximately 12 hours postrising, Negative Affect displays little variation at all, with mean values ranging between only –.10 and .10. In contrast, Positive Affect shows a clear and striking pattern. The level of Positive Affect is quite low (M = –.29) within the first hour of rising. After that it increases steadily and begins to approach its

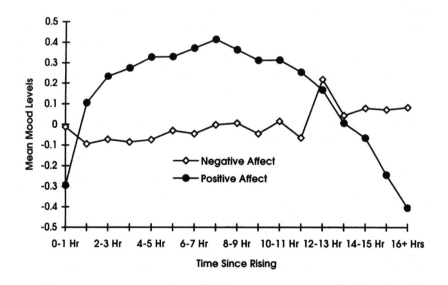

FIGURE 4.3. General affect levels as a function of time since rising.

maximum level at approximately 3 hours. Positive Affect continues to increase for several more hours, however, until it reaches its acrophase roughly 8 hours after rising. It then begins to decline but still remains relatively high until approximately 12 hours after rising, at which point it commences a much sharper decline. Note that Positive Affect scores again are remarkably low ($M = -.41$) beyond 16 hours postrising.

These data strikingly confirm Clark et al.'s (1989) suggestion that positive mood scores are at least partly a function of the proximity of sleep. In this regard, it is especially noteworthy—assuming again that the average waking day for these students was slightly less than 17 hours long—that the acrophase for Positive Affect was at the approximate midpoint between the termination of the previous night's sleep (i.e., rising) and the onset of the next night's sleep (i.e., retiring). In other words, Positive Affect falls to its lowest level at those times at which the person is closest to sleep (i.e., at rising and retiring) and reaches its zenith roughly at the point at which the individual is the farthest removed (temporally) from sleep. It therefore appears that one can predict momentary Positive Affect reasonably well as a function of the temporal proximity of sleep.

Individual Differences in Diurnal Variation

Some readers may suspect that these group data (which were collapsed across all respondents) mask important individual differences and, in fact, that different types of people may show different patterns of mood fluctuation over the course of the day. In particular, many of us would describe ourselves as "morning people" (also known as "larks"; see Coleman, 1986) or as "evening people" (also known as "owls"). One certainly might predict that morning and evening types would show substantially different patterns of diurnal variation. Morning types might be expected to be more enthusiastic, active, and alert early in the day and to report reduced levels of positive mood as the day wears on; conversely, one might anticipate that evening types would start the day quite slowly but eventually achieve relatively high levels of positive mood sometime at night.

However, the available data regarding morningness–eveningness actually are quite mixed. Some studies have found the expected patterns on measures of alertness/activity (Larsen, 1985; Monk et al., 1983), concentration (Patkai, 1971), self-reported arousal (Watts, Cox, & Robson, 1983), and general Positive Affect (Caminada & de Bruijn, 1992), whereas others have failed to obtain any strong or consistent differences in patterning between morning and evening types (e.g., Froberg, 1977). Thayer et al. (1988), for instance, reported that morning and evening types, as assessed by the Morningness–Eveningness Questionnaire (MEQ; Horne &

Ostberg, 1976) showed similar patterns of positive mood fluctuation over the course of the day. However, they did find that morning types reached their acrophase during the morning, whereas evening types achieved theirs much later in the day.

Moreover, even when significant effects are found, they typically reflect relatively subtle—rather than dramatic—differences in diurnal patterning across groups. For example, Caminada and de Bruijn (1992) examined momentary mood in 49 students (17 morning, 17 intermediate, and 15 evening types) at six times of the day across three different days. They found that morning types reported the highest levels of positive mood at 9 A.M., whereas evening types reported the most elevated positive mood at 9:30 P.M. Nevertheless, consistent with the data shown in Figures 4.1 and 4.2, all three groups showed marked increases in positive mood from 9 A.M. to 11:30 A.M.

Clark et al. (1989) have reported the most extensive analysis of morningness–eveningness. Students were classified as morning types ($N = 19$), evening types ($N = 57$), neither ($N = 14$), or both ($N = 33$), based on their own self-description. Overall, these students completed a total of 5,483 mood assessments ($M = 44.6$ per person). Surprisingly, the four groups failed to demonstrate significantly different diurnal patterns over the course of the day. Further analyses, however, revealed that they differed in their overall *level* of positive mood. That is, morning types had the highest overall levels of positive mood, followed by those who identified themselves as both, neither, and evening types, respectively. It is noteworthy that Froberg (1977) also found that morning types had significantly higher levels of positive mood than did evening types.

Clark et al. (1989) subsequently reran these analyses using only those students who classified themselves as either morning or evening types. Again, these groups showed broadly similar circadian patterns. Most notably, morning and evening types both reported their lowest levels of Positive Affect at the beginning (9 A.M.) and end (midnight) of the day and reached their peak sometime during the middle of the day. In fact, the only notable difference was that whereas the morning types reported significantly greater levels of positive mood early in the day, these differences tended to disappear at the later assessments (although the morning types still scored nonsignificantly higher).

More generally, although different people reach their acrophase at different times and show somewhat different curves over the course of the day, our analyses have demonstrated that this basic circadian rhythm— that is, low Positive Affect at the beginning and end of the day, with a peak occurring somewhere in the middle—is remarkably robust and generalizable across individuals. In our first diurnal study (Clark et al., 1989), for instance, we found that 153 students (78.1%) reported greater

Positive Affect at noon than at 9 A.M., and that 167 students (85.2%) had higher levels of positive mood at 9 P.M. than at midnight. Moreover, this effect persisted regardless of whether the students defined themselves as morning types, evening types, both, or neither: In each case, Positive Affect tended to be lower at the beginning and end of the day.

Similarly, I collapsed the data from our second diurnal study into five broad time periods: 6 A.M. to 9 A.M. (as shown in Figure 4.2, this is a time of very low Positive Affect), 9 A.M. to noon (a transitional period of intermediate Positive Affect), noon to 9 P.M. (the period of peak Positive Affect), 9 P.M. to midnight (another transitional period of intermediate mood), and midnight to 3 A.M. (another trough period of very low Positive Affect). Subsequent analyses (because of missing data, these results are based on $N = 200$) revealed that 77.5% of the students showed an increase in Positive Affect from the first period to the second, and that 79.0% reported an increase from the second to the third; even more strikingly, 90.5% of the respondents showed an increase in Positive Affect from the first period to the third. Conversely, 76.5% of the students experienced a decline in Positive Affect from the third period to the fourth, 71.5% showed a decrease from the fourth to the fifth, and 90.5% showed a decrease from the third to the fifth. Thus, this basic diurnal rhythm—Positive Affect is lowest at the ends of the day and is highest in the middle— is nearly universal among our respondents.

The robustness of this circadian rhythm is important for two reasons. First, it demonstrates that these diurnal mood fluctuations do not simply reflect idiosyncratic factors related to lifestyle. As noted earlier, the students in our samples showed widely varying sleep–wake cycles, as evidenced by the huge range in their rising and retiring times. Moreover, because our respondents also indicated whether they had recently engaged in various types of activities (e.g., socializing, exercising, eating, and studying), it is clear that their behavioral patterns varied dramatically as well. Accordingly, similar activity schedules or other factors related to lifestyle cannot account for the systematic diurnal effects we have identified (see Clark et al., 1989). On the contrary, the near universality of the observed rhythm strongly suggests that it results from endogenous biological processes, a point I consider subsequently.

Second, similar to the weather data discussed in Chapter 3, these results again suggest that people lack good insight into the nature of their mood fluctuations. The concepts of "morning people" and "evening people" are deeply ingrained in popular consciousness, and it is widely perceived that these two types of individuals show markedly different patterns of mood fluctuation over the course of the day. Many of the students in our two diurnal studies themselves believed this to be true. Indeed, several of our "owls" expressed the belief that they tended to experience their optimal mood state very late at night. In actuality, however, the daily rhythms of morning and evening types do not differ dramatically from one another; furthermore, *virtually no one* reaches his or her optimal mood state late at night.

Diurnal Variation in Specific Types of Affect

Analyses of the Positive Affects

Another important issue concerns the generality versus specificity of these diurnal effects. Thus far, we have seen that general Positive Affect shows a strong and systematic circadian rhythm but general Negative Affect does not. Do specific types of positive and negative mood behave similarly, or do we instead see evidence of content-specific effects?

To date, the most extensive published analysis of this issue was reported by Clark et al. (1989), who examined the robustness of the observed diurnal rhythm across different types of positive mood. Specifically, on the basis of earlier content analyses (Zevon & Tellegen, 1982), they divided the 10 terms comprising the general Positive Affect scale of the PANAS-X into four content-specific scales: Excited (enthusiastic, excited, inspired), Attentive (alert, attentive, interested), Proud (determined, proud) and Strong (active, strong). All four scales exhibited a systematic circadian pattern that closely paralleled that displayed by general Positive Affect (see Figure 4.1). Most notably, scores on all four content scales rose significantly from 9 A.M. to noon and fell significantly between 9 P.M. and midnight. Thus, these data demonstrated that various types of positive mood rise and fall together over the course of the day.

Because the students in our second diurnal study were assessed on the complete, 60-item PANAS-X, these data can be subjected to more extensive analyses of specificity. Again, standardized scores were collapsed across students to yield an overall mean score for each of seven periods. Figure 4.4 plots the resulting averages for the three basic positive mood scales of the PANAS-X: Joviality (e.g., cheerful, happy, lively, and enthusiastic), Self-Assurance (e.g., proud, confident, bold, and strong) and Attentiveness (e.g., alert, attentive, and determined). Also shown in the figure are the corresponding data for Fatigue (e.g., drowsy, sluggish, and tired). As discussed in Chapter 2, this scale is strongly negatively correlated with the positive affects in within-subject data; accordingly, I reversed the scores on this scale (so that they now represent "Low Fatigue") to facilitate comparison with the other measures.

Figure 4.4 indicates that the circadian cycles of these four scales are virtually identical. In each case, the scores initially are quite low and rise steadily from 6 A.M. to noon. They then increase more slowly until they reach their acrophase between 6 P.M. and 9 P.M., at which point they de-

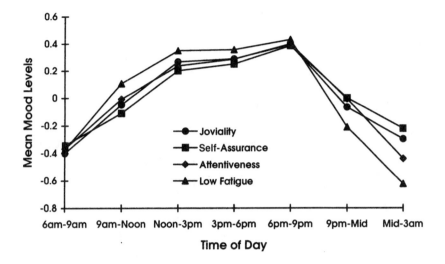

FIGURE 4.4. Diurnal variation in the basic positive affects and (low) fatigue (Sample 2).

cline steadily until another trough is achieved between midnight and 3
A.M. Clearly, we see no evidence of content specificity across these four
markers of the higher-order Positive Affect dimension.

We can explore this issue further in our third large-scale circadian
study. The participants in this study were 120 University of Iowa undergraduates who rated their current mood over the course of a week.
Each day, the students completed both a rising and a retiring mood rating. In between, they rated their momentary mood every 2 hours; note,
however, that each student was allowed to choose either an even-hour
(e.g., 10 A.M. and noon) or an odd-hour (e.g., 9 A.M. and 11 A.M.) schedule to accommodate differences in classes and lifestyle. Overall, these
students completed an average of 51.9 assessments (total $N = 6{,}233$ observations). Once again, I standardized these ratings on a person-by-
person basis and then collapsed them across all students. Finally, I computed mean affect scores for each 2-hour block (7 A.M. to 9 A.M., 9 A.M.
to 11 A.M., etc.).

Figure 4.5 presents the average scores for the same four scales at each
period. Once again, all four scales showed remarkably similar circadian
rhythms. Indeed, the only real difference is that Attentiveness reached its
acrophase much earlier (between 1 P.M. and 3 P.M.) than did the other
scales (which peaked between 5 P.M. and 7 P.M.). Thus, we again see that
the individual positive affects rise and fall together over the course of the
day, carried along by the power of the same circadian rhythm.

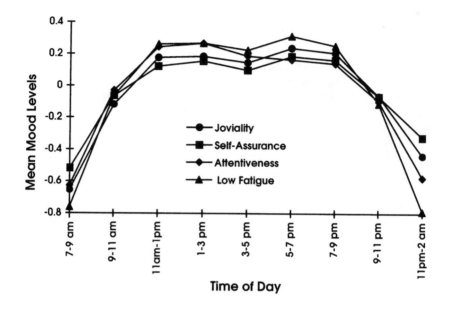

FIGURE 4.5. Diurnal variation in the basic positive affects and (low) fatigue (Sample 3).

Analyses of the Negative Affects

I now consider the specificity of circadian effects across different types of negative mood, using data from our second SMU sample. To address this issue, I standardized scores on the four basic negative mood scales of the PANAS-X: Fear (e.g., scared and nervous), Sadness (e.g., blue and lonely), Guilt (e.g., guilty and dissatisfied with self), and Hostility (e.g., irritable, scornful, and disgusted). I also examined Serenity (e.g., calm and re- laxed); as discussed in Chapter 2, this scale is strongly negatively cor- related with the negative affects in within-subject data. As in previous analyses of this data set, overall scores were computed for each of seven 3-hour periods.

Based on the results seen with general Negative Affect (see Figures 4.1 through 4.3), one would expect to find little systematic variation in these scales over the course of the day. In fact, two scales—Fear and Guilt—showed virtually no variation whatsoever: Across the time peri- ods, mean scores on these scales ranged from a low of only –.051 (Fear be- tween noon and 3 P.M.) to a high of only .066 (Guilt between midnight and 3 A.M.). Consequently, these scales will not be considered further.

Figure 4.6 plots the mean scores on the three remaining scales. The

range of diurnal variation in these scales is far less than that observed earlier for Fatigue and the positive affects; thus, even at the specific affect
level, we see clear evidence that positive mood displays a much stronger
circadian rhythm than does negative mood. Nevertheless, these three
measures all show some systematic diurnal variation. Hostility scores are
relatively high early in the day (a mean of .168 between 6 and 9 A.M.), low
during the middle of the day, and then slightly elevated late at night. In
contrast, Sadness and Serenity both are relatively low early in the morning and tend to increase over the rest of the day: Sadness is lowest between 9 A.M. and noon ($M = -.127$) and reaches its zenith between 9 P.M.
and midnight ($M = .229$), whereas levels of Serenity are lowest between 6
A.M. and 9 A.M. ($M = -.202$) and highest between midnight and 3 A.M.
($M = .163$). This latter finding perhaps explains why many "owls" believe
that they attain their optimal mood state late at night. That is, it appears
that many individuals do experience a pleasant state of relaxation (i.e.,
high Serenity) at this time; these pleasant feelings may be overgen-
eralized into the perception that positive mood is broadly elevated late at
night.

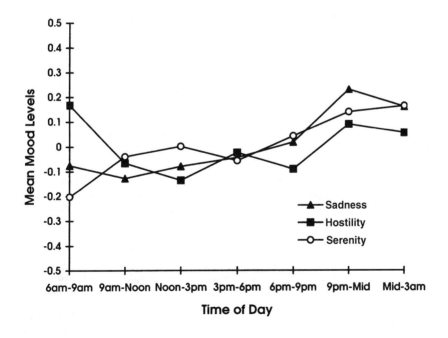

FIGURE 4.6. Diurnal variation in Hostility, Sadness, and Serenity (Sample 2).

Mechanisms Underlying the Observed Diurnal Variation in Positive Affect

What factors are responsible for these recurring cycles in positive mood? We currently lack sufficient data to answer this question definitively. However, as noted earlier, the near universality of the observed rhythm strongly suggests that it results from endogenous biological processes. In this regard, it is noteworthy that many biological variables (e.g., body temperature, the sleep–wake cycle, and hormonal secretion) have been shown to have endogenous circadian rhythms (e.g., Moore-Ede, Czeisler, & Richardson, 1983a, 1983b). It therefore seems plausible to suggest that our current, momentary feelings of enthusiasm, energy, and alertness reflect these biological rhythms as well.

The existing data suggest that there are two biological regulatory systems that emanate from the suprachiasmic nucleus of the hypothalamus (e.g., Moore & Eichler, 1972); these typically work in synchrony, but each is more closely linked to a particular subset of variables. One system (the "strong oscillator") regulates body temperature, rapid eye movement (REM) sleep, certain hormonal secretions, and so on, whereas the other (the "weak oscillator") more strongly influences the sleep–wake cycle and associated functions (Stroebel, 1985; Wehr & Wirz-Justice, 1982). Suggestive evidence links diurnal variation in positive mood to both of these regulatory systems. For instance, a number of studies have reported average body temperature curves that bear a striking resemblance to the diurnal rhythm for Positive Affect: In both cases, there is a sharp rise early in the morning, followed by a more gradual increase until late afternoon, then a leveling off until early evening, and finally a rapid decline (Blake, 1967; Folkard, 1975; Froberg, 1977).

Furthermore, studies jointly investigating the circadian cycles of positive mood and body temperature find a close correspondence between the two rhythms (Aschoff, Giedke, Poppel, & Wever, 1972; Monk et al., 1983; Thayer, 1978b). We have replicated these findings in our own data. Specifically, the students in our third (Iowa) sample measured their body temperature after completing their mood ratings at each assessment (see Watson et al., 1999). As before, these measures were standardized on a person-by-person basis and then collapsed across all students. Figure 4.7 plots the overall mean scores for Negative Affect, Positive Affect, and body temperature at hourly intervals over the course of the day. Consistent with previous research, Positive Affect and body temperature showed similar cycles: Both tended to be quite low in the morning and late at night, with elevated levels during the day (note, however, that Positive Affect rose more sharply in the morning and reached its acrophrase earlier in the day). Indeed, across the 18 hourly intervals, the correlation between Positive Affect and body temperature was .79.

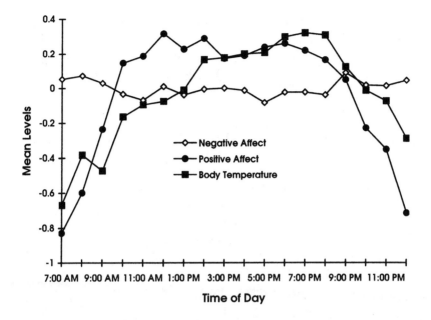

FIGURE 4.7. Diurnal variation in general affect and body temperature (Sample 3).

These results certainly suggest that Positive Affect is systematically linked to the strong oscillator. Note, however, that these data were collected under conditions in which the two regulatory systems would be expected to be in synchrony; accordingly, one cannot rule out the influence of the weak oscillator. Froberg (1977), however, examined variations in subjective alertness in women who were sleep deprived. Although the overall level of alertness gradually declined as the time without sleep lengthened, a clear periodicity remained in both alertness and body temperature, with alertness rising from early morning to late afternoon even after several days of sleep deprivation. In this case, the circadian rhythm of alertness was not simply the result of its association with the sleep–wake cycle but appeared to reflect the direct influence of the strong oscillator.

On the other hand, the data shown in Figure 4.3—together with the earlier findings of Clark et al. (1989)—indicate that Positive Affect also varies as a function of the proximity of sleep. As we have seen, positive mood levels were highest when the respondent was the farthest removed temporally from sleep and was lowest when the individual was closest to sleep. Moreover, these effects persisted regardless of the time of day (and, hence, of the individual's position on the body temperature cycle). On the basis of these results, it appears that positive mood levels do not simply follow the body temperature rhythm, independent of the sleep–wake cycle. Accordingly, it seems most likely that the circadian rhythm in Positive Affect reflects some interaction between the strong and weak oscillators (see also Clark et al., 1989).

MOOD FLUCTUATIONS ACROSS THE DAYS OF THE WEEK

Earlier Studies of Weekly Variation

I now consider mood fluctuations across the days of the week. The week is a peculiar unit of time that is unlike the others we are considering in this chapter. Whereas the day, the month, and the year all are associated with distinct astronomical phenomena involving either the sun or the moon, the week is marked by no clear astronomical event (Larsen & Kasimatis, 1990; Zerubavel, 1985). Moreover, the week is strangely out of synchrony with the other major units of time measurement. It typically is the case that each lower unit must complete a given number of cycles before a higher unit advances; that is, there are 60 seconds in a minute, 60 minutes in an hour, 24 hours in a day, a fixed number of days in each month, and 12 months per year. The week fails to conform to this pattern, however, in that it does not fit neatly into either the month or the year; indeed, it is quite possible to begin a new month—or a new year—in the middle of a week (Campbell, 1986; Larsen & Kasimatis, 1990; McGrath & Kelly, 1986).

Why, then, did the week emerge as an important unit of time? It is noteworthy that recent research has identified several biological processes that follow a 7-day "circaseptum" rhythm. For instance, 7-day rhythms have been found in immune system response (Campbell, 1986; Levi & Halberg, 1982), red blood cell counts and hemoglobin concentration in the blood (Haus, Lakatua, Swoyer, & Sackett-Lundeen, 1983), oral temperature and reaction times (Hildebrandt & Geyer, 1984), and calcium and sodium concentration in the urine (Halberg, 1983). On the basis of such evidence, several writers have suggested that the 7-day week is based on an endogenous biological rhythm (see Larsen & Kasimatis, 1990).

Whatever its origins, the week clearly plays a crucial role in organizing our lives and activities. Indeed, our lives typically are scheduled around the days of the week. For instance, during the academic year, I may teach on Mondays, Wednesdays, and Fridays; pursue research and scholarly interests on Tuesdays and Thursdays; and perform household tasks and engage in leisure activities on Saturdays and Sundays. Note, moreover, that this regularity in scheduling creates a consistent, predictable pattern that recurs again and again. Because of this, the week "is an excellent framework on which to build predictability and periodicity into one's life" (Larsen & Kasimatis, 1990). It is hardly surprising, therefore, that mood demonstrates a systematic circaseptum rhythm. Larsen and Kasimatis (1990), in fact, found that a sine wave with a period of 7 days accounted for 40% of the variance in daily mood data.

Although the 7-day week may reflect an endogenous biological rhythm, mood fluctuations across the individual days of the week surely must result from lifestyle and sociocultural factors. This is because the days of the week (unlike the hours of the day or the months of the year) do not bear any systematic relation to important astronomical or environmental phenomena. For instance, it is not consistently warmer or sunnier on Friday than on Tuesday; similarly, foraging for food is not more likely to be rewarded on Saturday than on Wednesday. The days of the week, therefore, are arbitrary in an evolutionary sense. Accordingly, there is no reason to believe that humans are biologically preprogrammed to feel better on certain days of the week than on others.

What patterns of mood fluctuation might be expected across the days of the week? First, as noted earlier, the dominant pattern in U.S. culture is for people to work and study from Monday through Friday (indeed, this period is commonly referred to as the workweek), with Saturdays and Sundays off. Consequently, we might expect to find a strong "weekend effect," such that people report a generally better mood (i.e., higher positive mood, lower negative mood, or both) on Saturdays and Sundays than during the rest of the week. Second, most individuals in our society believe that Monday is the emotional nadir of the week (see Farber, 1953; Stone, Hedges, Neale, & Satin, 1985). In fact, when I have asked the student participants in our mood studies to identify their worst day of the week, virtually everyone—and with little hesitation—names Monday. Accordingly, we would expect to find evidence of what has been termed the "blue Monday" phenomenon—that is, mood levels on Monday should be significantly worse (lower positive mood, higher negative mood, or both) than on other days.

The available evidence provides reasonably good support for the first of these expectations (although the days that actually constitute the subjective "weekend" have varied from study to study) but little for the second. The first large-scale analysis was reported by Rossi and Rossi (1977), who examined daily mood in 82 college students over a period of 40 days (a total of nearly 2,900 observations). Rossi and Rossi obtained clear evidence of a significant weekend effect. Specifically, positive mood was higher on Friday, Saturday, and Sunday than during the rest of the week; conversely, negative mood was lower on Saturday and Sunday than on other days. It is interesting to note, however, that positive mood actually reached its zenith on Friday and its nadir on Tuesday. More generally, Rossi and Rossi found no evidence that mood on Mondays was worse than on any of the other weekdays.

Stone et al. (1985) reported two intensive within-subject studies that focused in particular on the "blue Monday" phenomenon. In the first study, 46 married couples rated the husband's mood each day over 42 consecutive days. In the second study, 58 married couples rated the husband's daily mood over the same period. Both studies found a significant weekend effect: Levels of positive mood were higher—and negative mood was lower—on Saturday and Sunday than during the rest of the week. Consistent with Rossi and Rossi (1977), however, neither study yielded any indication that mood was worse on Monday than on Tuesday, Wednesday, or Thursday. Nevertheless, when the investigators later contacted 57 of the Study 2 husbands, 65% indicated that their mood was worst on Monday (the runner-up, incidentally, was Tuesday at only 9%). Thus, we again see a clear disjunction between people's beliefs and their actual affective experience.

Largely similar results were reported by McFarlane, Martin, and Williams (1988), who studied daily mood fluctuations in 62 college students over a period of 60 to 70 days. Mood was assessed using the Affect Grid (Russell, Weiss, & Mendelsohn, 1989), which yields global measures of pleasantness and arousal. McFarlane et al. found that levels of pleasantness were higher on Friday and Saturday than on Monday through Thursday; these latter days did not differ from each other. In contrast, ratings of arousal peaked on Friday and were higher on that day than on Sunday through Wednesday; they actually reached their lowest level on Sunday. Again, there was no suggestion that mood was worst on Mondays.

The results I have considered thus far are relatively clear and easy to summarize: Briefly put, these studies demonstrate a consistent weekend effect but fail to show that mood on one weekday is consistently worse than on any of the others. In contrast, the findings of Kennedy-Moore, Greenberg, Newman, and Stone (1992) are more complex and difficult to interpret. The authors examined daily mood variation in two samples of adult men. One group consisted of 94 men who rated their mood each day for an average of 75 days (a total of more than 7,000 observations) on the general Positive and Negative Affect scales of the PANAS-X. The second sample was composed of 77 men who rated their daily mood over a period of approximately 3 months (more than 8,500 observations). The men in this second group rated themselves on a modified version of the MACL (Nowlis, 1965), which also yields general measures of Positive and

Negative Affect. The negative mood scale consists of the terms "angry," "clutched up," "concentrating," "skeptical," and "sad," whereas positive mood is composed of the terms "playful," "elated," "energetic," "kindly," "self-centered," and "leisurely." Watson (1988b) found that these MACL scales correlated strongly with their PANAS-X counterparts.

This convergence would lead one to predict that the two samples would generate similar patterns across the days of the week. The two negative mood measures, in fact, did yield essentially identical patterns that were entirely consistent with those found in earlier studies: In both cases, negative mood levels were lower on Saturday and Sunday (especially the latter) than during the rest of the week; among the remaining days, the only notable finding was that Negative Affect peaked on Wednesday in the PANAS-X sample. However, positive mood variations were markedly different in the two samples. Specifically, the men in the MACL sample showed a typical weekend effect, such that they reported greater positive mood on Saturday and Sunday (particularly the latter) than during the rest of the week; the remaining days did not differ substantially from one another. In marked contrast, the men in the PANAS-X sample reported a moderately high level of positive mood that remained relatively stable from Tuesday through Saturday. Positive Affect was somewhat lower on Mondays, however, and—contrary to all expectation—was substantially lower on Sunday than on any other day.

The reasons for this marked discrepancy are unclear. Kennedy-Moore et al. (1992) attributed it to content differences between the two positive mood scales (for a related discussion, see Egloff, Tausch, Kohlmann, & Krohne, 1995). Specifically, they argued that "the best descriptor of positive affect on the PANAS may be 'engagement,' whereas positive affect on the MACL may more accurately be described as 'pleasantness' " (p. 153). Although it probably is true that the PANAS-X Positive Affect scale contains a stronger activation/engagement component than does its MACL counterpart, there are two problems with this argument. First, item-level analyses demonstrated that MACL terms reflecting high activation/engagement (e.g., "energetic" and "elated") and pleasantness (e.g., "leisurely" and "playful") both showed the same basic weekly pattern (i.e., greater positive mood on the weekend compared to weekdays). Hence, it is not the case that terms reflecting pleasantness consistently show the expected weekend effect, whereas descriptors representing high activation do not. Second, our own data using the PANAS-X Positive Affect scale (to be discussed shortly) have demonstrated a markedly different weekly pattern (although this finding of low positive mood on Sunday has persisted). Consequently, it appears that the anomalous findings in the PANAS-X sample must reflect other factors.

Finally, I noted earlier that sociocultural rhythms should give rise to patterns that are reasonably consistent across different individuals within the same culture but might differ dramatically cross-culturally. Clark and I found some suggestive evidence along these lines when we examined daily mood variation in 18 Japanese college students over a period of approximately 3 months (a total of 1,613 observations; see Clark & Watson, 1988). The results were quite unlike any collected in the United States. Specifically, negative mood was lower on Sunday than during the rest of the week but showed no other effects; furthermore, positive mood failed to display any systematic variation whatsoever. These results clearly need to be replicated using larger and more diverse samples. Nevertheless, they provide preliminary evidence that the patterns observed in the United States might not generalize well across cultures.

Our Own Studies of Weekly Variation in U.S. College Students

Higher-Order Analyses

If we exclude the anomalous results in the PANAS-X sample of Kennedy-Moore et al. (1992), the data from the U.S. studies can be summarized as follows: First, the so-called blue Monday phenomenon simply appears to be a cultural myth. To be sure, no one who has worked in this area would suggest that Mondays are particularly enjoyable; indeed, mood on this day tends to be noticeably worse than on the weekends. Nevertheless, the data consistently have shown that Mondays are no worse than Tuesdays or Wednesdays.

Second, negative and positive mood both show a clear weekend effect. Researchers consistently have found that negative mood is significantly lower on Saturday and Sunday than during the rest of the week. Moreover, most studies have identified Sunday as the point of lowest Negative Affect. Conversely, positive mood is substantially higher during the weekend than during the workweek. It is noteworthy, however, that college students and adults appear to show somewhat different weekly patterns. Specifically, studies of adults have reported that positive mood is elevated on Saturday and Sunday relative to the rest of the week (Kennedy-Moore et al., 1992, MACL sample; Stone et al., 1985, Studies 1 and 2); in these data, Fridays appear to be indistinguishable from other weekdays. In contrast, Friday appears to be the time of peak Positive Affect in college students. Rossi and Rossi (1977), for instance, found that positive mood scores were elevated from Friday through Sunday and that they reached their highest level on Friday. Similarly, McFarlane et al. (1988) reported that students' mood was more pleasant on Friday and Saturday than during the period from Monday through Thursday; in this sample, pleasantness levels were intermediate on Sunday.

On the basis of these results, we may speculate that the "subjective weekend" of adults corresponds to the formal, traditional period of Saturday and Sunday, whereas that of college students is shifted forward to include Friday. In fact, the data of McFarlane et al. (1988) might suggest further that the subjective weekend of college students actually consists of Friday and Saturday only, with Sunday acting more as a transitional period prior to the commencement of the workweek.

These speculations may prove helpful in interpreting my own weekly mood data, which are derived from two large college student samples. The first data set includes a total of 20,818 observations from 478 SMU students, each of whom rated his or her mood on a daily basis for at least 30 days. As in previous analyses, scores on the general Positive and Negative Affect scales were standardized on a person-by-person basis and then collapsed across all individuals. Figure 4.8 presents the overall mean affect scores for each day of the week; note that each data point represents more than 2,900 observations.

These data are broadly consistent with those of previous studies, especially those based on college students. Once again, there is no evidence of a "blue Monday" effect: Mood levels on Monday did not differ significantly from those of Tuesday or Wednesday on either mood scale. In addition, we again see a significant weekend effect, with students reporting the best mood on Fridays and Saturdays. Negative Affect shows less overall variation than Positive Affect, ranging from a low of only –.094 (on Monday) to a high of .094 (on Saturday). Nevertheless, it displays a clear and systematic weekly trend. Negative mood levels are highest on Monday and Tuesday and then show a gradual decline, reaching their lowest point on Fridays and Saturdays.

Consistent with the diurnal data, Positive Affect shows much more variability overall, ranging from a minimum of –.194 (on Sunday) to a maximum of .206 (on Friday). Its weekly course is quite systematic: Positive mood ratings are quite low on Sunday and are somewhat higher— but still below average—during the period Monday through Wednesday. After that, they rise markedly and are elevated from Thursday through Saturday, with a clear peak on Friday. Thus, with regard to positive mood, the subjective weekend of these SMU students seems to last from Thursday through Saturday.

We can assess the replicability of these findings by examining a second large data set consisting of 6,629 observations from 136 students at the University of Iowa, each of whom provided a minimum of 30 daily ratings. Again, scores on the general Positive and Negative Affect scales were standardized on a person-by-person basis and then collapsed across all individuals. Figure 4.9 presents the overall mean affect scores for each day of the week; in this sample, each data point represents more than 900 observations.

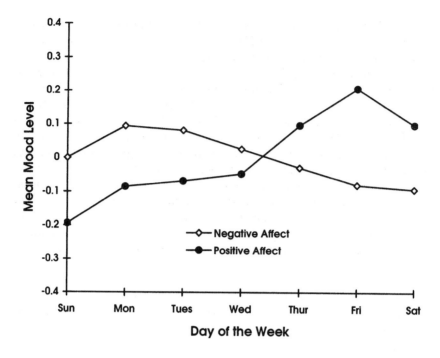

FIGURE 4.8. General Positive and Negative Affect across the days of the week (SMU sample).

Overall, the Iowa data closely replicate the SMU results. Once again, negative mood levels are highest at the beginning of the workweek and then show a gradual decline, reaching their lowest point on Fridays and Saturdays. The one notable difference is that Negative Affect scores in this sample are much higher on Monday (with a mean of .201) than on any other day, thus showing evidence of a "blue Monday" effect. Paralleling the SMU findings, positive mood ratings are quite low on Sunday and are somewhat higher—but still below average—during the period Monday through Wednesday. After that, they rise markedly and are elevated from Thursday through Saturday; in this sample, however, Positive Affect peaked on Saturday rather than Friday. Once again, the subjective weekend of college students seems to last from Thursday through Saturday.

However, the most striking aspect of these data is that positive mood levels reached their nadir on Sunday in both samples (the Positive Affect means were –.194 and –.207 in the SMU and Iowa samples, respectively).

This replicated finding was unexpected and its interpretation is unclear. One of my student assistants offered an interesting explanation, namely, that our respondents were so busy enjoying themselves from Thursday through Saturday—and, these being college students, much of their enjoyment results from drinking and carousing—that they were completely worn out by Sunday! Although this would seem to be a plausible interpretation of our own results, it seems less adequate in explaining the parallel finding reported by Kennedy-Moore et al. (1992) in their PANAS-X sample. Considering that the respondents in this group were middle-aged (*M* = 42.6 years) married men—most of them with children—it seems unlikely that their consistently low levels of positive mood on Sunday can be attributed to excessive partying.

Other possible explanations for this effect include (1) the pressure to finish tasks that have been put off but must completed before the end of the weekend, (2) a relative dearth of stimulating and engaging activities,

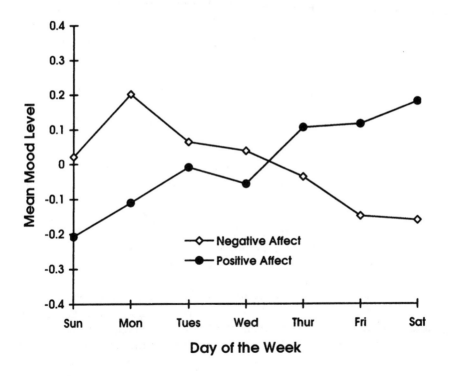

FIGURE 4.9. General Positive and Negative Affect across the days of the week (Iowa sample).

and (3) an anticipatory dread of the coming work week (Gregory, 1994). Whatever its explanation, it appears that this is not an isolated effect. Gregory (1994), for instance, has noted that the "Sunday night blahs" are relatively common among working adults. It also should be recalled, however, that several studies have found positive mood scores to be *elevated* on Sundays (Moore-Kennedy et al., 1992, MACL sample; Stone et al., 1985, Studies 1 and 2). We therefore are left with an intriguing inconsistency that warrants much closer attention in the future.

Lower-Order Analyses

Things may become a bit clearer if we examine specific types of affect. Daily mood ratings on the complete 60-item PANAS-X are available from 248 SMU students who generated a total of 11,323 observations ($M = 45.7$ per person), that is, roughly 1,600 assessments for each day of the week. Figure 4.10 plots standardized means for the three basic positive mood scales. Unlike the circadian data, these scores provide clear evidence of content-specific effects. On the one hand, Joviality and Self-Assurance show extremely similar patterns. Both affects remained low from Sunday through Wednesday; in fact, none of these mean scores differed significantly from one another on either scale. Scores on both scales increased significantly on Thursday, however, followed by even higher scores on Friday and Saturday. The variation in Joviality was particularly dramatic, ranging from a trough of −.165 on Monday to a peak of .280 on Friday; similarly, Self-Assurance scores ranged from a low of −.117 on Monday to a high of .229 on Friday. Thus, both scales showed a substantial weekend effect, with the period of Thursday through Saturday defining the subjective weekend.

However, Attentiveness displayed a pattern that was quite different from the others. Attentiveness scores initially were quite low on Sunday ($M = −.168$) and rose steadily over the course of the week until they reached their zenith on Thursday ($M = .106$); they then declined across both Friday and Saturday. In other words, our student respondents may have been extremely happy, enthusiastic, energetic, and confident on Fridays and Saturdays, but they were not particularly alert or attentive.

Again, we can attempt to replicate these findings by examining data from the Iowa sample; all these students completed the full PANAS-X. Figure 4.11 depicts the standardized means on the basic positive affects across the days of the week. Replicating the SMU findings, Joviality and Self-Assurance scores remain low from Sunday through Wednesday; they then show a significant increase on Thursday, followed by even higher scores on Friday and Saturday. Joviality displayed a particularly dramatic weekend effect, ranging from a trough of −.242 on Monday to peaks of

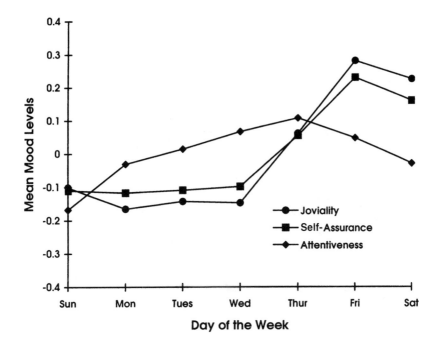

FIGURE 4.10. The basic positive affects across the days of the week (SMU sample).

.276 and .339 on Friday and Saturday, respectively. Once again, Attentiveness showed a fundamentally different pattern: Scores were elevated from Monday through Thursday and then were substantially lower from Friday through Sunday. Thus, similar to SMU students, Iowa undergraduates are not particularly alert as they enjoy themselves on Fridays and Saturdays.

These replicated differences highlight the importance of examining day-of-the-week effects at the specific, lower-order level. Having said this, however, I also should add that scores on all three positive affect scales were well below average on Sunday (with means ranging from −.101 to −.177) in both samples. Thus, the "Sunday blahs" noted earlier are not confined to one type of positive mood but seem to be more generally characteristic of the higher-order Positive Affect dimension. Again, this is an intriguing finding that merits further research.

I now examine specificity among the individual negative affects. Figure 4.12 plots the standardized means for the four basic negative mood scales of the PANAS-X in the SMU sample. Consistent with earlier data,

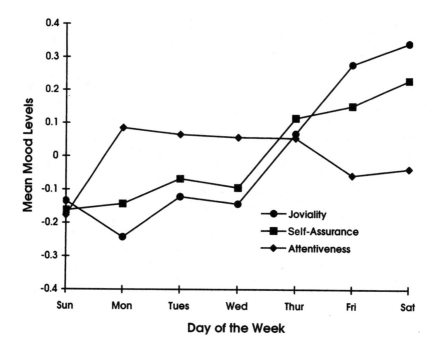

FIGURE 4.11. The basic positive affects across the days of the week (Iowa sample).

these scales showed much less variation overall; in fact, across the four measures, the means ranged from only −.111 (Sadness on Friday) to .128 (Fear on Tuesday). Again, we also see evidence of content-specific effects. On the one hand, Sadness, Guilt, and Hostility all display generally similar patterns: Each is elevated on Monday and then shows a gradual, continuous decline until it reaches its trough on Friday, followed by higher levels on Saturday and Sunday. Fear, however, displays a rather different pattern, reaching its peak on Tuesday and its nadir on Saturday and Sunday.

To assess the replicability of these effects, Figure 4.13 presents parallel data in the Iowa sample. Sadness, Guilt, and Hostility again show very similar patterns, although the pattern here is somewhat different from that seen in the SMU data. In this case, scores are elevated on Sunday and Monday and then show a gradual decline until they reach their nadir on Friday and Saturday. Fear shows a similar pattern in these data except that it (1) displays a much sharper peak on Monday and (2) is low— rather than elevated—on Sunday. The broadest generalization that can be drawn from these data (as well as those discussed earlier) is that negative mood scores show a steady and pervasive decline across the work week from Monday through Friday.

Summarizing across all these findings, we can provide a preliminary sketch of the days of the week, at least as they are typically experienced by U.S. college students. Mondays and Tuesdays both are relatively dysthymic, characterized by elevated levels of negative mood and reduced amounts of positive mood. Wednesday is a transitional day defined by low levels of Positive Affect (except for Attentiveness, which is slightly elevated) and average levels of Negative Affect. Thursday is marked by relatively high levels of Attentiveness and by more moderate elevations in other positive mood states; again, negative mood levels essentially are average. Fridays and Saturdays are the most euthymic days, characterized by high levels of Positive Affect (except for Attentiveness) and low to moderate Negative Affect. Finally, Sunday—which is emerging as the most enigmatic of days—is defined by relatively high levels of Sadness and Guilt and by relatively low levels of Fear and Positive Affect.

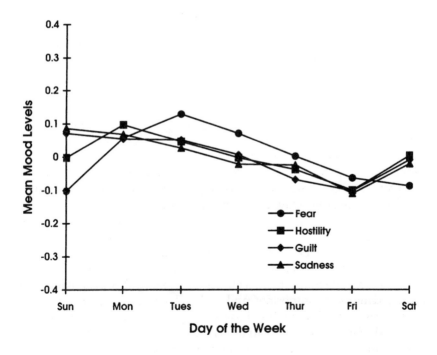

FIGURE 4.12. The basic negative affects across the days of the week (SMU sample).

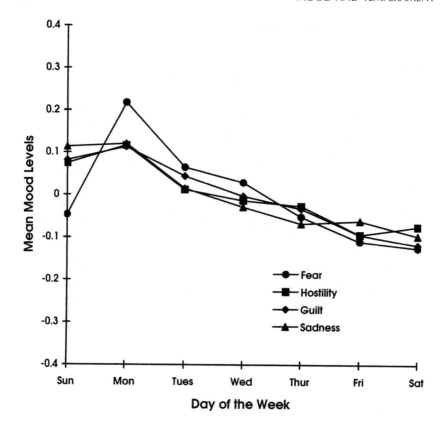

FIGURE 4.13. The basic negative affects across the days of the week (Iowa sample).

This pattern suggests that many students experience a relatively disengaged and anhedonic state on Sundays.

MOOD AND THE MENSTRUAL CYCLE

I now consider the mood-related effects of the monthly menstrual cycle in women. This is an important and somewhat controversial topic. It is widely believed in our culture that women experience profound affective changes due to hormonal fluctuations over the course of this monthly cycle (e.g., Ruble, 1977; McFarland, Ross, & DeCourville, 1989). These beliefs focus particularly on the premenstrual and menstrual phases, which are thought to be associated with increased irritability, tension, and emotional lability.

The issue of menstrual effects is politically sensitive and has aroused considerable passion. Ironically, this sensitivity has two quite opposite sources. On the one hand, many investigators have been concerned that menstrual effects not be *exaggerated* or overstated. This concern reflects a justifiable fear that menstrual effects might be used as a rationalization for discriminating against women in the workplace and in other areas of society (see Thayer, 1989). On the other hand, some researchers have been concerned that menstrual effects not be *minimized* or dismissed altogether. This concern also is quite justifiable: Male physicians long have shown a disturbing tendency to dismiss the physical complaints of women as manifestations of "hysteria" or "malingering" (e.g., Loevinger, 1987), and it would be truly unfortunate if legitimate physical and emotional complaints were callously disregarded. Consequently, it is extremely important that one be cautious and circumspect in interpreting findings in this area.

Unfortunately, this is an extremely difficult literature to summarize accurately. The basic problem is that although an enormous number of studies have provided indirect or suggestive evidence, relatively few investigators have analyzed this issue in a thorough and compelling manner. It is easy to understand why: Such research is extremely difficult to conduct. To examine menstrual mood effects properly, one really needs to perform intensive, within-subject analyses in a large sample of respondents (see McFarlane et al., 1988; Rossi & Rossi, 1977; Thayer, 1989). Moreover, it is important to examine women across several complete menstrual cycles to control for idiosyncratic characteristics of any single month (see McFarlane et al., 1988; Thayer, 1989). Furthermore, it is highly desirable to include appropriate comparison groups. For instance, because one inevitably sees a certain amount of fluctuation over time, it is useful to compare the monthly cycles of women and men to determine whether women actually show a more pronounced effect (see McFarlane et al., 1988). In addition, some evidence indicates that women taking oral contraceptives experience less menstrual mood fluctuation than do normally cycling women (Paige, 1971; Rossi & Rossi, 1977); accordingly, it is important to compare the ratings of women who are taking oral contraceptives with those who are not.

Regrettably, most researchers have used cross-sectional designs (i.e., a group of women currently in one phase is compared to a second group that is currently in another) or have examined women over only a few isolated points in the cycle (see McFarlane et al., 1988; Rossi & Rossi, 1977; Thayer, 1989). In addition, three other common problems can be noted. First, researchers have been extremely inconsistent in subdividing the cycle into phases. Rossi and Rossi (1977), for example, reviewed 23 studies that examined multiple, explicitly defined phases. Of these, one used eight phases, two used seven, five used four, nine used three, and six used two. Moreover, even among those using the same number of phases, researchers assigned specific days to each phase in highly idiosyncratic ways.

Second, the results of many studies may be biased due to expectancy effects. Especially in the early research conducted in this area, it was not uncommon to inform women explicitly that they were participating in a study of menstrual mood effects, and to do so prior to the collection of the mood ratings. Unfortunately, the available evidence suggests that women who are aware of the true purpose of the research show greater mood fluctuations than do those who are not (Parlee, 1974; Ruble, 1977).

The most serious problem, however, has been an overreliance on retrospective mood reports. That is, many researchers have asked women to recall how they felt during various phases of their most recent (or, alternatively, their worst) menstrual cycle (e.g., Coppen & Kessel, 1963; Moos, 1968, 1969). Investigators have favored this method because it is quicker and easier than measuring current, ongoing mood repeatedly over time. Unfortunately, considerable evidence indicates that retrospective reports differ systematically from concurrent daily ratings (Boyle & Grant, 1992; May, 1976; McFarlane et al., 1988; McFarland et al., 1989; Parlee, 1974; Ruble, 1977; Slade, 1984) because retrospective ratings are strongly influenced by the respondents' beliefs and stereotypes regarding their affective experience. In other words, people do not simply recall their actual experience; to a considerable extent, they distort their ratings to conform to their preexisting expectations. Because most people in our culture believe that there are substantial menstrual effects, retrospective reports consistently exaggerate the true magnitude of mood changes over the course of the menstrual cycle.

Are there, in fact, significant concurrent mood changes over the various phases of the menstrual cycle? The few studies employing intensive, within-subject designs have yielded extremely inconsistent results: Whereas some investigators have reported significant menstrual effects (Boyle & Grant, 1992; Rossi & Rossi, 1977), others have not (Almagor & Ben-Porath, 1991; Mansfield, Hood, & Henderson, 1989; McFarlane et al., 1988; McFarland et al., 1989). The earliest study was reported by Rossi and Rossi (1977), who obtained daily mood ratings from 67 college women over a period of 40 days (roughly 3,000 observations). Assuming a standardized 28-day menstrual cycle, Rossi and Rossi grouped these ratings into five phases: menstrual (days 1 through 4), follicular (days 5–11), ovulatory (days 12–16), luteal (days 17–24) and premenstrual (days 25–28). Analyses indicated that negative mood levels were significantly elevated during the menstrual and luteal phases whereas positive mood peaked during the ovulatory phase.

In contrast, neither Almagor and Ben-Porath (1991) nor Mansfield et al. (1989) found significant changes across the menstrual cycle. Almagor and Ben-Porath (1991) obtained 45 daily ratings of general Positive and Negative Affect from each of 50 Israeli women. These data were grouped into the same five phases used by Rossi and Rossi (1977), although specific days were subdivided differently (e.g., the follicular phase now consisted of days 6–10). The only significant effect was that women who used oral contraceptives reported higher levels of Positive Affect than those who did not. Mansfield et al. (1989) studied daily mood in nine married couples over a 3-month period. Again, these responses were divided into five phases (menstrual, follicular, luteal, premenstrual I, premenstrual II). The only significant effect was that the *husbands* reported greater positive mood during their wives' menstrual phase than during the follicular phase.

Three other studies have directly compared concurrent and retrospective ratings across the menstrual cycle. McFarlane et al. (1988) obtained daily assessments on the Affect Grid (Russell et al., 1989) from 42 undergraduate women over a period of 60 to 70 days. These data were subdivided into the five phases used by Rossi and Rossi (1977). At the conclusion of the daily rating period, the women also were asked to indicate their average mood over the previous 2 months in each of the five phases. The concurrent ratings yielded essentially negative results. In fact, the only notable finding was that women who were taking oral contraceptives reported a less pleasant mood during the menstrual and follicular phases. The normally cycling women showed no such effect, and neither group displayed any systematic variation on reported arousal. In marked contrast, the retrospective reports produced significant effects on both pleasantness and arousal. Most notably, women recalled that they experienced their best mood during the follicular and menstrual phases and their worst mood during the premenstrual phase.

McFarland et al. (1989) obtained daily negative mood ratings from 70 women over a 4 to 6 week period. These responses were grouped into three phases: premenstrual (the 3 days immediately preceding the onset of menstruation), menstrual (the first 3 days of the menstrual period), and intermenstrual (all other days). These concurrent ratings did not vary systematically across the three phases. Nevertheless, women recalled experiencing significantly greater negative mood during the premenstrual and menstrual phases than during the intermenstrual period. Furthermore, McFarland et al. (1989) found that women who believed more strongly in the existence of menstrual-related distress also showed a more pronounced tendency to exaggerate the extent of their negative mood fluctuations retrospectively.

Finally, Boyle and Grant (1992) examined daily mood in 103 undergraduate women over one complete menstrual cycle. As in McFarland et al. (1989), responses were divided into three phases: premenstrual (the 5 days preceding menstruation), menstrual (the first 2 days of the period), and intermenstrual (days 13 through 8 prior to menstruation). These ratings yielded significant concurrent effects for both positive and negative mood. Specifically, positive mood was higher during the intermenstrual period than during the other two phases, whereas negative mood was greatest during the premenstrual phase, intermediate during the menstrual phase, and lowest during the intermenstrual period. Retrospective judgments yielded similar findings, except that those for negative mood indicated stronger phase-related effects than actually occurred. That is, these retrospective ratings exaggerated the true extent of the menstrual effect.

In light of this confusing and contradictory evidence, it is impossible to reach any definite conclusions. At this point, enough supportive evidence exists to suggest that there are some systematic changes in mood as a function of the menstrual cycle, but the nature and magnitude of these effects currently cannot be ascertained with any confidence. Nevertheless, one important finding already has emerged in this literature: The available data clearly indicate that the actual, ongoing mood changes are not nearly as strong or as systematic as people widely believe them to be. Indeed, even women who have just completed an intensive daily study (and who should be quite sensitized, therefore, to their mood) tend to exaggerate the extent to which their mood varies across the phases of the menstrual cycle. Thus, we have further, dramatic evidence that people lack good insight into the true nature of their affective experience.

MOOD ACROSS THE SEASONS OF THE YEAR

I turn now to seasonal variations in mood. This examination is necessarily brief in that there is little evidence directly pertaining to this issue. As was the case with menstrual effects, it is easy to understand why: Good seasonal research is extraordinarily difficult to conduct. To examine this issue properly, one ideally should assess a large group of respondents at least once or twice a month for a minimum of 2 or 3 years. Again, this last provision is necessary to control for any idiosyncratic characteristics of individual years. For example, in the midwestern United States, the summer of 1993 was marked by incessant rain and extremely destructive floods; if, by chance, a researcher had been studying seasonal effects in this population during this period, it is unlikely that he or she would have found the summer to be a time of elevated mood.

Not surprisingly, no study of this scope and quality has ever been conducted. We therefore must content ourselves with indirect evidence.

Earlier, I suggested on theoretical grounds that Positive Affect should display a marked seasonal pattern, with greater positive mood being reported in the spring and summer than in the late fall and winter. Two lines of evidence suggest that this argument has some merit. First, recent research has established the existence of seasonal affective disorder (SAD; Rosenthal et al., 1984), a striking clinical syndrome that is particularly prevalent in northern latitudes (Booker & Helleckson, 1992; Rosen, Targum, Terman, & Bryant, 1990). As noted earlier, SAD is characterized by an episode of depression during the late fall and winter, often accompanied by a hypomanic phase in the spring or summer (see Bauer & Dunner, 1993; Depue et al., 1987; Kasper & Rosenthal, 1989; Rosenthal et al., 1984; Wehr & Rosenthal, 1989). This winter depression is triggered by various time cues associated with the changing seasons, especially the shortening of the photoperiod (i.e., the length of the daylight hours) and a drop in temperature (Kasper & Rosenthal, 1989). The most effective treatment for SAD is phototherapy, in which patients are exposed to bright artificial light (Lafer, Sachs, Labbate, & Thibault, 1994; Wehr et al., 1986; Wirz-Justice, Graw, Krauchi, & Gisin, 1993).

Depression is a disorder that is characterized by marked disinterest, low energy, and general reductions in positive mood (see Chapter 8). Indeed, my colleagues and I have shown that anhedonia (i.e., the absence of pleasure) and low Positive Affect are unique, defining features of depression that serve to differentiate it from other disorders (Clark & Watson, 1991b; Mineka, Watson, & Clark, 1998; Watson, Clark, & Carey, 1988; Watson et al., 1995). Consequently, the evidence regarding SAD demonstrates that at least a significant minority of the population experiences a marked reduction in Positive Affect during the late fall and winter.

The second line of suggestive evidence comes from cross-sectional analyses in which different groups of individuals are assessed at various times of the year. Consistent with theoretical expectations, cross-sectional analyses have indicated that positive mood varies significantly across the year, whereas negative mood shows a less clear and systematic seasonal trend (Andrews & Withey, 1976; Bradburn, 1969; Rossi & Rossi, 1977; Smith, 1979). The most extensive analysis was reported by Smith (1979), who compared mood ratings taken at 12 different times of the year; each of these assessments represented more than 600 individual respondents. Smith found that positive mood levels were highest in the spring and then declined slightly in the summer and fall, eventually reaching their lowest point in the winter. In contrast, negative mood showed little seasonal variation.

Similarly, in their daily mood study, Rossi and Rossi (1977) assessed students either during the fall (from mid-September to mid-November) or during the spring (from mid-March to early May). Rossi and Rossi found that the spring respondents reported much higher positive mood levels than did the students assessed in the fall. However, negative mood levels did not differ appreciably between the two groups.

Finally, in addition to this indirect evidence, we have some very limited longitudinal data. Harris and Dawson-Hughes (1993) conducted a 1-year prospective analysis in 250 Boston-area women. The women completed the POMS (McNair et al., 1971) four times during the year; at each assessment, they rated how they had felt "the previous week, including today." All the women completed one rating during either December or January and a second during June or July. Unfortunately, the timing of the two remaining mood assessments differed more widely: One was completed sometime between February and May whereas the other was made from August to November.

Accordingly, in their principal analyses, Harris and Dawson-Hughes were forced to collapse the data into four rather unusual periods: December–January, February–May, June–July, and August–November. Analyses of these scores yielded results that are inconsistent with those discussed previously. Specifically, the negative mood scales all showed a significant seasonal pattern; in each case, negative mood levels were highest in August–November and lowest in either February–May or June–July. In contrast, the POMS Vigor-Activity scale (which is strongly correlated with our general Positive Affect scale; see Watson & Clark, 1994b) failed to show a significant seasonal pattern. In other words, Harris and Dawson-Hughes (1993) found significant seasonal variation in negative mood, but not positive mood.

However, these surprising findings largely result from the atypical, 4-month groupings that the authors employed. Note, for example, that one would not necessarily expect affect scores to be similar in February and May or in August and November. In fact, Harris and Dawson-Hughes (1993) also presented plotted scores divided into even 2-month intervals (December–January, February–March, April–May, June–July, August–September, October–November), and these results are far more consistent with previous research and with theoretical expectations. Specifically, positive mood now showed a clear seasonal effect, with higher levels being reported from April to September and lower levels occurring from October to March. In addition, the negative mood scales continued to display a marked seasonal trend, with a well-defined peak occurring in October through November and relatively low levels being reported from February to September.

Clearly, intensive within-subject research (involving many more than four data points per person) is badly needed in this area; in the absence of such research, no definitive conclusions can be drawn. At this point, however, we have enough supportive evidence to suggest tentatively that positive mood exhibits a significant seasonal trend, with scores being elevated from mid-spring to early fall (i.e., roughly from April to September) and somewhat lower from mid-fall to early spring (i.e., from October to March). The data regarding negative mood are much less clear, although the findings of Harris and Dawson-Hughes (1993) suggest a peak in October and November.

CONCLUSION

In summary, three key points have emerged in this chapter. First, consistent with my theoretical analysis, Positive Affect shows a strong and systematic circadian rhythm: Positive mood levels are low at the beginning and end of the day and reach their peak roughly at the midpoint between rising and retiring. Moreover, this pattern is highly robust across different individuals (including both morning and evening types) and highly generalizable across different types of positive mood. Furthermore, this diurnal pattern is influenced by both the "strong oscillator" (which regulates body temperature) and the "weak oscillator" (which regulates the sleep–wake cycle). In sharp contrast—and again consistent with my theoretical expectation—negative mood does not display a strong or systematic diurnal pattern.

Second, people report a generally better mood during the weekend than on weekdays. However, the specific days encompassed by this "subjective weekend" appear to vary across different types of respondents. Among U.S. college students, the "weekend" lasts from Thursday to Saturday, a period that is associated with generally elevated positive mood and low to moderate levels of negative mood. The most surprising aspect of our data, however, was the robust emergence of the "Sunday blahs." Indeed, the evidence suggests that many people (including both adults and college students) experience a relatively disengaged and anhedonic state on Sundays. Finally, it is noteworthy that our day-of-the-week analyses yielded replicable evidence of content specificity, indicating that future work in this area needs to examine daily mood fluctuations at the lower-order level.

Third, we encountered additional evidence that people lack good insight into the nature of their mood fluctuations. Among other things, we found that (1) "owls" do not experience their optimal state late at night, despite their protestations to the contrary; (2) mood levels on Monday generally are no worse than those on Tuesday, thereby destroying the myth of the "blue Monday"; and (3) menstrual cycle effects actually are much weaker than they are widely perceived to be.

5

THE DISPOSITIONAL BASIS
OF AFFECT

I now leave the topic of transient mood and enter the realm of temperament. The next three chapters explore the origins, nature, and significance of basic affective traits. As discussed in Chapter 1, affective traits are stable individual differences in the tendency to experience a corresponding mood state. For instance, the trait of fearfulness represents one's tendency to experience episodes of fear, worry, and apprehension, whereas the trait of hostility reflects one's proneness to feelings of anger, annoyance, and scorn.

The presentation in earlier chapters was based on a structural scheme emphasizing a fundamental distinction between positive and negative emotional experience. The same basic scheme characterizes trait affect as well. Hence, the two most important traits in this area are the dispositional counterparts of general Negative Affect and Positive Affect; these typically are labeled Negative Affectivity (or Negative Emotionality) and Positive Affectivity (or Positive Emotionality), respectively (Watson & Clark, 1984, 1992b; Watson et al., 1994). These two traits are a primary focus of this chapter. Specifically, I present extensive evidence demonstrating that there are important individual differences in positive and negative affective experience that (1) persist over time, (2) generalize across situations, and (3) are largely independent of one another.

However, one also can identify traits corresponding to many specific types of affect. In fact, my colleagues and I have amassed evidence establishing that—with one exception—the 11 lower-order PANAS-X scales also can be validly assessed as traits; I present much of the supporting data in this chapter. As we will see, the single exception is Surprise, which shows relatively poor convergent and discriminant validity (see Watson & Clark, 1994b). This finding was not unexpected: Whereas people frequently use a wide variety of affect terms (e.g., "hostile," "nervous," "guilty," "lonely," "shy," "happy," "confident," "determined," and "calm") to characterize the personalities of others, one rarely uses descriptors of surprise (e.g., "amazed" and "astonished") in this manner. Consequently, it seems likely that this affect does not have a meaningful dispositional counterpart.

My primary goal in this chapter is to establish that affective traits exist and, moreover, exert a profound influence on our subjective experience. Two characteristics are crucially important in establishing the existence of a trait. First, an individual's standing on the trait should be relatively stable over time. That is, people should maintain a relatively consistent rank order across assessments: Individuals who initially score relatively high on the trait should remain relatively high upon retest, whereas those who initially are low on the trait should remain relatively low in subsequent assessments. Second, scores on the trait should show a reasonable level of consistency or generality across different situations and contexts. For instance, people who are relatively happy when they are working also should be relatively happy when they are not; similarly, individuals who are happy when they are socializing should remain relatively happy when they are alone. I first consider the issue of temporal stability.

THE TEMPORAL STABILITY OF AFFECTIVE EXPERIENCE

Short-Term Evidence

A large body of evidence demonstrates that affective responses are stable over time. Not surprisingly, however, the bulk of this evidence is based on relatively short time spans of less than 6 months. This short-term evidence is of two basic types. The first type is derived from intensive within-subject analyses of momentary or daily mood. The earliest evidence of this sort was reported by Diener and Larsen (1984), who collected momentary mood ratings from 42 students twice a day over a 6-week period (a total of 3,512 assessments). Each student wore a watch with an alarm that was preset to go off at random times during the day.

These times were selected to ensure that every 10-minute interval of the waking day was assessed over the 6-week period. When the alarm went off, the students rated their current mood on brief measures of Negative and Positive Affect.

Diener and Larsen then computed separate mean affect scores for the first (i.e., Weeks 1 through 3) and second (i.e., Weeks 4 through 6) halves of the rating period; note that each mean score reflects approximately 42 individual assessments. The two mean Positive Affect scores correlated .79 with one another; the corresponding value for Negative Affect was .81. These data clearly demonstrate that ratings of Positive and Negative Affect are strongly stable across a 6-week period.

I have replicated and extended Diener and Larsen's (1984) findings using data from our own intensive studies of daily mood fluctuations in students at SMU. The students completed a single mood assessment in the evening, rating how they had felt over the course of the entire day. The analyses reported here were restricted to the 459 individuals who completed a minimum of 35 daily ratings. Moreover, for those students completing more than 35 ratings, only the first 35 were used. Consequently, these results are based on a total of 16,065 observations.

I began by correlating the students' general Negative and Positive Affect ratings on each individual day with the corresponding scores at each of the other daily assessments. For instance, I correlated the Negative Affect ratings on Day 1 with the corresponding scores on Day 2, the scores on Day 4 with those on Day 30, and so forth. Similarly, I correlated the Positive Affect scores on Days 1 and 6, on Days 12 and 35, and so on. Because each student completed 35 assessments, there are a total of 595 separate day-to-day correlations for each affect scale. The first row of Table 5.1 reports the mean correlations—together with the highest and lowest values in the distribution—across all 595 coefficients for both Negative and Positive Affect. It is noteworthy that both scales display a moderate level of stability (M correlation = .44 for Positive Affect, .37 for Negative Affect) *even at the level of the individual day.* Indeed, even the lowest correlations (.28 for Positive Affect, .22 for Negative Affect) are statistically significant and moderate in magnitude. These findings are quite striking, in that they demonstrate that *we can predict an individual's Positive or Negative Affect score on any given day simply by knowing how that individual responded on any other day.*

I next performed parallel analyses on composites reflecting increasing numbers of adjacent days. For instance, I formed 2-day composites by averaging responses on Days 1 and 2, Days 3 and 4, and so on, and then correlated these composites with one another; note that because there are 17 different 2-day composites (Day 35 was excluded from these analyses), there are a total of 136 separate stability correlations at this level. Simi-

TABLE 5.1. Effects of Aggregation on the Temporal Stability of General Positive and Negative Affect: Retest Correlations for Daily Mood Composites Based on Increasing Numbers of Days

No. of days in composite	Positive Affect			Negative Affect		
	Mean	Lowest	Highest	Mean	Lowest	Highest
1	.44	.28	.67	.37	.22	.61
2	.56	.42	.71	.47	.36	.64
3	.63	.51	.74	.54	.45	.68
4	.69	.58	.77	.59	.50	.71
5	.72	.62	.80	.62	.53	.73
6	.74	.66	.81	.65	.59	.70
7	.76	.69	.81	.67	.57	.75
14	.85	—	—	.77	—	—

Note. $N = 459$. All correlations are significant at $p < .01$, two-tailed.

larly, I formed 11 different 3-day composites by averaging responses on Days 1 through 3, Days 4 through 6, and so forth, and then correlated them with one another. This process was continued for all 4-, 5-, 6-, 7-, and 14-day composites that could be formed by averaging scores on adjacent days.

These results also are reported in successive rows of Table 5.1. Two aspects of these data are especially noteworthy. First, consistent with the broader literature on aggregation (Epstein, 1980; Rushton, Brainerd, & Pressley, 1983), the stability correlations increase systematically as larger and larger samples of data are analyzed. Thus, the 3-day composites yield higher stability estimates than did the 2-day composites, the 4-day composites generate higher estimates than the 3-day composites, and so on.

Second, these estimates increase rapidly; thus it takes relatively little aggregation to produce strong evidence of stability. In the case of Positive Affect, for instance, the 4-day composites already produce a mean stability correlation of .69. At the level of the 7-day (i.e., one week) composites, both scales are strongly stable, with mean correlations of .76 and .67 for Positive and Negative Affect, respectively. In other words, average mood levels are highly predictable from one week to another. Of course, further aggregation yields even more impressive evidence of stability; in fact, the 14-day composites yielded stability coefficients (.85 and .77 for Positive and Negative Affect, respectively) that are comparable to those reported by Diener and Larsen (1984).

The second type of short-term evidence comes from between-subject designs in which respondents complete general, trait versions of affect scales on two or more occasions, each of which is separated by an interval ranging from a few weeks to a few months. Studies of this type report moderate to strong levels of stability, with retest correlations typically in the .50–.85 range (e.g., Izard, Libero, Putnam, & Haynes, 1993; Watson, Clark, & Tellegen, 1988; Zuckerman & Lubin, 1985). For instance, Spielberger, Gorsuch, Lushene, Vagg, and Jacobs (1983) investigated the stability of the State–Trait Anxiety Inventory (STAI) in high school students; they reported 1-month retest correlations of .71 and .75 in men and women, respectively, and corresponding 60-day retests of .68 and .65, respectively.

To date, however, Clark and I have collected the most extensive data of this kind, using our own PANAS-X scales (see Watson & Clark, 1994b). Table 5.2 presents 2-month retest correlations for nine of the scales in one sample of college undergraduates ($N = 502$) and for all 13 scales in another student sample ($N = 399$). All students completed a general, trait version of the PANAS-X at both assessments. Several aspects of these data warrant comment. First, the correlations generally fall between .50

TABLE 5.2. Two-Month Retest Stabilities of the PANAS-X Scales (General Instructions)

Scale	Sample 1 ($N = 502$)	Sample 2 ($N = 399$)
General affect scales		
Positive Affect	.70	.64
Negative Affect	.71	.59
Basic negative affects		
Fear	.62	.57
Guilt	.68	.65
Sadness	.62	.60
Hostility	.65	.58
Basic positive affects		
Joviality	—	.64
Self-Assurance	—	.68
Attentiveness	—	.55
Other affective states		
Shyness	.70[a]	.64
Fatigue	.57[a]	.53
Surprise	.56	.52
Serenity	—	.51

Note. All correlations are significant at $p < .01$, two-tailed. Adapted from Watson and Clark (1994b, Table 20).
[a]Data are based on preliminary, three-item versions of these scales.

and .70, demonstrating moderate to strong temporal stability in affect across the 2-month retest interval. Second, the retest coefficients generally are quite similar for the negative and positive affects, indicating that they show comparable patterns over time. Finally, the stability estimates for Surprise are among the lowest for any scale, consistent with my earlier assertion that this affect lacks a meaningful dispositional component.

Long-Term Evidence

These data clearly demonstrate that affective experience is strongly stable over periods ranging from a few weeks to a few months. Although these results are quite encouraging, they certainly do not constitute a strong test of temporal stability: People must be assessed over much longer time intervals before we can conclude that affect shows trait-like stability. Accordingly, I now consider evidence regarding long-term stability. Before doing so, however, I need to mention two methodological points that complicate any interpretation of this literature. First, much of the relevant data is based on ad hoc measures lacking clear evidence of reliability or validity; it seems likely that many of these are psychometrically poor measures that underestimate the true level of stability.

Second, many of these scales were not actually designed to measure trait affect per se. I already have shown (see Table 5.1) that stability estimates increase systematically as larger and larger time samples are examined. This same effect can be obtained by varying the time instructions that are used to generate the ratings themselves. For instance, ratings of how one has felt "during the past year" will show greater temporal stability than ratings of how one has felt "during the past few days." Similarly, ratings of how one "generally" feels will be more stable than ratings of the "past week" (Watson & Clark, 1994b; Watson, Clark, & Tellegen, 1988). Because of this, many of the measures used in this literature will underestimate the level of stability that would be observed using a true trait scale. Most notably, the widely used Affect Balance Scale (ABS; Bradburn, 1969)—which typically is employed with "past few weeks" or "past month" instructions—is likely to yield lower retest coefficients than measures using "general" or "past year" instructions.

With these caveats in mind, let us examine the longer-term stability of affect. Several studies have assessed a single, global measure of emotionality (i.e., general well-being) over periods ranging from 6 months to 3 years. The retest correlations are significantly lower than those obtained across shorter intervals but still are moderate to strong in magnitude, typically falling in the .40 to .60 range (Adams, 1988; Shanahan, Finch, Mortimer, & Ryu, 1991; Susman, Dorn, & Chrousos, 1991; Tiggemann, Winefield, Winefield, & Goldney, 1991; Townsend, Noelker, Deimling, &

Bass, 1989). For example, using the ABS, Waltz and Badura (1988) obtained 6-month and 1-year stability correlations of .50 and .52, respectively, in a sample of 400 male cardiac patients. Similarly, Murrell, Norris, and Chipley (1992) obtained a 2-year stability coefficient of .54 on a general well-being measure in 1,031 older adults.

Other investigators have examined the stability of more specific affects across comparable time intervals and have reported similar results (e.g., Mechanic & Hansell, 1989; Phifer & Norris, 1989). For example, in a relatively small sample of mothers (N = 55), Izard et al. (1993) reported 2.5-year stability correlations ranging from .33 to .71 across the 12 DES-IV scales, with a median coefficient of .59. In a slightly larger sample of adult women, Nelson (1990) obtained 1-year and 18-month retest correlations of .64 and .42, respectively, for a measure of general negative affect and corresponding values of .48 and .30, respectively, for the Positive Affect subscale of the ABS.

Data are sparse for time spans longer than 3 years, but the available evidence indicates that affect continues to show a moderate level of stability even over extremely long periods, with retest correlations typically falling in the .30 to .50 range (e.g., Headey & Wearing, 1989; Newton & Keenan, 1991). For instance, Waltz and Badura (1988) obtained a 5-year stability correlation of .38 on the ABS in their cardiac patient group, and Costa, McCrae, and Zonderman (1987) reported a 9-year retest coefficient of .48 on a global well-being scale in a U.S. national sample. However, two studies have reported higher stability estimates. First, Ormel and Schaufeli (1991) obtained 7- and 8-year retest coefficients of. 57 and .52, respectively, on the Negative Affect subscale of the ABS in a sample of 226 Dutch adults. Second, in a smaller group of college students (N = 99), Magnus and Diener (1991) reported 4-year stability correlations in the .50 to .70 range on various measures of happiness and subjective well-being.

Do Negative and Positive Affect show similar patterns over long time spans, or is one more stable than the other? Unfortunately, few studies of long-term stability have assessed these two types of affect separately; furthermore, the available data are inconsistent. On the one hand, using the ABS, Stacey and Gatz (1991) obtained a significantly higher 14-year retest coefficient for Negative Affect (.44) than for Positive Affect (.30), which suggests that these two aspects of emotionality are differentially stable. On the other hand, Headey and Wearing (1989) reported 2- to 6-year retest correlations ranging from .36 to .42 for Negative Affect and from .31 to .39 for Positive Affect. These data (which also are based on Bradburn's ABS) suggest that positive and negative emotional experience are similarly stable over time.

This inconclusive evidence motivated Walker and me to investigate the long-term stability of trait affect (Watson & Walker, 1996). The 336 participants initially were assessed (Time 1) on trait versions of our general Negative and Positive Affect scales when they were undergraduates at SMU. These Time 1 scores were collected between January 1985 and September 1988. Virtually all the participants were enrolled in an introductory psychology class at the time, although a few were taking more advanced psychology courses; consequently, most were in their first or second year of college at the beginning of the study. Two-month retest scores (Time 2) also were available for a subset of these students, a point I return to later. Finally, all the respondents were mailed the Time 3 packet—which contained "general" versions of the Positive and Negative Affect scales—during March and April 1993. I should note that all participants graduated from college during the interval between Time 1 and Time 3.

At the initial Time 1 assessment, participants completed one of two trait forms of the affect scales. First, 99 respondents rated the extent to which they had experienced each affect term "during the past year" (Year sample). This sample had a mean retest interval of approximately 85 months (range = 80 to 87 months), that is, slightly more than 7 years.

Second, 237 respondents initially rated the extent to which they "generally" experienced each affect (General sample). The mean retest interval in this group was approximately 73 months (range = 56 to 99 months), that is, slightly more than 6 years. However, because of the wide variability in the retest interval, we also created two more homogeneous cohorts in order to examine the effects of different time spans. Specifically, 112 respondents initially were assessed between January 1985 and September 1986 (1985/1986 cohort); the mean stability interval in this group was approximately 91 months (range = 80 to 99 months), that is, roughly 7.5 years. The remaining 125 respondents all were assessed during the Fall 1988 semester (1988 cohort); the mean retest interval in this group was 56 months, that is, roughly 4.5 years.

Finally, as noted earlier, a subset of the respondents in the General sample ($N = 128$) were retested approximately 2 months after the initial Time 1 assessment. The average retest intervals in this subsample were 2 (Time 1 vs. Time 2), 60 (Time 2 vs. Time 3), and 62 (Time 1 vs. Time 3) months. These data offer an unusual opportunity to compare the short-term versus long-term stabilities of Positive and Negative Affect.

In examining these data, I first consider the issue of *mean level stability*, that is, whether or not the average affect levels of the respondents changed systematically over the course of the study. These analyses necessarily are restricted to respondents in the General sample because those in the Year sample completed different trait forms at Time 1 (Past Year instructions) and Time 3 (General Instructions). Our analyses indicated that average levels of Positive Affect did not change significantly over the retest interval (Time 1, M = 36.3; Time 3, M = 36.6); in contrast, Negative Affect scores declined significantly from Time 1 (M = 19.3) to Time 3 (M = 17.4). This finding replicates the results of Newton and Keenan (1991), who initially assessed engineers in the final year of college and subsequently retested them after graduation at 2- and 4-year follow-ups; these individuals reported significant decreases in anxiety at both of the follow-up assessments. It therefore appears that negative affect levels decline significantly during this stage of life.

I turn now to the more familiar issue of *rank-order stability*, that is, whether or not respondents maintained their relative position within the group. Before discussing these results, I should note two related reasons why we might expect rank-order stability to be somewhat lower in this group than in other samples. First, all the participants went through at least one major life transition over the course of the study in that they graduated from college during the interval between Times 1 and 3. In addition, approximately 30% of the sample got married—and roughly 70% began working full time—during the study, so that many respondents actually experienced several substantial changes in their lives. Furthermore, as noted earlier, most of the respondents initially were assessed early in their undergraduate experience, so that they still were adjusting to college life; thus, it seems likely that many of them experienced significant life changes even before graduation.

Second, several studies have demonstrated that personality continues to develop and evolve not only during the high school and college years but even throughout the 20s (Costa & McCrae, 1994; Finn, 1986; Haan, Millsap, & Hartka, 1986; Helson & Moane, 1987; McCrae & Costa, 1990). Haan et al. (1986), for example, concluded that the most striking shifts in personality "occur, not during adolescence, but at its end when most people make the profound role shifts entailed by entry into full-time work and marriage" (p. 225). In fact, on the basis of this stability evidence, McCrae and Costa (1990) suggested that from the perspective of the trait psychologist, true adulthood does not begin until the age of 30. Because our respondents still were only in their mid-20s (M age = 24.8) at the Time 3 assessment, one may anticipate that they will produce lower stability estimates than would general adult or older adult samples.

Table 5.3 presents correlations among the Time 1 and Time 3 affect measures in both the General and Year samples. The most important finding is that both affect scales were moderately stable over the course of the study, with retest correlations ranging from .36 to .46. Thus, trait affect exhibits significant stability even across 6- and 7-year retest intervals. It also is noteworthy that Negative Affect and Positive Affect showed roughly similar levels of stability. Finally, the retest correlations are comparable in the General and Year samples, indicating that the level of stability was not systematically influenced by the trait form used at Time 1.

TABLE 5.3. Long-Term Retest Stabilities of the General Negative Affect and Positive Affect Scales (Overall Samples)

Time 3 score	Time 1 score	
	Negative Affect	Positive Affect
General sample		
Negative Affect	.43**	−.18**
Positive Affect	−.24**	.42**
Year sample		
Negative Affect	.46**	−.02
Positive Affect	−.03	.36**

Note. N = 237 (General sample) and 99 (Year sample). Test–retest correlation is shown in **boldface**. Adapted from Watson and Walker (1996, Table 1). Copyright 1996 by the American Psychological Association. Adapted by permission. **p < .01, two-tailed.

Table 5.4 reports corresponding data for the two General sample cohorts. Again, the most important finding is that Negative and Positive Affect both showed a significant, moderate level of stability in both cohorts, with retest correlations ranging from .33 to .56. It is particularly striking that both scales were significantly stable in the 1985/1986 cohort across an average retest interval of slightly more than 7.5 years. Beyond this basic finding of moderate stability, however, the two scales clearly displayed different patterns across the two cohorts: That is, although the re-

TABLE 5.4. Long-Term Retest Stabilities of the General Negative Affect and Positive Affect Scales (General Sample Cohorts)

Time 3 score	Time 1 score	
	Negative Affect	Positive Affect
1985–1986 cohort		
Negative Affect	.33**	−.05
Positive Affect	−.07	.44**
1988 cohort		
Negative Affect	.56**	−.29**
Positive Affect	−.35**	.46**

Note. N = 112 (1985–1986 cohort) and 125 (1988 cohort). Test–retest correlation is shown in **boldface**. Adapted from Watson and Walker (1996, Table 2). Copyright 1996 by the American Psychological Association. Adapted by permission. **p < .01, two-tailed.

test coefficients for Positive Affect were essentially identical, Negative Affect exhibited a significantly higher level of stability in the 1988 cohort than in the 1985/1986 cohort. Without further data, however, it is impossible to know whether this represents a true time span effect (i.e., the temporal stability of Negative Affect decays across longer time intervals) or whether it instead reflects a chance cohort effect (i.e., by chance, the 112 individuals assessed in the earlier cohort were somewhat less stable than the 125 respondents assessed in the later cohort).

Finally, Table 5.5 presents the stability coefficients for the General sample respondents who also completed the short-term Time 2 retest. Note that the two affect scales showed similar patterns in these data. Specifically, Negative Affect ($r = .70$) and Positive Affect ($r = .74$) both were strongly stable over the 2-month retest interval and also showed a significant but more moderate level of stability across an extended time span of approximately 5 years, with long-term stability r's ranging from .35 to .45. In fact, the short-term retest correlation for each scale was significantly greater than both of its long-term stability coefficients. These findings closely corroborate those of Veenhoven (1994), who reviewed evidence regarding the stability of happiness over both short- and long-term intervals. Taken together, these data clearly demonstrate that the stability of affect decreases substantially as one moves from short-term to long-term time spans.

These long-term retest data have extremely important implications for our understanding of affective experience in that they indicate that trait measures of both Positive and Negative Affect are substantially stable, even across intervals as long as 7.5 years. Indeed, for reasons discussed earlier, these data provide an especially strong test of the temporal stability of trait affect. In addition to the long retest intervals, the respondents all had experienced at least one major life transition during the intervening period. The participants began the study as relatively new and inexperienced undergraduates; by its end they all had graduated, 30% had married, and roughly 70% were working full time. Clearly, their roles and responsibili-

TABLE 5.5. Comparison of the Short-Term versus Long-Term Stabilities of General Positive and Negative Affect in Individuals Who Completed All Three Assessments

Comparison	Mean retest interval	Negative Affect	Positive Affect
Time 1 vs. Time 2	2 months	.70	.74
Time 2 vs. Time 3	60 months	.35	.45
Time 1 vs. Time 3	62 months	.42	.43

Note. $N = 128$. All correlations are significant at $p < .01$, two-tailed. Adapted from Watson and Walker (1996, Table 3). Copyright 1996 by the American Psychological Association. Adapted by permission.

ties—as well as the daily structure of their lives—changed dramatically over the course of the study. Finally, the respondents' age also is a crucial consideration. Because the participants in this study still were largely in their mid-20s at the final Time 3 assessment, it seems likely that these results significantly underestimate the level of stability that would be obtained with older respondents (including these same individuals if they continued to be examined over the remainder of their lives).

On the other hand, one should not lose sight of the fact that long-term stability correlations are only moderate in magnitude, typically falling in the .35 to .55 range. Consequently, it also is true that many respondents show substantial change in their characteristic affect levels over time. Indeed, consistent with the results of Newton and Keenan (1991), our analyses of mean-level stability indicated that Negative Affect declined significantly from Time 1 to Time 3. Thus, one sees clear evidence of systematic change during this period of life. Along these same lines, it is noteworthy that the long-term stability correlations were significantly lower than the 2-month retest coefficients for both affect scales (see Table 5.5). In other words, affect appears to be much more stable in the short-term than in the long-term, at least in a relatively young sample such as ours. These results underscore the need for studies that examine both stability and change in emotional experience, especially during this critical, transitional period of life.

THE CROSS-SITUATIONAL CONSISTENCY OF AFFECTIVE EXPERIENCE

The data regarding cross-situational consistency are much more sparse, but the available evidence establishes that affective responding shows substantial consistency across various roles and contexts. The earliest investigation of this issue was reported by Diener and Larsen (1984). As discussed previously, the students who participated in this study rated their current, momentary mood twice a day over a period of 6 weeks. At each assessment, the students also indicated the current situation or activity in which they were engaged. For instance, they reported whether they were working, recreating, or maintaining themselves (e.g., by eating). Similarly, they noted whether they were socially engaged or alone. Diener and Larsen then computed mean Negative and Positive Affect scores for each student in each type of situation. For example, they calculated the students' mean affect levels across all occasions in which they were socializing, as well as all those times they were alone. Finally, they correlated the mean scores that were produced by *maximally dissimilar* situations. That is, they compared responses generated while socializing with those made when alone; similarly, they compared mean levels while working with those completed while recreating.

These analyses demonstrated a high level of consistency across these dissimilar situations. That is, mean affect levels while socializing correlated strongly with corresponding values obtained when the students were alone ($r = .70$ for Negative Affect, .58 for Positive Affect). Similarly, mean levels when working were highly predictive of average scores while recreating ($r = .74$ for Negative Affect, .70 for Positive Affect). Thus, the students differed in ways that were highly generalizable across diverse situations and contexts: Some students reported generally higher levels of Positive Affect and/or Negative Affect than others, and these differences persisted regardless of whether they were working or recreating, or were socializing versus alone.

As in the case of temporal stability, I have replicated and extended Diener and Larsen's (1984) findings using data from our own intensive studies of momentary mood in SMU students. As discussed in Chapter 3, in addition to rating their current mood, the students indicated whether or not they had interacted socially during the previous hour. Following the procedure of Diener and Larsen (1984), I computed separate mean Positive and Negative Affect scores for each student across (1) those occasions when they reported socializing versus (2) those when they reported no recent social activity. To ensure that the data reflected a reasonable sample of responding, these analyses were restricted to the 339 individuals who reported at least 10 observations of each type; the average number of observations per student were 24.5 (socializing) and 19.7 (alone). Finally, I calculated correlations among the mean Negative and Positive Affect scores across the socializing and nonsocializing occasions.

These correlations are reported in Table 5.6. Replicating the results of Diener and Larsen (1984), these data again establish that affective responding is highly consistent across dissimilar situations. In fact, the cross-situational correlations in these analyses (.83 for Negative Affect; .75 for Positive Affect) are even stronger than the corresponding values reported by Diener and Larsen. In other words, individuals who are more cheerful and enthusiastic when they are socializing also tend to be more cheerful and enthusiastic when they are alone. Note also that these results further demonstrate the relative independence of Positive and Negative Affect, in that the cross-scale correlations ranged from only .15 to .28.

These data obviously are more relevant to Positive Affect than to Negative Affect, in that interpersonal activity is more strongly and systematically associated with the former than with the latter. Accordingly, I repeated these analyses using a variable that is more consistently related to Negative Affect: perceived stress. Recall that the students in our momentary mood studies also rated their current level of stress on a 5-point

TABLE 5.6. Cross-Situational Consistency of Momentary Affect: I. Correlations between Mean Affect Ratings Made while Socializing versus Alone

Ratings	1	2	3
Negative Affect while			
1. Socializing	—		
2. Alone	.83	—	
Positive Affect while			
3. Socializing	.19	.23	—
4. Alone	.28	.15	.75

Note. N = 339. Mean number of ratings = 24.5 (socializing) and 19.7 (alone). Convergent correlations are shown in **boldface**. All correlations are significant at *p* < .01, two-tailed.

scale. I dichotomized each student's ratings into "low stress" (i.e., a rating of 1, 2, or 3) and "high stress" (i.e., a rating of 4 or 5) responses. For each student, I then computed separate mean Negative Affect and Positive Affect scores for the low-stress and high-stress conditions. As before, these analyses were restricted to the 218 individuals who produced at least 10 ratings of each type; the mean number of observations per person were 22.1 (low stress) and 21.1 (high stress). Finally, I computed correlations among the mean Negative and Positive Affect scores across the low stress and high stress conditions.

Table 5.7 displays the results, and they again demonstrate the exis-

TABLE 5.7. Cross-Situational Consistency of Momentary Affect: II. Correlations between Mean Affect Ratings Made during High-Stress versus Low-Stress Conditions

Ratings	1	2	3
Negative Affect during			
1. High stress	—		
2. Low stress	.65**	—	
Positive Affect during			
3. High stress	−.02	.13	—
4. Low stress	.10	.02	.67**

Note. N = 218. Mean number of ratings = 21.1 (high stress) and 22.1 (low stress). Convergent correlations are shown in **boldface**.
**p* < .01, two-tailed.

tence of a strong dispositional component in affective experience. As in the analyses of social activity, responding was highly consistent across contexts, with cross-situational correlations of .65 (Negative Affect) and .67 (Positive Affect). Thus, an individual's characteristic affect levels during episodes of stress can be predicted quite well from his or her typical responses in relaxed, baseline settings. Put another way, people who are more nervous and upset during times of stress also tend to be more nervous and upset in the absence of stress.

ASSOCIATION BETWEEN AFFECTIVITY AND JOB AND LIFE SATISFACTION

Another way to investigate the issue of cross-situational consistency is to examine people's affective responses to—and overall satisfaction with—the major roles of their lives. If there are broad and generalizable individual differences in affectivity, these differences should manifest themselves in myriad ways across diverse aspects of life. For instance, individuals who generally are happy and satisfied with their jobs also should tend to derive considerable enjoyment from their interpersonal relationships; conversely, individuals who tend to be dissatisfied and unhappy with their work also should report more conflict and strain in the interpersonal sphere. In other words, we would expect that some people simply tend to be more euthymic and satisfied than others, regardless of the general sphere (i.e., work vs. relationships) or the particular activity (i.e., a specific job or relationship) involved. Moreover, these individual differences in satisfaction should be systematically correlated with the general traits of Negative and Positive Affectivity.

These expectations are confirmed by a growing body of evidence. I first consider data related to job satisfaction, which itself has been shown to be trait-like in character. Schneider and Dachler (1978), for instance, found that various aspects of job satisfaction were moderately to strongly stable over a 16-month period. Staw and Ross (1985) also reported significant stability in job satisfaction over time spans of 3 to 5 years. Furthermore, they demonstrated that employee satisfaction was generalizable across situations—that is, consistent individual differences were observed even when workers changed employers and/or occupations (see also Blood, 1969; Staw, Bell, & Clausen, 1986). In other words, some individuals seem to be predisposed to enjoy their jobs more than others. In this context, it is noteworthy that Arvey, Bouchard, Segal, and Abraham (1989) found that approximately 30% of the variance in overall job satisfaction can be attributed to innate genetic factors.

In a related vein, Schmitt and his colleagues (Schmitt & Bedeian, 1982; Schmitt & Pulakos, 1985) have shown that job satisfaction is significantly correlated with general life satisfaction. Of course, these results can be interpreted in two fundamentally different ways. On the one hand, a bottom-up or situational explanation would argue that increased job satisfaction leads to greater life satisfaction; in other words, because work comprises a major portion of adult daily life, individuals who enjoy their jobs necessarily will report greater overall satisfaction with their lives. On the other hand, a top-down or dispositional explanation would argue that basic differences in affectivity and temperament predispose people to be differentially satisfied with various aspects of their lives, including their jobs (see Brief, Butcher, George, & Link, 1993; Diener, 1984).

Top-down and bottom-up models make opposite predictions regarding the relation between job satisfaction and later life satisfaction following retirement. On the one hand, the dispositional view argues that some individuals simply are predisposed to be more happy and satisfied, regardless of the particular situation or circumstances in which they find themselves. Consequently, this model would predict that the same individuals who most enjoyed their jobs would continue to report the greatest overall life satisfaction after retirement. In sharp contrast, the situational view posits that job satisfaction is a primary source of life satisfaction. Once this source of euthymia has been eliminated through retirement, the significant correlation between job and life satisfaction should vanish. One might even expect the correlation to become negative: In other words, the more people liked their jobs, the *less* happy and satisfied they might be following retirement.

Schmitt and Pulakos (1985) tested these competing hypotheses and reported evidence strongly supporting the dispositional view. That is, they found that greater job satisfaction predicted increased life satisfaction in retirement one year later. On the basis of these results, they concluded that "individuals may have a general, relatively stable predisposition towards satisfaction or dissatisfaction in a variety of situations" (p. 164; for similar views, see Blood, 1969; Schneider, 1976).

Other evidence links job satisfaction to general individual differences in affectivity. For example, Staw et al. (1986) examined the hypothesis that individual differences in emotionality would predict later job satisfaction. To test this notion, they constructed a 17-item Affective Disposition scale that was composed of both positive (e.g., "cheerful" and "satisfied with self") and negative (e.g., "hostile" and "irritable") mood terms; accordingly, it is best viewed as a complex mixture of Positive and Negative Affectivity. This scale—which was assessed in adolescence—was a significant predictor of job satisfaction nearly 50 years later, even after controlling for objective differences in work conditions. Similarly, Judge and Hulin (1993) found that general individual differences in happiness and subjective well-being were significantly related to job satisfaction.

In addition, several studies have demonstrated a more specific link between Negative Affectivity and job and life satisfaction (Brief, Butcher, & Roberson, 1995; Burke, Brief, & George, 1993; Chen & Spector, 1991). Brief, Burke, George, Robinson and Webster (1988), for instance, reported that a measure of Negative Affectivity correlated −.24 with job satisfaction, .32 with job-related stress, and −.46 with general life satisfaction. Moreover, Negative Affectivity scores were strongly correlated (r's in the .50 to .70 range) with various measures of depressive symptoms, job-related affect, and somatic complaints at work. Similarly, Levin and Stokes (1989) reported that Negative Affectivity correlated −.31 with an overall index of job satisfaction derived from the Job Diagnostic Survey (JDS; Hackman & Oldham, 1975), and −.29 with the Work Satisfaction subscale of the Job Descriptive Index (JDI; Smith, Kendall, & Hulin, 1969).

Although these studies clearly demonstrated that job satisfaction was significantly associated with Negative Affectivity, they failed to examine the role of Positive Affectivity. On the basis of some suggestive evidence reported by George (1989), however, my colleagues and I reasoned that job satisfaction would be significantly correlated with *both* of these general affective traits. Moreover, in light of the stability data discussed earlier, we predicted that trait affect would be significantly related to job satisfaction even when the two sets of measures were separated by a considerable time interval.

Slack and I designed a study to test these predictions (Watson & Slack, 1993). The participants were 79 full-time employees at SMU. The sample was quite diverse and reflected a broad range of work roles, including secretaries, library staff, clerical workers, maintenance staff, health center personnel, academic advisers, accountants, office managers, administrators, and faculty. The employees initially were assessed (Time 1) on trait measures of Negative and Positive Affectivity between 1984 and 1986. They again were assessed (Time 2) on measures of affectivity and job satisfaction between August 1987 and January 1988. The mean interval between the Time 1 and Time 2 assessments was 27 months (range = 9 to 39 months); virtually all the respondents (95.1%) had a time span of at least 21 months between their two sets of ratings.

At both assessments, Negative and Positive Affectivity were measured using the Negative Emotionality (Nem) and Positive Emotionality (Pem) scales, respectively, of the Multidimensional Personality Questionnaire (Tellegen, in press). In addition, two measures of job satisfaction were included in the Time 2 assessment. First, overall satisfaction was assessed using the 20-item short form of the Minnesota Satisfaction Questionnaire (MSQ; Weiss, Dawis, England, & Lofquist, 1967). Second, the respondents completed the JDI (Smith et al., 1969); the JDI assesses five aspects of satisfaction (Work, Pay, Promotion, Supervision, and Coworkers) that are only weakly to moderately intercorrelated (e.g., Schneider & Dachler, 1978; Smith et al., 1969).

Table 5.8 presents concurrent and time-lagged correlations between trait affectivity and job satisfaction. The most important finding is that Negative and Positive Affectivity both are significantly correlated with some facets of job satisfaction. Moreover, these significant associations generally were maintained across the study period. In fact, Nem and Pem showed similar relations with job satisfaction at the two assessments. For instance, Pem was significantly related to overall satisfaction on the MSQ both concurrently and prospectively. Similarly, both affectivity measures were moderately correlated with JDI Work Satisfaction at both assessments. In other words, Positive and Negative Affectivity both are significantly, moderately correlated with employee satisfaction, even when sat-

TABLE 5.8. Concurrent and Time-Lagged Correlations between Trait Affect and Job Satisfaction

	Correlations with	
Job Satisfaction Scale	Nem	Pem
Concurrent correlations		
JDI Work	−.40**	.38**
JDI Pay	−.27*	.22
JDI Promotion	−.10	.20
JDI Supervision	−.29**	.16
JDI Coworkers	−.22	.20
MSQ	−.19	.35**
Time–lagged correlations[a]		
JDI Work	−.36**	.44**
JDI Pay	−.20	.17
JDI Promotion	−.22*	.27*
JDI Supervision	−.21	.18
JDI Coworkers	−.30**	.08
MSQ	−.11	.30**

Note. $N = 79$. Nem, Negative Emotionality; Pem, Positive Emotionality; JDI, Job Descriptive Index; MSQ, Minnesota Satisfaction Questionnaire. Data from Watson and Slack (1993).
[a]Mean interval = 27 months.
*$p < .05$, two-tailed; **$p < .01$, two-tailed.

isfaction is assessed more than 2 years later. These findings strongly attest to both the temporal stability and predictive utility of trait affect scales.

It also is noteworthy that both emotionality scales were most strongly correlated with the JDI Work Satisfaction subscale, suggesting that general affective temperament is most highly predictive of the extent to which employees enjoy their various work-related activities. These data are consistent with other findings, suggesting that the "intrinsic" aspects of job satisfaction (e.g., the extent to which work is perceived as challenging and fulfilling) have a stronger dispositional component than do the "extrinsic" aspects (e.g., working conditions, supervision) (see Arvey et al., 1989).

Simple correlations between affectivity and job satisfaction may be confounded by objective differences in job quality; in other words, some individuals might be generally happier—and also like their jobs more—simply because their work tends to be more interesting and enjoyable (see Davis-Blake & Pfeffer, 1989; Gerhart, 1987). To examine this issue, Watson and Slack (1993) assessed various aspects of occupational quality (e.g., the cognitive complexity of the skills required on the job and the socioeconomic status of the occupational category). Not surprisingly, these objective measures of occupational quality accounted for a substantial amount of the variance in job satisfaction. Nevertheless, even after controlling for job quality, Time 1 affectivity still correlated significantly with the JDI Work and Coworkers subscales. Thus, these data clearly demonstrated that trait and environmental variables both play a crucial role in employee satisfaction (see also Locke, 1976; Staw & Ross, 1985).

Other investigators have subsequently replicated our basic finding that Positive and Negative Affectivity both are significantly correlated with job satisfaction (e.g., Iverson, Olekalns, & Erwin, 1998). Agho, Price and Mueller (1992), for instance, examined relations among Nem, Pem and a six-item job satisfaction scale in a sample of 550 employees of a Veterans Administration Medical Center. A confirmatory factor analysis identified three latent underlying dimensions that represented Job Satisfaction, Positive Affectivity, and Negative Affectivity, respectively. Subsequent analyses indicated that individual differences in Job Satisfaction correlated .44 with Positive Affectivity and –.26 with Negative Affectivity.

Taken together, these findings establish that some aspects of job satisfaction are moderately correlated with general individual differences in both Positive and Negative Affectivity. At a more fundamental level, these results indicate that individuals who are happy and satisfied with their jobs also tend to be happy and satisfied with other aspects of their lives. Consequently, these data further establish the cross-situational generality of affective experience.

ASSOCIATION BETWEEN AFFECTIVITY
AND MARITAL AND RELATIONSHIP SATISFACTION

As suggested earlier, if affective experience is consistent across different roles and contexts, then satisfaction in intimate relationships should be significantly correlated with more general differences in emotionality. Two related lines of research have established the existence of this predicted pattern. First, elevated levels of depression, maladjustment, and psychological symptomatology are significantly related to marital dissatisfaction and dissolution, both concurrently (Thompson, Sobolew-Shubin, Galbraith, Schwankovsky, & Cruzen, 1993; Weiss & Aved, 1978) and prospectively (Kurdek, 1991, 1993; Ulrich-Jakubowski, Russell, & O'Hara, 1988).

Second, trait measures of Negative Affectivity also are significantly associated with marital dissatisfaction and divorce (Eysenck, 1980; Eysenck & Wakefield, 1981; Karney, Bradbury, Fincham, & Sullivan, 1994; Lester, Haig, & Monello, 1989). The most striking evidence was reported by Kelly and Conley (1987), who studied 278 married couples from the mid-1930s through the early 1980s. The participants initially were assessed (Time 1) on measures of marital satisfaction and Negative Affectivity between 1936 and 1941; their marital satisfaction subsequently was retested in 1954–1955 (Time 2) and 1980–1981 (Time 3). The respondents who initially were high on Negative Affectivity were more likely to become divorced over the course of the study; moreover, this effect held for both early (i.e., between Times 1 and 2) and late (i.e., between Times 2 and 3) divorces. Furthermore, Time 1 Negative Affectivity was significantly correlated with current marital dissatisfaction among the husbands at Times 1 and 2, and among the wives at Times 2 and 3. Thus, Negative Affectivity scores showed significant predictive power even across time spans of more than 40 years.

Although these studies have established systematic links between Negative Affectivity and marital satisfaction, they did not include clear measures of Positive Affectivity. Accordingly, my colleagues and I decided to examine the correlates of both affective traits in two samples (Watson, Hubbard & Wiese, in press-a). The first sample consisted of 75 married couples from the St. Louis metropolitan area. The participants in this study had a mean age of 47.2 years, and had been married an average of 17 years. They all rated how they "generally" felt on the Negative and Positive Affect scales of the PANAS-X. In addition, they each rated their current level of marital satisfaction on four different measures: the Marital Adjustment Test (Locke & Wallace, 1959), the Quality Marriage Index (Norton, 1983), and scales assessing Conflict and Intimacy that were created by Jana Assenheimer and myself (Assenheimer & Watson, 1991). Scores on all these measures were strongly intercorrelated; we therefore standardized them and combined them into a single index of marital satisfaction.

The second sample consisted of 136 couples who currently were dating; at least one member of each couple was a student at the University of Iowa. On average, these couples had known each other approximately 3 years and had been dating for roughly 18 months. Again, both members of each couple rated how they "generally" felt on our Negative Affect and Positive Affect scales. In addition, each respondent also rated his or her current level of relationship satisfaction on our Intimacy and Conflict scales, as well as a modified version of the Dyadic Adjustment Scale (Spanier, 1976). Once again, these measures all were substantially interrelated; we therefore standardized them and combined them into an overall index of relationship satisfaction.

Table 5.9 presents the correlations between self-rated affectivity and relationship satisfaction in both of these samples; these data are reported separately for the men and women in each study. The most important finding is that relationship satisfaction is consistently correlated with both Positive and Negative Affectivity. Moreover, the overall magnitude of these associations is quite similar across the two traits; the coefficients with Positive Affectivity ranged from .24 to .47, whereas those for Negative Affectivity ranged from −.29 to −.50. Finally, it is noteworthy that significant, moderate correlations were obtained in both samples, attesting to the generality of these associations.

It could be argued, however, that these correlations are artifactually

TABLE 5.9. Correlations between Positive and Negative Affectivity and Measures of Relationship Satisfaction

Scale/sample	Man's satisfaction	Woman's satisfaction
Positive Affectivity		
Self-rated (married couples)	.47	.40
Self-rated (dating couples)	.40	.24
Spouse-rated (married couples)	.37	.44
Negative Affectivity		
Self-rated (married couples)	−.39	−.50
Self-rated (dating couples)	−.29	−.42
Spouse-rated (married couples)	−.35	−.40

Note. N = 74 (married couples) and 136 (dating couples). All correlations are significant at $p < .01$, two-tailed.

inflated because a single rater provided both the affectivity and the satisfaction data. One reason for this is that systematic response biases can artifactually raise correlations between variables that are collected from the same person. For example, as discussed in Chapter 1, some people may present a biased view of themselves based on the social desirability of the items they are rating; that is, they may overreport pleasant, socially acceptable characteristics and underreport socially undesirable qualities. In the current case, this might mean that some people would be highly motivated to (1) describe themselves as being high in Positive Affect and low in Negative Affect and (2) rate their marriages as happy and satisfying. If this bias were operating, it would tend to inflate the magnitude of observed correlations toward +1.00. Similarly, as discussed in Chapter 2, the acquiescence bias also can inflate observed correlations upward toward +1.00.

To control for the potential influence of these response biases, we also had the members of the married dyads rate their spouses' general level of affectivity on our Negative and Positive Affect scales. We then correlated these ratings with marital satisfaction. That is, we correlated the wife's ratings of her husband's affectivity with his ratings of marital satisfaction, and we correlated the husband's ratings of his wife's affectivity with her satisfaction scores. Thus, these correlations involve *two different raters*. These correlations (see Table 5.9) yielded results that are quite similar to those obtained using self-ratings. Most notably, spouse-rated Positive Affectivity (r's = .37 and .44) and Negative Affectivity (r's = −.35 and −.40) were moderately correlated with the marital satisfaction of both husbands and wives.

Thus, individuals who generally are upset and dissatisfied (i.e., high Negative Affectivity) also tend to have upsetting and unsatisfying relationships, whereas those who generally are cheerful and enthusiastic (i.e., high Positive Affectivity) tend to report more satisfying and fulfilling relationships. These data further establish the cross-situational generality of affective experience.

CONVERGENCE BETWEEN SELF- AND OTHER-RATINGS OF AFFECT

Thus far, I have demonstrated that emotionality scores are stable over time and consistent across situations and contexts. Note, however, that with some rare exceptions (e.g., objective evidence of divorce and correlations between spouse-rated affectivity and marital satisfaction), the data I have examined consist entirely of peoples' own self-reports. As discussed in Chapter 1, I believe that this focus is entirely appropriate in that self-report represents the most proximal and valid measure of affective experience. Nevertheless, in establishing the validity of a construct, it clearly is necessary to consider non–self-report data as well (Cronbach & Meehl, 1955; Loevinger, 1957). Accordingly, as another key step in establishing the existence of affective traits, I examine the convergence between self- versus other ratings of emotionality.

It is well established that affect self-ratings converge nicely with corresponding judgments made by others. Because subjective distress is a crucial component of many psychiatric disorders (American Psychiatric Association, 1994; Mineka, Watson, & Clark, 1998)—and because self-report affect scales are widely used in clinical settings—most of the relevant research has examined the agreement between self- and clinicians' ratings. Generally speaking, these data show a strong degree of convergence. For example, Clark and Watson (1991a) computed a weighted mean correlation of .72 across 16 studies that examined the relation between the self-rated BDI (Beck, Ward, Mendelson, Mock, & Erbaugh, 1961) and the clinician-generated Hamilton Rating Scale for Depression (HRSD; Hamilton, 1960). Similarly, in a review of anxiety measures, Clark and Watson (1991b) reported an average self-clinician correlation of .65 across eight studies that used reliable, psychometrically adequate clinical ratings.

These data are worth mentioning because they clearly establish the external validity of self-report measures of subjective distress. Furthermore, they demonstrate the clinical usefulness of these scales; that is, because self-ratings of depression and anxiety converge quite well with clinicians' judgments, the former can be used as a quick and easily obtainable complement to the latter. Nevertheless, most of the self-report scales studied in the clinical literature contain both affective and non-affective content, so that these data ultimately are of limited value for our purpose. For example, in addition to assessing depressed mood, the BDI examines many other depressive symptoms, including loss of energy and libido, sleep and appetite disturbance, and crying spells. Thus, these studies do not clearly establish the level of convergence that can be achieved using affect ratings per se.

Fortunately, a few studies have examined self-clinician convergence using pure mood scales. These correlations tend to be lower than those obtained using broader syndromal measures, but still are quite substantial. For instance, Clark and Watson (1991b) obtained mean convergent correlations of .69 and .57 for depressed and anxious affect, respectively, across three studies that used reliable clinical ratings.

Compared to this extensive clinical literature, relatively few studies have examined the convergent validity of affect scales using peers or spouses as raters. The paucity of research in this area probably reflects the internal, subjective nature of affective experience. Given the inherently subjective quality of affect ratings, most researchers apparently have assumed that it would be extremely difficult for peers to judge others with any degree of accuracy. This viewpoint is best summed up by Zuckerman and Lubin (1985), who stated, "While traits like sociability are almost entirely judged by public behavior alone, it is assumed that there is a private dimension to feelings that is only accessible through self-report data" (p. 12). This viewpoint is not unreasonable. Indeed, studies have consistently shown that highly observable personality traits (i.e., those with clearer and more frequent behavioral manifestations, such as extraversion) produce better interjudge agreement and higher self-peer correlations than do more internal, subjective traits (e.g., Funder & Colvin, 1988; Funder & Dobroth, 1987; Norman & Goldberg, 1966; Watson, 1989; Watson & Clark, 1991b).

Nevertheless, the few available studies have reported significant correlations between self- and peer-rated affect. Much of the relevant research has examined happiness or general well-being. For instance, Hartmann (1934) reported a .34 correlation between the happiness self-ratings of 195 students and average judgments made by four of their friends. Similarly, Andrews and Withey (1976)—using their single item Delighted–Terrible Scale—obtained a self-peer correlation of .33 in a sample of 222 adults. Finally, Kammann, Smith, Martin, and McQueen (1984) reported a self-peer correlation of .25 on the Affectometer 1 (a measure of general well-being) in a sample of 138 students.

In addition, a few studies have presented multitrait analyses of several different affects (Diener, Smith, & Fujita, 1995; Zuckerman & Lubin, 1985). McCrae and Costa have reported particularly interesting evidence of self–other convergence. McCrae (1982) obtained self- and spouse ratings (completed 6 months apart) from 281 adults on the Anxiety, Depression, Hostility, and Positive Emotions facet scales of the NEO Personality Inventory (NEO-PI; Costa & McCrae, 1985b). All these scales showed substantial self–spouse agreement, with convergent correlations ranging from .36 (Positive Emotions) to .58 (Anxiety). Moreover, a follow-up analysis conducted 6 years later indicated that the level of agreement did not decay over time (Costa & McCrae, 1988b).

The limited data in this area motivated my colleagues and me to conduct several multitrait studies of our own (e.g., Watson & Clark, 1991b, 1994b). I concentrate here on the best available evidence, which comes from our sample of 75 married couples (discussed previously in my examination of relationship satisfaction) who rated both themselves and their spouses on all 13 PANAS-X scales. Why do these data provide the best, most compelling evidence? Numerous studies have demonstrated that the reliability and convergent validity of peer judgments improves with increasing self–peer acquaintance (e.g., Funder & Colvin, 1988; Norman & Goldberg, 1966; Paulhus & Reynolds, 1995; Watson, 1989; Watson & Clark, 1991b). In other words, one obtains the best, most valid peer judgments when the judges know the people they are rating quite well. It is particularly important to use well-acquainted judges in studies of internal, subjective traits, which are especially difficult to rate (Watson & Clark, 1991b). Consequently, these couples—who had been married an average of 17 years—provide the best, most valid test of the convergent validity of affect ratings.

Table 5.10 presents convergent correlations between the self- and spouse ratings on each of the PANAS-X scales. Overall, these data clearly establish the convergent validity of these trait affect scales. The large majority of the correlations are in the .35 to .55 range, with a median value of .43; convergence is particularly impressive for Self-Assurance (.52), Fatigue (.52), Hostility (.50), Joviality (.49), Guilt (.49), and Sadness (.47). The one notable exception is Surprise, which produced a nonsignificant self–

TABLE 5.10. Correlations between Self- and Spouse Ratings on General, Trait Versions of the PANAS-X Scales

PANAS-X Scale	Correlation
General affect scales	
Negative Affect	.43**
Positive Affect	.38**
Basic negative affects	
Fear	.36**
Hostility	.50**
Guilt	.49**
Sadness	.47**
Basic positive affects	
Joviality	.49**
Self-Assurance	.52**
Attentiveness	.25**
Other affective states	
Shyness	.37**
Fatigue	.52**
Serenity	.37**
Surprise	.11

Note. N = 150.
**$p < .01$, two-tailed.

spouse correlation of only .11; this poor convergence supports my earlier assertion that this affect does not have a meaningful dispositional counterpart. For our purpose, however, the key point is that self-ratings on the PANAS-X scales generally showed a significant, moderate level of convergent validity when correlated with corresponding judgments made by spouses. Consequently, these data further establish the existence of meaningful affective traits (for a more complete discussion of these data, see Watson, Hubbard, & Wiese, in press-b).

INDIVIDUAL DIFFERENCES
IN CHARACTERISTIC VARIABILITY

Thus far, I have focused solely on individual differences in *mean-level experience*. For instance, I have demonstrated that some individuals report generally higher levels of positive mood than others, and that these differences are both stable over time and consistent across situations. Similarly, I have established the existence of stable, generalized individual differences in the tendency to experience negative mood. As discussed in Chapter 1, however, any comprehensive examination of affect-based dispositions also must consider individual differences in *characteristic variability*. By characteristic variability I mean that some individuals are consistently more labile, more variable than others.

Scientific interest in this topic is relatively recent and the phenomenon itself remains poorly understood. Nevertheless, it already is quite clear that trait-like individual differences in mood variability can be identified. Larsen (1987) obtained daily mood ratings from 62 college students over a 56-day period (a total of 3,472 observations); time series analyses of these data revealed "a stable pattern of change that repeats itself over time within a person" (p. 1202); in other words, the respondents displayed stable patterns of mood variability that persisted over the course of the study.

Penner, Shiffman, Paty, and Fritzsche (1994) explored three key dispositional properties of mood variability. Penner et al. (1994) collected more than 4,200 momentary mood assessments from a sample of 54 adults; at each assessment, the respondents rated themselves on 11 mood terms. First, to examine temporal stability, the authors correlated the respondents' variability across all odd-numbered days with the corresponding value computed over all even-numbered days. These odd–even stability coefficients were quite high, producing a mean correlation of .76 across the 11 mood terms. Next, Penner et al. (1994) investigated the issue of cross-situational generality by correlating the respondents' variability across two different activities, eating and working. These cross-situational coefficients also were strong, yielding an average correlation of .51. Finally, Penner et al. (1994) explored the issue of internal consistency by correlating variability scores across the individual mood terms. These interitem correlations also tended to be moderate to strong in magnitude, with an overall mean value of .41. Thus, Penner et al. (1994) demonstrated that individual differences in variability are stable over time, consistent across situations, and generalizable across different types of mood.

With regard to this last issue, it is especially noteworthy that variability was consistent across both positive and negative mood terms. In other words, those individuals who experienced greater variability in their positive mood also reported greater lability in their negative mood. Similarly, Emmons and King (1989) conducted two intensive within-subject studies of mood in college student samples. In both samples, Positive Affect was assessed using a four-item scale (e.g., "happy" and "joyful") and Negative Affect was measured with a five-item scale (e.g., "unhappy," "angry," and "anxious"). Overall variability scores were computed by calculating each respondent's standard deviation on each scale across all assessments. Analyses indicated that variability in Positive Affect was strongly positively correlated with variability in Negative Affect.

I have conducted additional analyses of mood variability based on our own studies of daily mood fluctuations in SMU students. These analyses were restricted to the 379 students who completed at least 42 daily ratings. Furthermore, for those students completing more than 42 ratings, only the first 42 were used. These restrictions enabled me to split each student's data into two equal halves, namely, Weeks 1 through 3 (i.e., observations 1–21) and Weeks 4 through 6 (i.e., observations 22–42). In separate analyses of each of these halves, I calculated each student's mean score and standard deviation on the general Positive Affect and Negative Affect scales. Finally, I computed correlations among these various means and standard deviations.

Table 5.11 shows the results. Several aspects of these data are noteworthy. First, consistent with data I presented earlier, mean levels on both affects were highly stable over time (r's = .82 and .86 for Negative Affect and Positive Affect, respectively). In addition, we again see that mean Negative Affect and Positive Affect levels are virtually independent of one another, with correlations ranging from only .03 to .08.

Next, replicating the results of Larsen (1987) and Penner et al. (1994), Table 5.11 shows that mood variability was strongly stable over time. Specifically, variability computed across Weeks 1–3 correlated .53 (Negative Affect) and .68 (Positive Affect) with variability computed over Weeks 4–6. Furthermore, consistent with the findings of Emmons and King (1989) and Penner et al. (1994), variability in Positive Affect was moderately cor-

TABLE 5.11. Correlations among Mean Level and Variability Scores for General Negative and Positive Affect

Variable	1	2	3	4	5	6	7
Mean level							
1. NA (Weeks 1–3)							
2. NA (Weeks 4–6)	.82**						
3. PA (Weeks 1–3)	.03	.06					
4. PA (Weeks 4–6)	.08	.07	.86**				
Variability							
5. NA (Weeks 1–3)	.67**	.45**	.00	.08			
6. NA (Weeks 4–6)	.51**	.66**	.00	.04	.53**		
7. PA (Weeks 1–3)	.16**	.11	−.05	.01	.43**	.29**	
8. PA (Weeks 4–6)	.10	.10	−.01	.08	.36**	.37**	.68**

Note. N = 379. NA, Negative Affect; PA, Positive Affect.
**$p < .01$, two-tailed.

related with variability in Negative Affect, with coefficients ranging from .29 to .43.

Finally, it is important to note that variability in Negative Affect is moderately to strongly correlated with mean-level scores on the same scale (r's ranged from .45 to .67). In other words, individuals who generally report high levels of negative mood also tend to show more variability on the dimension. This finding reflects the fact that virtually no one reports high levels of negative mood on a consistent basis, at least in nonpathological samples; in other words, it is extremely rare to find normal individuals who report feeling nervous (or angry or sad or guilty) most of the time. Consequently, high mean scorers also tend to be at least moderately variable: Sometimes they report elevated levels of negative mood (if they did not, then they could not be classified as a high scorer), but other times they do not. On the other hand, it is not uncommon for individuals to report consistently *low* levels of negative mood. Indeed, because negative mood levels generally are rather low (see Chapter 1), the only way that one can be classified as a low mean scorer is to report consistently low levels of Negative Affect. Accordingly, low mean scorers necessarily show little variability as well.

Thus, negative mood variability arises largely for mundane reasons. Note, moreover, that these strong correlations also demonstrate that negative mood variability is highly redundant with the mean-level score. Consequently, negative mood variability appears to yield little useful information beyond that already obtainable from existing trait and temperament measures, and probably is of little general interest.

In sharp contrast, variability in Positive Affect is virtually unrelated to mean-level scores on both scales; specifically, its correlations ranged from –.05 to .08 with mean-level Positive Affect, and from .10 to .16 with mean-level Negative Affect. These findings are consistent with preliminary evidence suggesting that the two basic dispositional parameters of the positive affective system—mean level and variability—vary independently of one another across individuals (Depue, Krauss, & Spoont, 1987).

Furthermore, it appears that this characteristic variability is an intrinsic feature of the positive affective system. As discussed earlier (see Chapters 1 and 4, this volume), positive mood is a component of the BFS (see also Depue & Iacono, 1989; Depue et al., 1987, 1994; Fowles, 1980, 1992, 1994). The essential function of the BFS is to ensure that the organism engages in approach and appetitive behaviors (e.g., eating, drinking, and social and sexual activity) that are necessary both for its own survival and for that of its species. In Chapter 4, I showed that the BFS in general—and positive moods specifically—are subject to preprogrammed, endogenous cycles. The purpose of these biological rhythms is to maximize the efficiency of these approach behaviors; that is, organisms are preprogrammed to be active and energetic when appetitive behaviors have a relatively high probability of success and to be sluggish and inactive when these behaviors are more likely to lead to failure and frustration.

Consequently, variability is a predesigned and innate feature of the BFS. This, in turn, suggests that over the course of evolution, control mechanisms have developed to regulate this variability and to ensure that it is maintained within reasonable bounds (Depue et al., 1987). If so, the characteristic variability of Positive Affect that we observe in Table 5.11 may reflect stable individual differences in the quality and functioning of these BFS control mechanisms.

In fact, the bipolar mood disorders (American Psychiatric Association, 1994) may arise from a pathological breakdown of these regulatory control mechanisms (Depue et al., 1987). Note that the bipolar disorders are marked by extraordinary variations in this positive affective system. On the one hand, manic episodes are characterized by heightened levels of energy, activity, interest, and alertness; a subjective mood state that tends to be elated, euphoric, and "elevated"; and enhanced feelings of confidence and optimism. On the other hand, depressive episodes are characterized by a sad, depressed, and "low" mood; marked reductions in interest, energy, and activity; poor concentration; and pervasive feelings of pessimism and ineffectuality. In light of these striking symptoms, it appears that the BFS regulatory mechanisms fail to function properly in affected individuals, thereby allowing this preprogrammed variation in the positive affective system to fluctuate wildly out of control.

CONCLUSION

In this chapter, I established the dispositional basis of affective experience by demonstrating that individual differences in Negative and Positive Affectivity are both stable over time and generalizable across different roles and contexts. In examining the latter issue, I showed that these affective traits are consistently, moderately associated with both (1) job satisfaction and (2) relationship satisfaction. I further established the validity of trait affect scales (with the exception of Surprise) by demonstrating that self-ratings on these scales converge moderately well with corresponding judgments made by well-acquainted peers, such as spouses. Finally, I established that people display trait-like differences in affective lability and argued that systematic variability in Positive Affect may have important theoretical and clinical implications, particularly with regard to the etiology of the bipolar disorders. In the following chapter, I build on this evidence by examining how individual differences in affectivity relate to more general dimensions of temperament, as well as to other types of personality traits.

6

TEMPERAMENT
AND PERSONALITY

In Chapter 5, I showed that people differ markedly in their characteristic levels of affect and, moreover, that these individual differences persist over time and generalize across different roles and contexts. What processes give rise to these marked individual differences in affective experience? The next two chapters seek to provide some basic, preliminary answers to this important question. In this chapter, I examine trait affect in relation to general dispositions of personality. As we will see, these data have fascinating implications for our understanding of personality. Chapter 7 then explores more basic issues—including the possible genetic and biological origins of these observed individual differences—and offers a general model of happiness and well-being.

THE STRUCTURE OF PERSONALITY

In exploring the association between affect and the basic traits of personality, we immediately are confronted with a formidable problem, namely: *Which traits* should be examined? This question may seem forbidding to many readers, considering the bewildering array of potential candidates. After all, personality psychologists have created hundreds—even thousands—of trait scales, with many new measures still being developed each year. Moreover, researchers in this area have created dozens of highly sophisticated omnibus inventories—some measuring 8 attributes, others 11, and still others 16 or 30—each of which purports to assess the most important traits of personality. These contradictory claims clearly must be viewed with considerable skepticism.

Fortunately, in recent years personality researchers have made tremendous strides toward developing a comprehensive structural model; thus it is now possible to offer some general assertions regarding the basic phenotypic traits of personality. Taxonomic interest has focused in particular on the widely influential five-factor model, or "Big Five." This line of research originated in Allport and Odbert's (1936) effort to compile an exhaustive list of trait-related terms in the English language (for historical reviews, see Block, 1995; Digman, 1990; Goldberg, 1993; John, 1990). Allport and Odbert (1936) eventually settled on a list of 4,504 terms that clearly described traits of personality (e.g., "aggressive," "introverted," and "sociable"). Cattell (1945, 1946) reduced this set to 35 bipolar scales through content sortings and cluster analyses. Cattell initially identified 12 to 15 factors in peer ratings of these scales. However, subsequent investigators consistently found that five robust factors—Neuroticism (vs. Emotional Stability), Extraversion (or Surgency), Conscientiousness (or Dependability), Agreeableness, and Openness (or Imagination, Intellect, or Culture)—were sufficient to represent the structure of these traits (Borgatta, 1964; Fiske, 1949; Norman, 1963; Tupes & Christal, 1992).

This five-factor model originally was identified in analyses of peer ratings. The robustness of the structure repeatedly has been demonstrated in diverse populations and under a wide range of conditions. For example, highly similar factors have emerged in ratings of both adults and children, and regardless of the degree or type of acquaintance between judge and target (e.g., Digman & Inouye, 1986; Fiske, 1949; Norman, 1963, 1969; Norman & Goldberg, 1966; Tupes & Christal, 1992). More recently, these same five factors have been observed in various types of self-report data, including several omnibus trait inventories (e.g., Costa & McCrae, 1988a, 1992; McCrae & Costa, 1985, 1987). Finally, closely parallel structures have been identified in other languages, establishing the cross-cultural replicability of the model (e.g., John, Goldberg, & Angleitner, 1984; McCrae & Costa, 1997). On the basis of these converging findings, McCrae and Costa (1986, 1987, 1997) have argued that the five-factor model provides a basic taxonomic structure for personality research.

Nevertheless, the five-factor model has been criticized on various grounds (see Block, 1995; Eysenck, 1992; McAdams, 1992; Tellegen, 1993). One recurrent criticism has come from researchers who favor more differentiated models of personality and who argue, therefore, that five factors are incapable of capturing the richness and complexity of human personality (see Block, 1995; Briggs, 1989). At first glance, this criticism may appear to be quite compelling. Its force is diminished, however, when one recognizes that personality traits are ordered hierarchically at different levels of breadth or abstraction (see Goldberg, 1993; Hampson, John, & Goldberg, 1986; John, 1990; Watson, Clark, & Harkness, 1994). Superfactors such as the Big Five traits are at the highest level of this hierarchy and, as such, represent the broadest, most general dimensions of individual differences. Note, however, that each of these higher-order dispositions can be decomposed into several distinct lower-order traits. For instance, the higher-order factor of Extraversion can be subdivided into more specific traits such as Dominance (i.e., extraverts tend to be forceful and assertive), Gregariousness (i.e., extraverts seek the company of others), and Exhibitionism (i.e., extraverts enjoy being the center of attention) (Watson & Clark, 1997a). In other words, the five-factor model is entirely compatible with more differentiated, multidimensional views, and it is fully capable of capturing the rich complexity of human personality.

The five-factor model also has been extensively criticized by researchers favoring some type of "Big Three" scheme (see especially Eysenck, 1992). These Big Three models grew out of the seminal work of Hans Eysenck. Starting in the late 1940s, Eysenck conducted an extensive series of analyses that identified two broad factors: Neuroticism and Extraversion (e.g., Eysenck & Eysenck, 1968). However, subsequent analyses led to the identification of a third broad trait dimension, which Eysenck called Psychoticism (Eysenck & Eysenck, 1975); despite this label, however, it is better characterized as a dimension of disinhibition (i.e., undercontrolled, "acting out" behavior) versus constraint (i.e., overcontrolled behavior) (see Digman, 1990; Watson & Clark, 1993). Several similar three-factor models have been proposed in recent years, including those of Tellegen (1985), Gough (1987), and Cloninger (1987).

Proponents of the Big Three have objected primarily to the relatively atheoretical nature of the five-factor model (Eysenck, 1992; Tellegen, 1993). Researchers working within the Big Five tradition have focused on articulating a comprehensive phenotypic description of personality without grappling with the issue of why these particular traits should have emerged. Put another way, they have focused on the *what* of personality rather than the *why*. In sharp contrast, Big Three theorists have labored long and hard to link their superfactors to basic biological and genetic processes (e.g., Cloninger, 1987; Eysenck, 1967; Fowles, 1992, 1994; Tellegen, 1985), a point to which I return in Chapter 7. Because of this biological grounding, many personality theorists find these Big Three models to be more compelling than the Big Five.

I entirely agree that these Big Three schemes provide a more compelling *genotypic* model of personality. In fact, Clark and I recently developed our own version of the Big Three (see Watson & Clark, 1993). For our present purposes, however, the comprehensive phenotypic description afforded by the five-factor model will be quite sufficient. Indeed, it is important to note that in a purely descriptive sense, the Big Five simply represent a slightly expanded version of the Big Three. Note that both models share a common "Big Two": Neuroticism and Extraversion. Moreover, the third Big Three dimension— Disinhibition (or Psychoticism) versus Constraint—is a complex combination of Conscientiousness and Agreeableness (Digman, 1990; John, 1990; Watson & Clark, 1992b; Watson et al., 1994). In other words, one essentially can transform the Big Three into the Big Five by (1) decomposing the third dimension into Conscientiousness and Agreeableness and (2) including the additional dimension of Openness. Thus, descriptive results based on one taxonomic scheme easily can be converted into the other.

GENERAL RELATIONS BETWEEN AFFECT AND PERSONALITY

In examining relations between affect and the Big Five, I make extensive use of six large student samples. Data from Samples 1 through 4 previously were reported in Watson and Clark (1992b); findings from Samples 5 and 6 are presented here for the first time. The respondents were undergraduates enrolled in various psychology courses at SMU (all samples) or the University of Texas at Dallas (Sample 2). They all completed a trait affect questionnaire in which they rated the extent to which they "generally" felt each of the mood terms. The students in Samples 1 and 2 were assessed only on our general Positive Affect and Negative Affect scales, whereas those in Samples 3 through 6 completed the full, 60-item PANAS-X. Several different measures were used to assess the Big Five traits, including the NEO-PI (Costa & McCrae, 1985b), the Revised NEO Personality Inventory (NEO-PI-R; Costa & McCrae, 1992), the NEO Five Factor Inventory (NEO-FFI; Costa & McCrae, 1992), and adaptations of scales originally developed by Goldberg (Watson & Clark, 1992b).

Before examining specific relations, it is instructive to consider the overall degree of overlap between these two domains. Consequently, I first conducted a series of analyses to determine the extent to which trait affect is predictable from the Big Five. Two separate multiple regression analyses were performed in each sample. In these analyses, the general Negative Affect and Positive Affect scales served as criteria and scores on the Big Five traits—entered simultaneously as a single block—were the predictors.

Table 6.1 reports the final multiple correlation (R) for each affect scale in each sample, as well as an overall weighted mean R computed across all six data sets. These data clearly establish that trait Negative Affect and Positive Affect scores both are *strongly* related to these higher-order traits of personality. Specifically, the overall mean R for Negative Affect was .62, indicating that approximately 38% of the variance in this scale was predictable from the Big Five traits. Similarly, the mean R for Positive Affect was .66, indicating that roughly 44% of the variance in positive affective experience is recoverable from the five-factor model. These findings establish that these general personality traits are strongly related to affect and have profound implications for our understanding of affective experience.

The second series of analyses examined these same relations from the opposite perspective, investigating the extent to which the Big Five traits are predictable from measures of affectivity. To explore this issue, I conducted five separate regression analyses in Samples 3 through 6. In these analyses, the Big Five scores were the criteria and the 11 specific PANAS-X scales (Fear, Hostility, Joviality, etc.)—entered simultaneously as a single block—served as predictors.

Paralleling the earlier analyses, Table 6.2 reports the final multiple R for each personality trait in each sample, as well as an overall weighted mean R calculated across all four data sets. The most striking finding is that four of the Big Five are strongly related to affectivity. An inspection of the mean R indicates that more than half the variance in Neuroticism (56%) and Extraversion (55%) is predictable from the affectivity scales; in

TABLE 6.1. Predicting Scores on the General Negative and Positive Affect Scales of the PANAS-X from Measures of the Five-Factor Model

	Criterion	
Sample	Negative Affect	Positive Affect
Final multiple R		
1	.57	.68
2	.66	.72
3	.57	.57
4	.67	.73
5	.64	.68
6	.62	.57
Weighted mean	.62	.66

Note. N = 532 (Sample 1), 236 (Sample 2), 225 (Sample 3), 325 (Sample 4), 500 (Sample 5), and 325 (Sample 6). All values are significant at $p <$ .01, two-tailed.

TABLE 6.2. Predicting Scores on Measures of the Five-Factor Model from the 11 Lower-Order PANAS-X Scales

Sample	N	E	O	A	C
			Criterion		
Final multiple *R*					
3	.67	.66	.34	.53	.54
4	.81	.84	.30	.69	.72
5	.77	.75	.29	.63	.66
6	.72	.66	.29	.59	.61
Weighted mean	.75	.74	.30	.62	.64

Note. N = 225 (Sample 3), 325 (Sample 4), 500 (Sample 5), and 325 (Sample 6). N, Neuroticism; E, Extraversion; O, Openness; A, Agreeableness; C, Conscientiousness. All values are significant at $p < .01$, two-tailed.

addition, approximately 40% of the variance in Conscientiousness (41%) and Agreeableness (38%) is recoverable from these scales. Only Openness is modestly related to trait affect: Its mean R of .30 indicates that only about 9% of its variance is predictable from the PANAS-X.

These data are important for two reasons. First, on a purely pragmatic level, they demonstrate that scores on Big Five measures—including the NEO-PI and NEO-PI-R—are highly predictable from a simple, brief affect questionnaire. Put another way, much of the interesting variance in the five-factor model is recoverable from simple ratings of affectivity. This finding suggests, in turn, that affect questionnaires may offer a useful complement to more traditional personality inventories.

More fundamentally, these findings challenge traditional views of personality that have minimized the importance of affective processes. Note that these data demonstrate that four of the Big Five traits *are strongly affective in character.* In the case of Neuroticism and Extraversion, this is no longer new or surprising. The essentially affective nature of Neuroticism has been recognized for some time, and it is now quite clear that affect-related processes lie at the very core of the trait (e.g., Allik & Realo, 1997; McCrae & Costa, 1987; Watson & Clark, 1984; Watson et al., 1994). Similarly, although traditional models of Extraversion focused primarily on the interpersonal aspects of the trait, more recent views have strongly emphasized the centrally defining role of affect (e.g., Tellegen, 1985; Watson & Clark, 1992b, 1997a).

In contrast, the affective nature of Agreeableness and Conscientiousness generally has been unrecognized in the literature. For instance, Costa and McCrae (1992) state that Agreeableness "is primarily a dimension of interpersonal tendencies. The agreeable person is fundamentally altruistic. He or she is sympathetic to others and eager to help them, and believes that others will be equally helpful in return. By contrast, the disagreeable or antagonistic person is egocentric, skeptical of others' intentions, and competitive rather than cooperative" (p. 15). In discussing Conscientiousness, Watson et al. (1994) argue that the dimension "is centered around the basic issue of impulse control. Conscientious individuals are less swayed by the immediate sensations of the moment and are controlled more strongly by the broader, longer term implications of their behavior. . . . Conversely, low scorers are oriented primarily toward the feelings and sensations of the immediate moment and are relatively unaffected by more remote or abstract considerations" (p. 27). I am not suggesting that these general characterizations are wrong; my point, rather, is that these statements would not lead one to predict that roughly 40% of the variance in these traits is predictable from the PANAS-X. We clearly need to reexamine the basic meaning of these traits so as to capture their affective quality more satisfactorily.

NEUROTICISM AND EXTRAVERSION

Relations with General Negative and Positive Affect

I turn now to an examination of specific relations between individual trait and affect scales. Following from the pioneering work of Costa and McCrae (1980a, 1984) and Tellegen (1982, 1985), most of the research in this area has focused on Neuroticism and Extraversion and their relation to general Negative and Positive Affect. The findings have been highly robust, and they have been quite striking. Simply put, measures of Negative Affect are strongly correlated with Neuroticism but are more weakly related to Extraversion whereas Positive Affect scores are substantially correlated with Extraversion but not Neuroticism (Costa & McCrae, 1980a, 1984; Emmons & Diener, 1985, 1986; Tellegen, 1982, 1985; Watson & Clark, 1984). The clarity and replicability of this striking differential pattern led Tellegen (1985) to argue that Neuroticism and Extraversion should be relabeled "Negative Emotionality" and "Positive Emotionality," respectively (see also Watson & Clark, 1984, 1997a; Watson et al., 1994). In Tellegen's view, Neuroticism and Extraversion represent basic dimensions of temperament that reflect individual differences in the propensity to experience negative and positive mood states, respectively. I return to this issue subsequently.

These initial studies used state affect measures that asked respondents to rate how they had felt during the recent past (e.g., "during the past few weeks"). Because of this, the correlations were only moderate in magnitude, generally falling in the .20 to .50 range. More recent studies have used trait affect measures, however, and have demonstrated an even stronger level of convergence between personality and affectivity. For instance, Meyer and Shack (1989) reported that Neuroticism correlated .63 with trait Negative Affect but only −.17 with trait Positive Affect; conversely, Extraversion had correlations of .66 and −.22 with trait Positive and Negative Affect, respectively.

To date, my colleagues and I have amassed the most extensive evidence relevant to this issue. Table 6.3 reports correlations between Neuroticism and Extraversion and the general Negative and Positive Affect scales in each of the six samples; also shown are weighted mean correlations averaged across all six data sets. We consistently have obtained the same striking differential pattern. As expected, Negative Affectivity is strongly associated with Neuroticism, generating a mean correlation of .58 across the six samples; this value indicates that Neuroticism and Negative Affectivity scores share roughly 34% of their variance. In contrast, trait Negative Affect scores are much more weakly related to Extraversion, showing an average coefficient of only −.22 (5% shared variance). Conversely, Positive Affectivity is much more strongly related to Extraversion; the mean correlation of .54 indicates that these measures share approximately 29% of their variance. Finally, as expected, Positive Affect is more modestly correlated with Neuroticism, yielding an average correlation of −.32 (approximately 10% shared variance). Thus, we again see a clear and strong affinity between Neuroticism and Negative Affect on the one hand and between Extraversion and Positive Affect on the other.

TABLE 6.3. Correlations between General Negative and Positive Affect and Measures of Neuroticism and Extraversion

	Negative Affect		Positive Affect	
Sample	Neuroticism	Extraversion	Neuroticism	Extraversion
1	.52**	−.21**	−.25**	.62**
2	.64**	−.23**	−.24**	.64**
3	.56**	−.13	−.30**	.48**
4	.65**	−.21**	−.35**	.54**
5	.57**	−.30**	−.36**	.54**
6	.59**	−.20**	−.41**	.40**
Weighted mean	.58	−.22	−.32	.54

Note. N = 532 (Sample 1), 236 (Sample 2), 225 (Sample 3), 325 (Sample 4), 500 (Sample 5), and 325 (Sample 6). Correlations of |.30| or greater are shown in **boldface**.
**p < .01, two-tailed.

Consistent with previous research (e.g., Costa & McCrae, 1992; Digman, 1997; Meyer & Shack, 1989), Extraversion and Neuroticism were moderately negatively correlated in these data sets, with coefficients ranging from −.20 to −.36. I therefore computed partial correlations between (1) Negative Affect and Extraversion, controlling for the influence of Neuroticism; and (2) Positive Affect and Neuroticism, eliminating the influence of Extraversion. As before, I calculated these correlations separately in each sample and then computed weighted mean values across all six data sets. The average partial correlations were only −.09 and −.22, respectively, indicating modest levels of association. Consequently, we can conclude that individual differences in negative affective experience are strongly correlated with Neuroticism but are essentially unrelated to Extraversion; conversely, individual differences in positive affective experience are strongly correlated with Extraversion but only weakly related to Neuroticism.

The results reported in Table 6.3 all are based on a classic between-subjects design in which the affect and personality scores were collected in a single session. Our extensive studies of daily mood in SMU students provide another—and rather different—way of examining these affect–personality relations. The students who participated in these studies rated their mood once a day over a period of several weeks. At each assessment, they rated the extent to which they had experienced each mood term that day; all the assessments were completed in the evening, so that the ratings would provide a reasonable estimate of the students' mood over the course of the entire day. General Negative and Positive Affect scores were available from 379 students, each of whom completed a minimum of 30 daily assessments; overall, these students completed a total of 16,514 daily mood ratings (mean = 43.6 per person). These ratings were averaged to yield overall mean Negative Affect and Positive Affect scores for each student across the entire rating period.

The students also were assessed on two measures of Neuroticism and Extraversion. First, they completed the Neuroticism and Extraversion scales of the NEO-FFI (Costa & McCrae, 1992). Second, they were assessed on the Negative Temperament and Positive Temperament scales of the General Temperament Survey (GTS; Clark & Watson, 1990). The GTS consists of three factor-analytically derived scales (the third scale measures disinhibition vs. constraint) that were designed to assess the higher-order traits of the Big Three model. Previous research has shown that Negative Temperament and Positive Temperament are very strongly correlated with Neuroticism and Extraversion, respectively (Watson & Clark, 1992b; Watson et al., 1992, 1994). Similarly, in the current sample Negative Temperament correlated .73 with NEO-FFI Neuroticism, whereas Positive Temperament correlated .64 with NEO-FFI Extraversion. Accordingly, I created overall indexes of Neuroticism and Extraversion for each student by standardizing the scales and then averaging the two markers of each trait.

Table 6.4 reports correlations among Neuroticism, Extraversion, and mean daily Negative and Positive Affect. The convergent correlations are somewhat lower, but these results otherwise closely replicate those shown in Table 6.3. As expected, mean daily Negative Affect correlated moderately with Neuroticism but was entirely unrelated to Extraversion. Conversely, average daily Positive Affect was moderately correlated with Extraversion but was more weakly related to Neuroticism.

Relations with Specific Types of Affect

Thus far, I have established strong connections between Neuroticism and the general Negative Affect dimension and between Extraversion and general Positive Affect. It is important to ask, however, whether these relations remain consistent at the specific affect level. Note that Tellegen's (1985) temperamental reformulation of Neuroticism and Extraversion leads to the prediction that these traits are broadly related to the negative and positive affects, respectively. Is this view correct? For instance, do all of the basic negative affects (fear, guilt, sadness, hostility) correlate comparably with Neuroticism? Similarly, is Extraversion comparably related to all types of positive mood?

To address these issues, Table 6.5 presents weighted mean correlations—averaged across Samples 3 through 6—between Neuroticism and Extraversion and the 11 specific affect scales of the PANAS-X. The table displays both simple, zero-order correlations and partial correlations that control for the influence of the other trait (i.e., the influence of Extra-

TABLE 6.4. Correlations between Neuroticism and Extraversion and Average Daily Mood Scores on the General Negative Affect and Positive Affect Scales

Score	1	2	3	4
Personality trait scores				
1. Neuroticism	—			
2. Extraversion	–.32**	—		
Mean daily mood scores				
3. Mean Negative Affect	.43**	–.07	—	
4. Mean Positive Affect	–.18**	.36**	.09	—

Note. N = 379.
**p* < .01, two-tailed.

TABLE 6.5. Mean Zero-Order and Partial Correlations (Controlling for the Influence of the Other Trait) between Neuroticism and Extraversion and Specific Types of Affect

Affect scale	Simple correlations		Partial correlations	
	Neuroticism	Extraversion	Neuroticism	Extraversion
Basic negative affects				
Fear	.52	−.18	**.49**	−.04
Guilt	.57	−.25	**.54**	−.10
Sadness	.59	−.36	**.54**	−.24
Hostility	.41	−.22	**.36**	−.12
Basic positive affects				
Joviality	−.33	**.64**	−.19	**.59**
Self-Assurance	−.43	**.45**	−.36	**.37**
Attentiveness	−.28	.25	−.23	.19
Other affective states				
Shyness	.36	−.46	.27	−.40
Fatigue	.33	−.22	.28	−.14
Surprise	.04	.18	.09	.20
Serenity	−.46	.13	−.44	−.01

Note. These are weighted mean correlations averaged across Samples 3 through 6. The analyses are based on a combined *N* of 1,375. Correlations of | .30 | or greater are shown in **boldface.**

version is removed from the correlations with Neuroticism, and the influence of Neuroticism is eliminated from the correlations with Extraversion).

These data clearly establish that Neuroticism is broadly related to negative affective experience. Neuroticism is moderately to strongly correlated with all four basic negative affects, with simple *r*'s ranging from .41 to .59. Moreover, the partial correlations demonstrate that these associations persist after the influence of Extraversion has been removed. The only evidence of specificity is that Neuroticism correlates less strongly with Hostility than it does with Sadness, Guilt, and Fear; its relations with these other three negative affects are essentially identical. I return to this association between Neuroticism and Hostility when I consider the affective correlates of the remaining Big Five traits. For present purposes, however, the key point is that Neuroticism is substantially related to all four negative affects.

Beyond this basic finding, Neuroticism is more moderately related to several other PANAS-X scales, including Serenity, Fatigue, and Shyness. As was discussed in Chapter 2, these scales all tend to be moderately positively (Fatigue, Shyness) or negatively (Serenity) correlated with the basic negative affects and, therefore, also reflect the influence of the general Negative Affect dimension. Accordingly, these correlations are most parsimoniously viewed as further evidence of the broad and nonspecific relation between Neuroticism and Negative Affect. In contrast, the moderate negative correlation with Self-Assurance is unexpected and indicates that Neuroticism is associated with lowered levels of self-confidence and daring.

Putting these findings together, we can conclude that Neuroticism is associated with pervasive feelings of distress and dissatisfaction. Individuals high in neuroticism report elevated levels of nervousness, fear, guilt, shame, dissatisfaction, self-loathing, sadness, loneliness, anger, irritability, fatigue and timidity, and lowered levels of relaxation and confidence. These results demonstrate the profoundly affective nature of Neuroticism, and they are entirely consistent with Tellegen's (1985) reformulation of this trait as reflecting general individual differences in the propensity to experience negative mood states (see also Allik & Realo, 1997; Watson & Clark, 1984).

The data for Extraversion are more ambiguous; depending on one's viewpoint, these findings could be construed as demonstrating either extremely specific or broadly general relations with the positive affects. On the one hand, Extraversion's correlations with the three basic positive affects differ dramatically in magnitude. That is, Extraversion is very strongly correlated with Joviality (simple $r = .64$, partial $r = .59$), moderately correlated with Self-Assurance (simple $r = .45$, partial $r = .37$), and only modestly correlated with Attentiveness (simple $r = .25$, partial $r = .19$). These results clearly establish at least some degree of specificity in these relations.

On the other hand, this evidence for specificity must be balanced against two other considerations that argue for at least a certain amount of generality in these relations. First, despite these widely varying levels of association, it nevertheless remains true that Extraversion is significantly related to all three basic positive affects. Note, moreover, that its correlations with both Joviality and Self-Assurance are relatively strong, and that only its association with Attentiveness is weaker than might be expected. Viewed in this light, it is reasonable to conclude that Extraversion is broadly related to individual differences in positive affective experience.

Second, it is noteworthy—and probably is not coincidental—that Extraversion is most strongly correlated with Joviality. Our analyses of the PANAS-X scales consistently reveal that Joviality is more highly saturated with variance from the general Positive Affect dimension than are either Self-Assurance or Attentiveness (e.g., Watson & Clark, 1994b). This finding makes perfect sense, as the descriptors comprising this scale (e.g., "happy," "cheerful," "enthusiastic," and "lively") seem much more centrally related to the experience of positive mood than do those comprising either Self-Assurance (e.g., "bold" and "proud") or Attentiveness (e.g., "alert" and "determined"). Furthermore, Joviality is the longest (eight items) and broadest of the lower-order PANAS-X scales and, as such, comes the closest to representing a general—rather than a specific—construct. Viewed in this context, the data in Table 6.5 indicate that Extraversion is broadly related to those mood terms that lie at the very core of the general Positive Affect dimension. This, in turn, suggests that Tellegen's (1985) reinterpretation of Extraversion as Positive Emotionality is not inappropriate.

In addition, Extraversion is moderately negatively correlated with both Shyness and Sadness. The former finding is hardly surprising, as it indicates that introverts report being more bashful and shy than extraverts. The latter finding also is not unexpected and reflects the fact that among the negative affects, Sadness has the strongest inverse relation with Joviality and the other positive affects (see Chapter 2).

Once again, we can assess the robustness of these relations by considering parallel data derived from our intensive studies of daily mood. Ratings on the complete, 60-item PANAS-X were available from 256 of the 379 students who were described earlier. As before, each student completed a minimum of 30 daily mood assessments; overall, they completed a total of 11, 281 daily mood ratings (mean = 44.1 per person). These ratings were averaged to yield overall mean scores on the 11 specific PANAS-X scales for each student across the entire rating period.

Table 6.6 presents simple and partial correlations (controlling for the influence of the other personality trait) between Neuroticism and Extraversion and these average daily affect scores. Not unexpectedly, the convergent correlations are somewhat lower in these analyses, but these data otherwise replicate the pattern seen in Table 6.5. Neuroticism again correlates substantially (and quite similarly) with Fear, Guilt, and Sadness and more moderately with Hostility and Shyness; we also see a modest negative correlation with Serenity. It is noteworthy, moreover, that once the effects of Extraversion are eliminated, Neuroticism is entirely unrelated to average daily levels of positive mood.

Conversely, Extraversion again is moderately to strongly correlated with the various positive affects and is entirely unrelated to average daily negative mood once the effects of Neuroticism are removed. Note, moreover, that Extraversion again is more strongly related to Joviality (simple $r = .48$, partial $r = .45$) than it is to either Self-Assurance or Attentiveness (r's range between .24 and .32). Thus, these data are quite consistent with my earlier conclusion that Extraversion is broadly associated with individual differences in positive affective experience.

TABLE 6.6. Mean Zero-Order and Partial Correlations (Controlling for the Influence of the Other Trait) between Neuroticism and Extraversion and Average Daily Mood Scores on the 11 Lower-Order PANAS-X Scales

Affect scale	Simple correlations		Partial correlations	
	Neuroticism	Extraversion	Neuroticism	Extraversion
Basic negative affects				
Fear	.38**	−.02	.39**	.12
Guilt	.42**	−.08	.42**	.07
Sadness	.41**	−.15*	.39**	−.01
Hostility	.30**	−.12	.27**	−.02
Basic positive affects				
Joviality	−.18**	.48**	−.02	.45**
Self-Assurance	−.15*	.28**	−.06	.24**
Attentiveness	−.12	.32**	−.02	.30**
Other affective states				
Shyness	.34**	−.17**	.30**	−.06
Fatigue	.17**	−.08	.15*	−.02
Surprise	.14*	.10	.19**	.15*
Serenity	−.25**	.16*	−.22**	.08

Note. N = 256. Correlations of |.30| or greater are shown in **boldface**.
*p < .05, two-tailed; **p < .01, two-tailed.

The Temperamental Basis of Neuroticism and Extraversion

Why are Neuroticism and Extraversion so strongly related to Negative and Positive Affect, respectively? Two general models have been proposed to explain these striking associations; perhaps not surprisingly, one model emphasizes the importance of environmental factors, whereas the other argues for the salience of endogenous biological processes (see Larsen & Ketelaar, 1991; McCrae & Costa, 1991). First, the environmentally oriented *instrumental view* argues that personality traits such as Neuroticism and Extraversion give rise to actions and circumstances that have important affective consequences and, therefore, generate marked individual differences in emotionality. For instance, we saw in Chapter 3 that social interaction is associated with marked elevations in Positive Affect. If extraverts socialize more extensively than introverts, this could explain the observed associations between this trait and Positive Affectivity. More generally, the instrumental view would argue that extraverts experience greater Positive Affect *simply because they engage in more pleasurable activities.* Many readers will recognize that this instrumental view represents another example of a bottom-up theory of well-being (see Chapter 5).

Instrumental relations of this sort surely are at least partly responsible for the strong associations between affect and personality. For instance, my colleagues and I have collected data demonstrating that extraverts do engage in more frequent and extensive socializing than do introverts (Watson, 1988a; Watson et al., 1992). Watson et al. (1992) reported two studies relevant to this issue. In Study 1, 85 students rated the number of times they engaged in each of 15 different social activities (e.g., dating, having a discussion, and going out for a drink or meal) over the course of the previous week; these ratings were collected once a week over a period of 13 weeks (a total of 1,037 assessments). The ratings were summed across activities and weeks to produce an overall social activity score for each student; this overall index of socializing correlated .35 with Extraversion. In Study 2, 127 students rated the amount of time they spent in each of 21 different social activities over the course of that day; these ratings were completed on a daily basis over a period of several weeks (a total of 5,424 observations). As before, the ratings were summed across days and activities to yield an overall socializing index for each student; in this analysis, overall social activity correlated .28 with Extraversion.

The data regarding Neuroticism are more sparse, but the available evidence again suggests that the instrumental view has merit. For instance, Headey and Wearing (1989) conducted a four-wave panel study over a period of 6 years. Neuroticism and Extraversion scores were obtained in the first wave (1981). In the subsequent waves (collected in 1983, 1985 and 1987), respondents indicated whether or not they had experienced various life events during the 2-year interval since the last assessment. These events later were subdivided into those that were relatively subjective and open to interpretation (e.g., "made lots of new friends") and those that were highly objective (e.g., "got married" and "child died"). It is noteworthy that Extraversion scores predicted the subsequent occurrence of favorable life events at all three later assessments but were entirely unrelated to the frequency of unfavorable events; conversely, Neuroticism predicted the subsequent occurrence of adverse life events but was unrelated to the frequency of favorable events. Moreover, the results remained largely unchanged when the subjective life events were dropped from the analyses. Finally, consistent with other research (e.g., Stone, 1981; Warr, Barter, & Brownbridge, 1983; Zautra & Reich, 1983), the occurrence of adverse events was moderately correlated with Negative Affect but was unrelated to Positive Affect; conversely, the frequency of favorable events was more strongly associated with Positive Affect than with Negative Affect.

Simply put, the data of Headey and Wearing (1989) show that (1) good things tend to happen to extraverts, and (2) these good things tend to make people feel better (i.e., they experience higher levels of Positive Affect); conversely, (3) bad things are more likely to happen to those high in Neuroticism, and (4) these bad things tend to make people feel worse (i.e., they experience higher levels of Negative Affect). These data are entirely consistent with an instrumental view. Moreover, Ormel and Wohlfarth (1991) subsequently replicated these Neuroticism–life events findings in a similar three-wave study. It is especially noteworthy that life events were demonstrated to be partly responsible for the observed association between Neuroticism and Negative Affect.

Before proceeding further, I should comment on an aspect of these data that may be puzzling to some readers. It seems perfectly reasonable that good things tend to happen to extraverts; that is, that extraverts are actively responsible for generating favorable events (such as pleasurable social activities) that give rise to elevated levels of Positive Affect. But why are bad things more likely to happen to those high in Neuroticism? The reason this may be puzzling is that stress and trauma often are viewed as external, environmentally based events that befall unfortunate souls who simply happen to be in the wrong place at the wrong time. This commonsense model implies that the occurrence of stress is entirely unrelated to the personality characteristics of the affected individual. This model seems quite appropriate for certain types of stressful and traumatic events (e.g., rape and natural disaster), but it is highly implausible when applied to others (e.g., divorce and being fired from a job). This is because maladaptive personality characteristics (e.g., being demanding, hostile, hypercritical, and morose or unpleasant) undoubtedly influence the likelihood that certain types of stressful life events—such as being divorced or fired—will occur. Viewed in this context, it is quite understandable that those high in Neuroticism may actively generate stressful events and adverse life circumstances that are at least partly responsible for their elevated levels of negative mood.

The data I have reviewed demonstrate that—consistent with the instrumental view—Neuroticism and Extraversion each are associated with significant affect-producing life circumstances. Nevertheless, the available evidence also indicates that the instrumental view is incapable of completely explaining the observed relations between affect and personality. One problem is that the instrumental view itself leads to further, troublesome questions. For example, even if one assumes that extraverts report greater Positive Affect simply because they socialize more, this inevitably leads to a further, unresolved question: Why exactly do they socialize more?

A more fundamental problem for the instrumental view, however, is that these substantial affect–personality relations persist even after controlling for the effects of activity or life circumstances. For instance, Ormel and Wohlfarth (1991) demonstrated that Neuroticism had a strong, direct relation with Negative Affect that was entirely independent of adverse life circumstances. Similarly, Watson et al. (1992) computed partial correlations between Extraversion and Positive Affect that controlled for individual differences in social activity. These partial correlations remained substantial and highly significant (.43 and .39 in Studies 1 and 2, respectively). In other words, extraverts reported higher levels of Positive Affect even after the effects of social activity had been eliminated. Clearly, life circumstances alone are insufficient to account for the observed links between Neuroticism and Negative Affect, and between Extraversion and Positive Affect.

Consequently, the biologically based *temperamental view* has found increasing support among researchers in recent years (e.g., Larsen & Ketelaar, 1991; McCrae & Costa, 1991; Tellegen, 1985; Watson & Clark, 1992b). According to this view, Neuroticism and Extraversion represent basic dimensions of affective temperament. Put another way, affectivity is an intrinsic aspect of these traits, so that individual differences in affect and personality ultimately reflect the same common, underlying processes. That is, extraverts are naturally endowed with a more lively, cheerful, and enthusiastic temperament than are introverts, so that individual differences in Positive Affectivity are an innate component of this trait. Conversely, individuals high in Neuroticism are naturally predisposed to experience higher levels of subjective distress and dissatisfaction.

In the following chapter, I examine the possible genotypic origins of these two general temperaments. For now, I concentrate instead on their phenotypic manifestations. In particular, I want to focus on two key points that have emerged from recent research into the nature of Extraversion and Neuroticism. First, this emerging temperamental view establishes that individual differences in Negative and Positive Affectivity must form an important component in the phenotypic descriptions of these traits. As noted earlier, the essentially affective nature of Neuroticism has been recognized for quite some time (e.g., McCrae & Costa, 1987; Watson & Clark, 1984), so these data simply have clarified the precise nature of the affective component (i.e., Neuroticism is strongly linked to Negative Affect but not to Positive Affect). In contrast, most traditional models of Extraversion focused almost exclusively on the highly salient interpersonal aspects of the trait and discussed its affective component much more cursorily (see Watson & Clark, 1997a, for an historical review). Consequently, recent data have led to a major reconceptualization of this trait; contemporary views now explicitly recognize that it also is strongly affective in character (see Costa & McCrae, 1992; John, 1990; Tellegen, 1985; Watson & Clark, 1992b, 1997a).

I must emphasize, however, that a temperamental reconceptualization of Neuroticism and Extraversion does *not* mean that these traits simply can be reduced to individual differences in Negative and Positive Affect. Both of these general traits are, in fact, associated with a wide range of cognitive, attitudinal, and behavioral characteristics that are systematically related to, but certainly not reducible to, trait affectivity (e.g., Costa & McCrae, 1985b, 1992; McCrae & Costa, 1987; Tellegen, 1985; Watson & Clark, 1984, 1997a; Watson et al., 1994). In this regard, it may be useful to consider briefly the nature and range of the attributes that are subsumed under the broad concepts of Neuroticism and Extraversion. With this in mind, Table 6.7 presents a proposed set of component traits (adapted from Watson et al., 1994, Table 3) for each dimension.

Taken together, these primary traits yield intriguing psychological portraits of the sorts of individuals who are prone to experience negative and positive mood states. Note that in the case of Neuroticism, several of the component traits simply represent individual differences in various types of Negative Affectivity. Beyond this, however, high scorers on this trait also report suffering from a wide variety of problems (including minor somatic problems such as headaches, dizziness, and nausea) and generally blame themselves for these problems; thus, they generally feel inadequate and inferior to others. Interestingly, although they are highly self-critical, they also tend to be overly sensitive to perceived criticism from others, so that they easily feel slighted. Those high in Neuroticism report elevated levels of life stress and indicate that they cope poorly with this stress, causing pronounced emotional lability. As we already have seen, these elevated stress appraisals are veridical to some degree, apparently because these individuals actively create problems for themselves (Headey & Wearing, 1989; Ormel & Wohlfarth, 1991). In addition, however, these individuals are prone to negativistic appraisals of their environment and, therefore, tend to see threats, crises, and problems where others do not.

Putting these characteristics together, we have a group of individuals who experience the world as threatening and problematic and who perceive themselves as entirely inadequate to meet this challenge; not surprisingly, they also report pervasive feelings of subjective distress and dissatisfaction. In contrast, low scorers on this dimension generally are self-satisfied and view the world as essentially benign; they report few problems, low levels of negative mood, and little ongoing stress.

Markedly different attributes are associated with individual differences in positive affective experience. Generally speaking, the Extraversion dimension involves a willingness to engage and confront the environment, including the social environment (see also Watson & Clark, 1997a). At the high end of the trait, extraverts actively approach life with

TABLE 6.7. The Component Traits Comprising the General Dispositions of Neuroticism and Extraversion

Primary trait	Description of a high trait scorer
	Neuroticism (Negative Emotionality)
Anxiety	Prone to fear, tension, worry, nervousness, and apprehension
Depression	Experiences high levels of sadness, loneliness, and hopelessness
Anger	Prone to episodes of anger, irritability and frustration
Guilt/Self-blame	Frequently experiences guilt; blames self for mistakes and failures
Self-consciousness	Prone to embarrassment and shame and feelings of inferiority
Oversensitivity	Sensitive to criticism and ridicule; feels slighted easily
Self-criticism	Dissatisfied with self; sees self as having many undesirable qualities
Stress overreactivity	Copes poorly with stress; easily upset by even small disturbances
Emotional lability	Experiences sudden, marked mood swings
Negativistic appraisal	Tends to view events as threatening and problematic
Somatic complaints	Frequently experiences troublesome somatic symptoms
	Extraversion (Positive Emotionality)
Gregariousness	Seeks out and enjoys the company of others
Dominance	A leader; forceful, assertive and persuasive in social situations
Exhibitionism	Enjoys being the center of attention in social situations
Energy	Feels lively and energetic; leads a full, fast-paced, and active life
Positive Affectivity	Is cheerful, enthusiastic, and confident
Excitement seeking	Seeks out interesting, intense, and vivid experiences

Note. Adapted from Watson, Clark, and Harkness (1994, Table 3). Copyright 1994 by the American Psychological Association. Adapted by permission.

energy, enthusiasm, cheerfulness, and confidence. They seek out and enjoy the company of others and are confident and comfortable in their social interactions. They also seek out exciting and intense experiences, and they do not shrink from the social limelight. At the low end of the dimension, introverts lack this same level of confidence, energy, and enthusiasm. They tend to be reserved and socially aloof and to avoid intense experiences.

   Both of these temperaments encompass a very wide range of psychological characteristics. The range seems especially great for Extraversion, which includes interpersonal, experience seeking, and purely affective components. What common factor do these diverse personality attributes share that leads them to be related at a higher-order level? In other words, what causes individual differences in Anxiety, Anger, Self-Criticism, Negativistic Appraisal, and so on, to be positively correlated with one another, thereby creating a more general disposition of Neuroticism? In a related way, why do gregarious individuals also tend to be dominant, exhibitionistic, energetic, and enthusiastic, thereby forming the higher-order trait of Extraversion?

This brings me to the second key point that has emerged from the recent literature. Similar to the model originally proposed by Tellegen (1982, 1985), Clark and I have argued that individual differences in Negative and Positive Affectivity, respectively, comprise the central cores of these traits; that is, they represent the unifying "glue" that forms these higher-order dispositions and maintains them as integrated wholes (Watson & Clark, 1984, 1992b, 1997a). Accordingly, I believe that Tellegen's (1985) proposed alternatives of "Negative Emotionality" and "Positive Emotionality" are entirely appropriate labels for these traits and have included them in Table 6.7. I should add that we view the affective core of Extraversion as comprising both the Positive Affectivity and Energy components (see Watson & Clark, 1997a). Note that each of these traits reflects content that is contained in the general Positive Affect and Joviality scales of the PANAS-X.

The reconceptualization of Neuroticism as "Negative Emotionality" is no longer controversial: It now is generally acknowledged that individual differences in Negative Affectivity lie at the very heart of the trait (Watson & Clark, 1984, 1992b). Costa and McCrae (1992), for instance, state that "the general tendency to experience negative affects such as fear, sadness, embarrassment, anger, guilt, and disgust is the core of the N[euroticism] domain" (p. 14). More generally, McCrae and Costa (1987) conclude that "virtually all theorists would concur in the centrality of negative affect to neuroticism . . . " (p. 87). Because of this, the terms "Neuroticism," "Negative Emotionality," and "Negative Affectivity" now are used more or less interchangeably in the personality literature.

However, recasting Extraversion as Positive Emotionality clearly constitutes a more radical reformulation of the construct. As I discussed previously, traditional models of this trait emphasized the centrality of its interpersonal component (see Watson & Clark, 1997a). What evidence suggests that positive affective experience actually comprises the central core of the dimension?

First, we already have seen that individual differences in (1) general Positive Affect and (2) Joviality are strongly correlated with Extraversion. Furthermore, *all* the component traits of Extraversion are significantly related to these affect scales. For instance, Watson and Clark (1992b) found that all six NEO-PI Extraversion facet scales were significantly correlated with both general Positive Affect (mean $r = .31$) and Joviality (mean $r = .37$). I reconducted these analyses on the six NEO-PI-R Extraversion facets in the current Sample 6 and obtained similar results, with mean correlations of .28 and .34, respectively. The consistency of these relations is especially impressive when one considers that these facet scales themselves are only moderately intercorrelated; in fact, the mean correlation among the NEO-PI and NEO-PI-R facet scales tends to fall in the .30-to-.35 range (Botwin & Foley, 1988; Costa & McCrae, 1992; Watson & Clark, 1992b). In other words, the various components of Extraversion correlate as highly with Positive Affect and Joviality as they do with one another.

In exploring the core of Extraversion, it is particularly instructive to examine correlations among the interpersonal and affective components of the trait. Consistent with Table 6.7, all the major conceptualizations of Extraversion have included two basic interpersonal traits: Gregariousness (i.e., seeking out and enjoying the company of others) and Dominance (i.e., being forceful, assertive and persuasive in social settings). Not coincidentally, these two traits also represent the two major dimensions that consistently emerge in analyses of interpersonal behavior (e.g., LaForge & Suczek, 1955; Wiggins, 1979, 1982; Wiggins & Trapnell, 1997).

Watson and Clark report two analyses examining relations among these interpersonal traits and various measures of Positive Affectivity (1997, Tables 1 and 2). In the first analysis, 234 psychiatric patients completed single measures of Gregariousness, Dominance, and Positive Affectivity. Consistent with previous research in this area (e.g., Hogan, 1983; Wiggins, 1979), Dominance and Gregariousness were significantly but only weakly related to one another ($r = .17$). Both traits, however, were more strongly correlated with Positive Affectivity (for Dominance, $r = .36$; for Gregariousness, $r = .37$). Furthermore, after the underlying influence of Positive Affectivity had been eliminated using partial correlation, the association between Dominance and Gregariousness vanished entirely. In other words, the modest correlation between Gregariousness and Dominance—the two basic interpersonal traits of Extraversion—resulted from the underlying influence of Positive Affectivity; once this influence had been eliminated, the two traits no longer were related at all. This finding supports my argument that positive affective experience constitutes the unifying "glue" that holds the higher-order trait together.

The second analysis was conducted on 254 undergraduates; the design was quite similar to the first except that the students were assessed on three different measures of positive affective experience (in terms of the classification scheme used in Table 6.7, two were measures of Positive Affectivity per se, whereas the third assessed Energy). Replicating the results of the first analysis, Dominance and Gregariousness correlated only

.16 with one another. Again, however, they both were more strongly and consistently correlated with the Positive Affectivity scales, with mean correlations of .42 and .21, respectively. Finally, as in the first analysis, when the influence of Positive Affectivity was eliminated, the association between Gregariousness and Dominance disappeared. Thus, we again see clear evidence that Positive Affectivity is the common element that binds Dominance and Gregariousness together.

CONSCIENTIOUSNESS, AGREEABLENESS, AND OPENNESS

Simple and Partial Correlations with Affect

As I noted earlier, researchers in this area have focused primarily on Neuroticism and Extraversion; in comparison to this large and burgeoning literature, remarkably few studies have investigated the affective correlates of the other Big Five traits. Carp (1985) conducted the first study assessing affect in relation to the complete five-factor model. Carp examined data from two samples of elderly adults who were adjusting to life in a public housing facility. Respondents completed an eight-item happiness scale and also were rated on the Big Five by several staff members. Measures of happiness and contentment are affectively complex—that is, they tend to be mixtures of high Positive Affect and low Negative Affect (Watson, 1988b; Watson & Clark, 1997b; Watson & Tellegen, 1985). Because of this, one would expect Extraversion to be positively correlated—and Neuroticism to be negatively correlated—with rated happiness, and this is, in fact, what Carp found. In addition, Agreeableness was positively correlated with happiness in both samples; indeed, its correlations were comparable in magnitude to those obtained for Extraversion and Neuroticism. Conscientiousness and Openness, however, generally were unrelated to affect in these data.

McCrae and Costa (1991) obtained self-ratings on Negative and Positive Affect as well as self- and spouse-rated scores on each of the Big Five traits. It is noteworthy that the self- and spouse ratings generally yielded similar findings. As expected, Neuroticism and Extraversion were substantially correlated with Negative Affect and Positive Affect, respectively. In addition, Conscientiousness and Agreeableness showed a similar pattern to each other: Both had low positive correlations with Positive Affect (range = .10 to .15 in the self-report data) and generally comparable negative correlations with Negative Affect (range = −.11 to −.24). Finally, Openness again displayed weak positive correlations with both types of affect (range = .08 to .14 in the self-report data). Thus, McCrae and Costa obtained at least some evidence linking all of the Big Five traits to rated affect. However, the correlations with Conscientiousness, Agreeableness, and Openness all tended to be rather low.

Although these studies are interesting and suggestive, they are limited in two basic ways. First, they included only global, nonspecific measures of emotionality (i.e., global happiness; general Negative and Positive Affect), and so were unable to examine relations between the Big Five and specific types of affect. As we will see shortly, global assessments of affect mask the existence of strong and potentially important relations at the lower-order level. Second, the five-factor markers that were used in these studies were not completely independent. I already have discussed the fact that Neuroticism and Extraversion scores tend to be moderately negatively correlated. More generally, measures of the Big Five tend to have low to moderate correlations with one another (e.g., Botwin & Foley, 1988; Costa & McCrae, 1992; Digman, 1997; Norman, 1963). This means that scores on Conscientiousness, Agreeableness, and Openness all are significantly correlated with Neuroticism and/or Extraversion. Consequently, the fact that these other three traits correlate significantly with affect does not necessarily demonstrate that they have significant *independent* relations with emotionality that would persist if the influence of Neuroticism and Extraversion were removed. Put another way, the possibility remains that these other traits provide no useful incremental information beyond that already obtainable from Neuroticism and Extraversion.

Of these earlier studies, only McCrae and Costa (1991) examined this issue of incremental validity. They found that Agreeableness and Conscientiousness both contributed significantly to the prediction of global well-being (as with rated happiness, such measures typically are a combination of high Positive Affect and low Negative Affect), even after controlling for Neuroticism, Extraversion, and Openness. However, Negative and Positive Affect were not examined separately in these analyses; accordingly, it is not clear which traits added significantly to the prediction of Negative Affect and which contributed to the prediction of Positive Affect.

My colleagues and I have collected extensive data to address these unresolved issues. Table 6.8 reports weighted mean correlations between Conscientiousness, Agreeableness, and Openness and all 13 PANAS-X scales; as with the earlier data for Neuroticism and Extraversion, correlations with the general Negative Affect and Positive Affect scales are averaged across Samples 1 through 6, whereas those for the specific scales are computed over Samples 3 through 6. For each affect–personality scale pair, the table displays both simple, zero-order correlations and partial correlations that control for the influence of Neuroticism and Extraversion. These partial correlations demonstrate the predictive/ explanatory power of the remaining Big Five traits over and beyond that attributable to the "Big Two" of Neuroticism and Extraversion.

I previously showed that four of the Big Five were strongly predictable from the PANAS-X scales; the sole exception was Openness, which was only modestly related to affect (see Table 6.2). On the basis of these earlier data, one would predict that Conscientiousness and Agreeableness each would have strong affective correlates but that Openness would not. The data presented in Table 6.8 strongly confirm this prediction. Note that Openness has only one simple correlation above | .20 |, and no partial correlation greater than | .15 |. In light of these unimpressive results, the most parsimonious conclusion is that individual differences in Openness are unrelated to affective experience.

TABLE 6.8. Mean Zero-Order and Partial Correlations (Controlling for Neuroticism and Extraversion) between Measures of Conscientiousness, Agreeableness, and Openness and the PANAS-X Scales

Scale	Conscientiousness		Agreeableness		Openness	
	Simple	Partial	Simple	Partial	Simple	Partial
General affect scales						
Negative Affect	−.21	−.06	−.25	−.17	−.12	−.09
Positive Affect	**.40**	**.35**	.18	.07	.24	.09
Basic negative affects						
Fear	−.13	.02	−.12	−.04	−.08	−.08
Guilt	−.29	−.15	−.22	−.14	−.06	−.05
Sadness	−.17	.02	−.19	−.06	−.02	.06
Hostility	−.21	−.10	**−.48**	**−.44**	−.14	−.13
Basic positive affects						
Joviality	.21	.12	.29	.15	.11	−.07
Self-Assurance	.21	.08	−.10	**−.32**	.10	.01
Attentiveness	**.59**	**.54**	.17	.09	.09	.04
Other affective states						
Shyness	−.08	.06	−.04	.13	−.17	−.07
Fatigue	−.21	−.12	−.20	−.13	−.11	−.09
Surprise	.02	.02	.05	.02	.00	−.06
Serenity	.07	−.08	.15	.09	.06	.06

Note. These are weighted mean correlations; those for the general affect scales are averaged across Samples 1 through 6 (overall N = 2,143); those for the specific affect scales are averaged across Samples 3 through 6 (overall N = 1,375). Correlations of | .30 | or greater are shown in **boldface.**

The findings for Conscientiousness and Agreeableness, however, are strikingly different. Table 6.8 indicates that Conscientiousness is moderately correlated (mean $r = .40$) with general Positive Affect. It is noteworthy, moreover, that this association persists even after eliminating the influence of Extraversion and Neuroticism (partial $r = .35$). In other words, Conscientiousness demonstrates a unique and independent association with Positive Affect that cannot be attributed to the hidden influence of the Big Two.

However, it is somewhat misleading to speak of a relation between Conscientiousness and Positive Affect: This statement is overly broad and ignores important evidence from the lower-order scales. An inspection of these scales indicates that Conscientiousness is strongly correlated with Attentiveness ($r = .59$), a relation that remains substantial even after controlling for the influence of the Big Two. Indeed, Attentiveness is much more strongly related to Conscientiousness than it is to Extraversion. In contrast, Conscientiousness is only weakly related to Joviality and Self-Assurance ($r = .21$ for each); moreover, these associations essentially vanish when the influence of Extraversion and Neuroticism is removed. The specificity of these lower-order relations is astonishing: Conscientiousness has a partial correlation of .54 with Attentiveness, but no other partial correlation exceeds |.15|. Thus, rather than concluding that Conscientiousness is associated with Positive Affect, we can state with far greater precision that this trait has a specific affinity with Attentiveness: Highly conscientious individuals report elevated levels of determination, concentration and alertness (Attentiveness).

Agreeableness shows a somewhat similar pattern. This trait has relatively modest correlations with the general affect scales, but displays more substantial associations at the lower-order level. Most notably, Agreeableness is associated with substantially lower levels of Hostility (mean $r = -.48$), a relation that is maintained after controlling for the influence of the Big Two (partial $r = -.44$). Again, the specificity of this relation is quite striking: Although Agreeableness is strongly negatively correlated with Hostility, it is essentially unrelated to the other negative affects. The only other finding of note is that Agreeableness yielded a moderate negative partial correlation ($-.32$) with Self-Assurance. This finding must be viewed with some caution, however, because the simple correlation between these scales was only $-.10$. That is, this significant association emerged only after the influence of Neuroticism and Extraversion was removed.

Once again, we can assess the robustness of these relations by examining parallel data from our intensive studies of daily mood. As noted earlier, ratings on the general Negative and Positive Affect scales were available from 379 students who completed a minimum of 30 daily mood assessments; data on the lower-order scales were obtained from a subset of 256 students who completed the full, 60-item PANAS-X. These ratings were averaged to yield overall mean scores on the various PANAS-X scales for each student across the entire rating period. Table 6.9 presents simple and partial correlations (again controlling for both Neuroticism and Extraversion) between these average daily scores and Conscientiousness, Agreeableness, and Openness.

These results clearly replicate those shown in Table 6.8. Once again, Openness was not strongly related to any of the PANAS-X scales; this trait simply is unrelated to affective experience. As expected, Conscientiousness was moderately correlated with Attentiveness (simple $r = .36$, partial $r = .29$) but only weakly related to the other positive affects. Finally, Agreeableness again showed a moderate inverse association with

TABLE 6.9. Zero-Order and Partial Correlations (Controlling for Neuroticism and Extraversion) between Conscientiousness, Agreeableness, and Openness and Average Daily Mood Scores on the PANAS-X Scales

	Conscientiousness		Agreeableness		Openness	
Scale	Simple	Partial	Simple	Partial	Simple	Partial
General affect scales						
Negative Affect	−.19**	−.12*	−.28**	−.17**	.03	.02
Positive Affect	.21**	.13*	.05	−.06	.07	.01
Basic negative affects						
Fear	−.17**	−.14*	−.17**	−.10	.07	.03
Guilt	−.23**	−.19**	−.21**	−.12	.04	.01
Sadness	−.19**	−.11	−.20**	−.09	.01	.00
Hostility	−.21**	−.16*	**−.35****	−.29**	−.04	−.06
Basic positive affects						
Joviality	.19**	.06	.16**	−.01	.02	−.07
Self-Assurance	.23**	.15*	−.04	−.17**	.07	.04
Attentiveness	**.36****	.29**	.17**	.07	.11	.06
Other affective states						
Shyness	−.23**	−.16*	−.17**	−.06	−.11	−.13*
Fatigue	−.21**	−.19**	−.17**	−.12	−.02	−.03
Surprise	−.06	−.07	−.15*	−.16*	−.03	−.07
Serenity	.12	.05	.12	.02	−.08	−.09

Note. For the general Negative Affect and Positive Affect scales, $N = 379$. For the specific affect scales, $N = 256$. Correlations of |.30| or greater are shown in **boldface**.
*$p < .05$, two-tailed; **$p < .01$, two-tailed.

Hostility (simple $r = -.35$, partial $r = -.29$) but was unrelated to the other negative affects.

Allik and Realo (1997) recently demonstrated the cross-cultural replicability of these effects in a non–Indo-European language (Estonian). Consistent with the results I have reported, Allik and Realo found that Neuroticism and Extraversion were strongly and broadly associated with individual differences in negative and positive emotional experience, respectively. As expected, Agreeableness and Conscientiousness instead displayed specific, lower-order associations with affect. Replicating the data reported in Tables 6.8 and 6.9, Agreeableness showed a moderate negative correlation with Hostility but was weakly related to other types of negative affect, whereas Conscientiousness was strongly related to Pertinacity (which was defined by terms such as "determined" and "tenacity"; it therefore appears to be similar to the PANAS-X Attentiveness scale) but was unrelated to other types of positive emotional experience. Finally, consistent with our data, Openness was weakly related to affect.

Instrumental versus Temperamental Views of These Lower-Order Relations

Why are Conscientiousness and Agreeableness so strongly related to affect? McCrae and Costa (1991) have argued for an instrumental interpretation of these relations. That is, individual differences in these traits are assumed to create differential situations and life experiences that, in turn, have powerful affective consequences. Thus, McCrae and Costa argue that "the interpersonal bonds that A[greeableness] fosters and the achievements and accomplishments that C[onscientiousness] promotes may contribute to greater quality of life and higher life satisfaction" (p. 228). As discussed earlier, these authors did, in fact, find that high levels of Conscientiousness and Agreeableness were associated with increased Positive Affect and decreased Negative Affect; furthermore, high scorers on these traits reported greater overall well-being and a higher level of life satisfaction. Consistent with their instrumental view, McCrae and Costa (1991) interpreted these significant associations as demonstrating that "loving and hardworking people have more positive experiences and fewer negative experiences *because these traits foster social and achievement-related successes*" (p. 231, emphasis added).

It certainly seems plausible that higher levels of Agreeableness and Conscientiousness should promote the types of interpersonal and achievement-related experiences that lead, in turn, to greater life satisfaction. Nevertheless, there is a problem with McCrae and Costa's (1991) interpretation: It is based exclusively on results viewed at the nonspecific, higher-order level. That is, their data indicated simply that conscientious and agreeable individuals reported greater Positive Affect, well-being, and life satisfaction—and less Negative Affect—than those low on these traits. From this limited perspective, an instrumental model provides the most compelling interpretation of the data.

The situation changes markedly, however, when we examine affect at the lower-order level. Conscientiousness really has only one significant lower-order correlate: It is strongly correlated with Attentiveness and is essentially unrelated to all of the other specific affects. Consequently, the real finding to be explained is that conscientious individuals report higher levels of determination, concentration, and alertness. Are these affective tendencies merely the *result* of real-world accomplishments and achievement-related successes? Perhaps, but it is much more plausible to argue that they are an important *cause* of such outcomes. In other words, it seems likely that individuals who are alert and determined ultimately will accomplish more than those who are not. More fundamentally, the patterning of these lower-order relations suggests that these affective tendencies should be viewed as an intrinsic feature of the Conscientiousness dimension. That is, an important part of what it means to be "conscientious" is to be driven, determined, and attentive to detail (see also Watson & Clark, 1992b). Viewed in this way, Conscientiousness begins to display some of the essential properties of a temperament.

Similarly, our data indicate that the affective correlates of Agreeableness are quite narrow. Among the basic negative affects, Agreeableness is substantially correlated only with Hostility: Not surprisingly, agreeable individuals experience lower levels of anger, irritability, and scorn than do those who are more antagonistic. Among the basic positive affects, Agreeableness only showed a moderate negative correlation with Self-Assurance, indicating that agreeable individuals report *lower* levels of confidence and daring. As with Conscientiousness, one must wonder whether McCrae and Costa's (1991) model really offers a plausible interpretation of these findings. Are disagreeable, antagonistic individuals more hostile simply because they have had more negative life experiences? Perhaps this is so, but it also seems likely that they have had more negative life experiences precisely because they are disagreeable and antagonistic. Rather than arguing over which variable causes the other, however, it makes more sense to conclude that Agreeableness and Hostility reflect the same underlying dispositional construct. Put another way, it is difficult to imagine antagonistic and disagreeable individuals who are not at least somewhat angry and hostile. Thus, individual differences in hostility form an intrinsic component of the Agreeableness dimension. As in the case of Conscientiousness, Agreeableness now seems to show some of the essential characteristics of a temperament.

McCrae and Costa's (1991) interpretation made perfect sense *given the limited data that were available to them.* Perhaps the most important conclusion that can be drawn from these results is that restricting assessment to the nonspecific, higher-order level may lead to inaccurate or mislead-ing interpretations of the data. Clearly, it is important to assess affect at both the higher-order and lower-order levels.

Neuroticism, Agreeableness, and Hostility

Hostility is unique among the specific affects in that it is substantially re-lated to two different Big Five traits (Neuroticism and Agreeableness). This pattern reflects the dualistic nature of the Hostility scale (see also Watson & Clark, 1992b). That is, because Hostility is a negative affect, the Hostility scale of the PANAS-X is strongly saturated with variance attrib-utable to the general Negative Affect dimension. As was discussed in Chapter 2, this general factor reflects the variance that is common to all of the negative affects; as such, it accounts for the strong observed correla-tions among scales assessing these affects (e.g., Fear, Sadness, and Hostil-ity). In other words, to some extent hostility is a negative affect that is just like any other negative affect.

Clearly, however, there is something specific to the experience of hos-tility that differentiates it from fear, sadness, and guilt. In other words, hostility is not simply interchangeable with other types of negative affect. Thus, the PANAS-X Hostility scale actually contains two distinct sub-components: (1) a nonspecific component that reflects the contribution of the general Negative Affect dimension and (2) a specific component that represents the unique qualities of this affect. Incidentally, each of the basic affect scales of the PANAS-X can be decomposed in this same manner.

Once the dualistic nature of the Hostility scale is recognized, it is a relatively simple matter to explain its associations with Neuroticism and Agreeableness. The key consideration is that *all* the negative affects corre-late substantially with Neuroticism but *only Hostility* is significantly asso-ciated with Agreeableness. Clearly, therefore, it is the nonspecific compo-nent of Hostility that is responsible for its significant correlation with Neuroticism, whereas it is the specific, unique component that gives rise to its negative association with Agreeableness. Thus, Hostility correlates with Neuroticism *because it is a negative affect,* but it correlates with Agree-ableness *because it is Hostility.*

The importance of this pattern becomes readily apparent when one considers the links between hostility and health. Health researchers now distinguish between two different types of anger/hostility (Bushman, Cooper, & Lemke, 1991; Costa, McCrae, & Dembroski, 1989; Musante, MacDougall, Dembroski, & Costa, 1989; Smith & Williams, 1992). The first type ("anger experience") represents the subjective component of hostility and includes feelings of anger, frustration, and resentment. The second type ("anger expression") reflects the behavioral or expressive component of hostility and includes tendencies toward verbal and physical aggression; individuals high in anger expression also may view the world in a suspicious and cynical manner.

Interestingly, anger experience is primarily related to Neuroticism and so reflects the nonspecific component of Hostility; whereas anger expression is primarily related to (dis)Agreeableness, and so appears to represent the specific, unique aspects of the trait. A growing body of evidence indicates that anger expression (i.e., the specific component) is a much better predictor of coronary heart disease than is anger experience (i.e., the nonspecific component) (see Dembroski, MacDougall, Costa, & Grandits, 1989; Siegman, Dembroski, & Ringel, 1987; Smith & Williams, 1992). These data again demonstrate the importance of assessing affect at both the higher-order and lower-order levels.

CONCLUSION

In this chapter I explored the links between affectivity and the traits comprising the five-factor model of personality. I began by showing that affect is strongly related to four of the Big Five traits; the sole exception is Openness, which consistently displays little relation to emotional experience. I then demonstrated that Neuroticism and Extraversion are strongly and broadly correlated with individual differences in negative and positive emotional experience, respectively. I further argued that individual differences in Negative and Positive Affectivity, respectively, comprise the central cores of Neuroticism and Extraversion; that is, they represent the unifying "glue" that forms these higher-order dispositions and maintains them as integrated wholes.

In contrast, Conscientiousness and Agreeableness show specific, lower-order associations with affectivity. Conscientiousness is strongly related to Attentiveness, whereas Agreeableness displays a consistent negative correlation with Hostility. The specific nature of these links suggests that individual differences in determination and hostility, respectively, are intrinsic components of the Conscientiousness and Agreeableness dimensions. Accordingly, these two general traits also show some of the essential characteristics of a temperament.

Chapters 5 and 6 have established the existence of individual differences in affectivity that persistent over time and across situations and that are related to general dimensions of personality. However, they failed to confront the basic issue of *why* these individual differences arise in the first place. Why are some people happier and more enthusiastic—or more nervous and distressed—than others? This is the focus of Chapter 7.

7

UNDERSTANDING INDIVIDUAL DIFFERENCES IN AFFECT AND WELL-BEING

In this chapter, I conclude my survey of affective traits and temperament by examining the fundamental issue of *why* people differ so widely in their characteristic levels of affect and well-being. After exploring possible sociocultural and biological factors that give rise to individual differences in affectivity, I offer a general model of happiness and well-being.

THE DEMOGRAPHICS OF HAPPINESS

A huge body of research has examined how numerous demographic variables—age, gender, marital status, ethnicity, income, socioeconomic status, and so on—are related to individual differences in affect and well-being (for recent reviews, see Argyle, 1987; Diener, 1996; Diener & Diener, 1996; Lykken & Tellegen, 1996; Myers & Diener, 1995; Veenhoven, 1991, 1994). This research is extremely relevant to any general exploration into the origins of well-being, as it can identify possible sociocultural factors that make happiness more or less likely. For instance, if studies show that married people tend to be happier than those who are single, this would suggest that stable, intimate relationships play a key role in maintaining a euthymic mood and a sanguine outlook on life. Similarly, a link between income and well-being would suggest that lifestyle-related factors are partly responsible for manifest individual differences in affectivity.

I must emphasize, however, that most of the relevant evidence is cross-sectional (i.e., measuring different individuals at the same point in time) rather than longitudinal (i.e., measuring the same individuals at different points in time). Accordingly, the direction of causality cannot be determined in most cases. Suppose, for instance, that a researcher finds a significant positive correlation between income and well-being, indicating that individuals who make more money also tend to report elevated levels of happiness. The commonsense interpretation of this finding would be that money helps to create certain conditions—increased opportunities for travel, better living conditions, improved health care, and so on—that are conducive to happiness. This may well be true; nevertheless, it also is true that causality may flow in the opposite direction. That is, happiness and well-being may lead to certain conditions—such as increased levels of confidence, energy and enthusiasm, and enhanced social popularity—that facilitate the earning of money (Veenhoven, 1991). Consequently, even when significant correlations are observed, they may not necessarily demonstrate that sociocultural factors influence happiness. Wherever possible, I emphasize longitudinal data that help to clarify causal issues.

Happiness across the Lifespan

Several popular beliefs assume that affect levels vary systematically over the lifespan (Myers & Diener, 1995). For instance, one widely held idea is that people experience a "midlife crisis" of angst and uncertainty during their 40s. Another popular notion is the "empty-nest syndrome"—that is, the feelings of depression and despondency that parents supposedly feel as their grown-up children leave home. In a related vein, many people associate the postretirement years with feelings of depression and aimlessness.

It is surprising, therefore, that affect and well-being show virtually no age-related effects (see Adelmann, Antonucci, Crohan, & Coleman, 1989; Argyle, 1987; Diener, 1984; Myers & Diener, 1995). For example, Inglehart (1990) examined the reported life satisfaction of 169,776 respondents sampled across 16 countries. Overall levels of life satisfaction were virtually identical across the six analyzed age groups (15–24, 25–34, 35–44, 45–54, 55–54, 65 and older). Similarly, a meta-analysis of earlier research yielded a near-zero correlation between age and well-being (Stock, Okun, Haring, & Witter, 1983).

The one well-replicated age-related effect—discussed previously in Chapter 5—is that negative mood levels show a small but significant decline from late adolescence to early adulthood. Using longitudinal designs, Newton and Keenan (1991) and Watson and Walker (1996) both found that respondents who initially were assessed as college students reported significantly lower levels of negative mood after graduation. Other researchers have reported parallel declines on trait measures of Neuroticism between the ages of 20 and 30 (McGue, Bacon, & Lykken, 1993; Viken, Rose, Kaprio, & Koskenvuo, 1994); it is noteworthy, moreover, that Helson and Klohnen (1998) recently extended these findings by demonstrating a significant decrease in Neuroticism between the ages of 27 and 43. Finally, cross-sectional analyses indicate that college students score significantly higher on measures of Neuroticism and trait Negative Affect than do general adult samples (Costa & McCrae, 1992; Spielberger et al., 1983; Watson & Clark, 1994b).

Thus, we do see some evidence supporting the popular notion that adolescence is a time of heightened stress and anxiety. Beyond that, however, it appears that happiness does not vary as a function of age, and that popular beliefs in the "midlife crisis," the empty-nest syndrome, and late-life depression are largely unfounded.

Affect and Well-Being in Men and Women

Women are widely viewed as being more "emotional"—with wider, more intense mood swings and a more frequent episodes of dysphoria—than men (e.g., Eysenck, 1990). This view is not entirely unfounded, as women are approximately twice as likely to develop a major depression than are men (Kessler et al., 1994; Nolen-Hoeksema, 1987, 1990; Robins & Regier, 1991). In addition, women show significantly higher lifetime prevalence rates for dysthymic disorder, generalized anxiety disorder, panic disorder, and agoraphobia (American Psychiatric Association, 1994; Kessler et al., 1994). Thus, women do report elevated rates of clinically significant forms of distress.

However, studies in general population samples consistently find that men and women show few—if any—differences in happiness and life satisfaction (Argyle, 1987; Diener, 1984; Myers & Diener, 1995). For instance, in his analysis of 169,776 respondents across 16 nations, Inglehart (1990) found that 80% of men and 80% of women said that they were at least "fairly satisfied" with life. Similarly, Michalos (1991) examined the responses of 18,032 students from 39 different countries and found that men and women reported virtually identical levels of happiness and life satisfaction. Finally, in a meta-analysis of 146 studies, Haring, Stock, and

Okun (1984) found that gender accounted for less than 1% of the variance in global reports of well-being.

Clearly, men and women are indistinguishable on global measures of happiness, well-being, and life satisfaction. What happens, however, when we examine more specific affect measures? Interestingly, some evidence suggests that women tend to report slightly greater levels of both Positive and Negative Affect (Argyle, 1987; Diener, 1984; Fujita, Diener, & Sandvik, 1991; Myers & Diener, 1995; Wood, Rholes, & Whelan, 1989). It may be these two countervailing elevations tend to cancel each out, thereby eliminating gender differences on more global measures of well-being. It must be emphasized, however, that even when these gender differences are found, they tend to be quite small. Moreover, these gender differences do not consistently emerge in the data. For example, Watson and Clark (1994b) compared men and women on the general Negative and Positive Affect scales of the PANAS-X in 10 large data sets (overall, they included 3,322 men and 4,709 women). Analyses of the general Negative Affect scale revealed no significant gender differences in any sample. The general Positive Affect scale yielded significant gender differences in 2 of the 10 data sets; however, men reported greater Positive Affect in one case whereas women reported elevated positive mood in the other. Clearly, men and women reported comparable levels of both Positive and Negative Affect in these data.

It is possible that these analyses of general affect mask significant gender differences at the specific affect level. Do men and women differ significantly in their experience of fear, sadness, anger, joy, and other feelings? Unfortunately, few studies have systematically examined gender differences at the specific affect level. One notable exception is Watson and Clark (1994b), who compared men and women on the 11 lower-order PANAS-X scales in the same 10 data sets noted earlier. Consistent gender differences could be identified on only three scales. Specifically, men reported higher levels of Hostility (i.e., feelings of anger, scorn, and disgust), Self-Assurance (i.e., feelings of fearlessness, confidence, and pride) and Serenity (i.e., feelings of relaxation) than did women. However, these differences tended to be quite small.

To provide a better sense of these gender effects, Table 7.1 reports data from 2 of the 10 data sets analyzed in Watson and Clark (1994b). The first is a very large sample of college students (660 men, 989 women) who completed a general, trait form of the PANAS-X; the second is a smaller sample of Dallas-area adults (142 men, 186 women) who rated how they had felt "during the past week." The table reports correlations between gender and scores on all 13 PANAS-X scales separately for each sample. Note that a positive correlation indicates that women tended to have

TABLE 7.1. Correlations between Gender and Affect (Single Assessments)

Affect scale	College students	Adults
General dimension scales		
Negative Affect	−.04	.06
Positive Affect	.07**	−.14*
Basic negative affects		
Fear	.02	.04
Guilt	−.07	.06
Sadness	−.03	.12*
Hostility	−.20**	.03
Basic positive affects		
Joviality	.15**	−.07
Self-Assurance	−.13**	−.23**
Attentiveness	.11**	−.14**
Other affective states		
Shyness	−.11**	−.01
Fatigue	−.04	.11
Surprise	−.02	−.06
Serenity	−.08**	−.12*

Note. N = 660 men, 989 women (college students) and 142 men, 186 women (adults). Gender is coded as male = 0 and female = 1. Hence, a positive correlation indicates that women had a higher mean score and a negative correlation indicates that men had a higher mean score.
*p < .05, two-tailed; **p < .01, two-tailed.

higher scores on the scale, whereas a negative correlation indicates that men generally had higher scores.

Consistent with my earlier discussion, these data indicate that scores on the general Negative and Positive Affect scales are essentially unrelated to gender. It also is noteworthy that only 2 of the 22 lower-order correlations are as high as |.20|. Specifically, Hostility correlated −.20 with gender in the college student sample, whereas Self-Assurance correlated −.23 with gender in the adult sample. Overall, these data suggest that large, consistent gender differences cannot be identified even at the specific affect level.

One limitation of these data, however, is that they are based on a classic between-subject design in which each respondent was assessed only once. It might be argued that single, global assessments are subject to retrospective biases and other distortions and, therefore, may not accurately reflect online judgments of emotional experience. We can bypass this potential problem by making use of our intensive, longitudinal analyses of daily mood. As discussed in previous chapters, we conducted a series of studies in which SMU students rated their mood once a day over a period of several weeks. Collapsing across all these studies, we have 30 or more daily mood assessments from 475 students (144 men, 331 women) on the general Negative and Positive Affect scales; overall, these data represent 6,325 ($M = 43.9$) and 14,414 ($M = 43.6$) observations from our male and female respondents, respectively. In addition, 267 of these students (64 men, 203 women) completed the full 60-item PANAS-X, thereby yielding data on the 11 lower-order scales; analyses of these scales are based on 2,845 ($M = 44.5$) and 8,896 ($M = 43.8$) observations, respectively.

I began by computing an overall mean daily mood score for each respondent on all relevant PANAS-X scales. I then conducted separate *t*-tests for each scale, comparing the overall mean scores of the male and female students. Table 7.2 reports the results of these analyses—together

TABLE 7.2. Mean Daily Mood Scores for Male and Female College Students

Affect scale	Men	Women	*t*
General dimension scales			
Negative Affect	16.02	16.68	−1.60
Positive Affect	28.38	28.39	−0.01
Basic negative affects			
Fear	9.28	9.83	−1.44
Guilt	8.94	8.99	−0.11
Sadness	8.19	8.21	−0.06
Hostility	9.80	9.20	1.80[†]
Basic positive affects			
Joviality	21.81	23.05	−1.83[†]
Self-Assurance	14.63	14.67	−0.09
Attentiveness	10.86	11.42	−1.71[†]
Other affective states			
Shyness	5.73	5.49	1.07
Fatigue	8.78	8.51	0.83
Surprise	5.56	5.54	0.08
Serenity	8.68	8.17	2.07[*]

Note. For the general dimension scales, $N = 144$ (men) and 331 (women). For all other scales, $N = 64$ (men) and 203 (women).
[†]Difference between means is significant at $p < .10$, two-tailed.
[*]Difference between means is significant at $p < .05$, two-tailed.

with the grand scale means across the entire sample. Once again, these data indicate that men and women report extremely similar levels of general Positive and Negative Affect: The small gender difference on Negative Affect only approached significance, whereas the mean Positive Affect scores of the two groups were essentially identical. At the lower-order level, men reported higher daily levels of Serenity, thereby replicating the findings of Watson and Clark (1994b). Men also reported marginally higher levels of Hostility, whereas women reported slightly greater amounts of Joviality (i.e., feelings of joy, enthusiasm, and energy) and Attentiveness (i.e., feelings of alertness and determination).

Overall, one sees few differences between men and women in nonclinical samples. Thus, although women do show elevated rates of clinically significant distress, they are not generally prone to increased levels of unhappiness or ill-being.

Income and Education

Income

The relation between wealth and well-being has fascinated people for centuries, and it continues to exert a strong—and seemingly paradoxical—hold on the popular consciousness. On the one hand, an old and honored saying reminds us that "money can't buy happiness." On the other hand, when I have lectured on this topic, I have found that a great many people are skeptical of this traditional view. Indeed, when confronted with this old saying, a common audience response is: "All I ask is a chance to prove than money can't buy happiness!" Clearly, the accumulation of wealth remains a tremendously important motive in our society, even among those who already are relatively affluent; and it is apparent that many people continue to believe that increased wealth somehow will lead to greater happiness (see Myers & Diener, 1995).

Three distinct lines of research have examined the relation between wealth and happiness. First, investigators have compared average levels of well-being across countries differing in per capita income. The data are not entirely consistent, but they generally reveal a substantial association between national wealth and well-being. For example, Veenhoven (1991) compared mean happiness levels across seven world regions. The four regions with the greatest wealth (North America, Australia, western Europe, and Japan) all reported substantially greater levels of happiness than two much poorer regions (Africa and Asia). Unexpectedly, however, Latin America—another relatively poor region—reported levels of well-being comparable to Japan and western Europe. On the basis of his findings, Veenhoven (1991) suggested that people require minimally sufficient economic conditions before they can be happy; once these minimal conditions are satisfied, further increases in wealth have little effect on well-being.

Diener, Diener, and Diener (1995) examined this issue in a more comprehensive manner, analyzing the responses of more than 120,000 individuals from 55 different countries (jointly representing roughly 75% of the world's population). Their analyses yielded a .64 correlation between national wealth and average reports of well-being. It is noteworthy, moreover, that the association was linear, rather than curvilinear, indicating that increases in national income continued to predict higher levels of happiness and life satisfaction even after basic life needs (e.g., food, water, and sanitation) clearly had been met. Thus, it is not simply the case that happiness requires the fulfillment of certain minimal economic conditions.

Again, however, there were some anomalous findings that could not be explained by wealth per se; for instance, the Irish report greater happiness than do the more affluent Germans (see Myers & Diener, 1995). Clearly, other forces must at work in producing these manifest cross-national differences in well-being. In this regard, Diener, Diener, and Diener (1995) found that even after controlling for income and other factors, people in individualistic countries (e.g., the United States and Australia) tended to report greater satisfaction than do those in collectivist societies (e.g., Japan and China).

A second line of research has examined—within a single country—whether an individual's income is related to his or her rated happiness; for example, do rich Americans tend to be happier than poor Americans? When analyzed in this manner, income shows extremely weak correlations with happiness and life satisfaction. In the United States, Diener, Sandvik, Seidlitz, and Diener (1993) found that income correlated only .13 with well-being in a national probability sample of nearly 5,000 adults; similarly, Lykken and Tellegen (1996) reported that income accounted for no more than 1–2% of the variance in well-being in analyses of more than 2,000 U. S. twins (see also Argyle, 1987; Crohan, Antonucci, Coleman, & Adelmann, 1989; Diener, 1984, 1996; Myers & Diener, 1995). Diener, Horwitz, and Emmons (1985) examined reported happiness, life satisfaction, and Positive and Negative Affect in a sample taken from *Forbes* magazine's list of wealthiest Americans. This group reported only slightly greater well-being than average; indeed, 37% of these respondents rated themselves as less happy than the average American. Studies conducted in other parts of the world have yielded essentially identical results (e.g., Inglehart, 1990).

The third line of evidence analyzes longitudinal trends in happiness as a function of changing income. These data indicate that even profound changes in wealth have virtually no impact on happiness and well-being. For instance, Myers and Diener (1995) examined trends in the United States between 1957 and 1993. During this time span, per capita income roughly doubled, from $8,000 to $16,000 (in constant 1990 dollars). Nevertheless, levels of well-being stagnated during this period. Indeed, analyses of large national samples indicated that 35% of Americans rated themselves as very happy in 1957, compared to 32% in 1993. Subsequent analyses demonstrated that levels of happiness in the United States, Japan, and France have remained largely unchanged since 1946, despite dramatic increases in wealth (Diener, 1996; Diener & Diener, 1996). Finally, it is noteworthy that the same pattern emerges at the individual level; thus, Diener et al. (1993) showed that individuals whose income had risen or declined over the previous decade did not differ in their rated happiness.

Education

Taken together, these data reveal that wealth and income are relatively weak predictors of happiness. Analyses of educational attainment yield a similar conclusion, consistently demonstrating that education tends to be only weakly correlated with various indicators of well-being (see Argyle, 1987; Campbell, 1981; Diener, 1984; Glenn & Weaver, 1981). For instance, in their large twin sample, Lykken and Tellegen (1996) found that educational attainment accounted for only 2–3% of the variance in two different indicators of well-being. It should be noted, however, that earlier U.S. studies tended to find stronger associations, suggesting that the mood-enhancing effects of education have diminished over time (see Argyle, 1987; Campbell, 1981). In addition, some evidence suggests that education may interact with income, such that education only is related to happiness in low-income groups (Argyle, 1987; Campbell, 1981).

These weak correlations are surprising in that education is associated with better, more interesting work opportunities, improved access to resources, and other advantages. In attempting to explain these data, Campbell (1981) speculated that although education tends to be associated with increasing resources, it also may lead to higher aspirations in an individual, thereby minimizing any overall effects on happiness. Aspiration level is an important consideration in this area, and I return to it subsequently.

Work and Socioeconomic Status

In Chapter 5, I reviewed data indicating that job satisfaction is moderately correlated with individual differences in general life satisfaction and trait affectivity. Of course, these data can be interpreted as showing either that (1) people with a euthymic temperament are predisposed to like their jobs or (2) having a good job tends to make one happier. To investigate this issue further, it is interesting to examine how objective aspects of work relate to affect and well-being. For instance, is it true that people with better jobs tend to be happier? Moreover, does work per se tend to increase levels of happiness and life satisfaction; that is, are people who work happier than those who do not?

One relevant body of research has examined how affect relates to socioeconomic status (SES). SES typically is defined in terms of the status or desirability of a person's occupation, ranging from unskilled labor at the lowest end to professional employment at the highest (e.g., Veroff, Douvan, & Kulka, 1981). Somewhat surprisingly, studies consistently have found that SES is essentially unrelated to happiness and life satisfaction. For instance, Warr and Payne (1982) found small differences in well-being across varying levels of SES in a British sample; Cantril (1965) reported similar results in several countries, including India, Cuba, Brazil, and Israel. Crohan et al. (1989) reported that SES correlated .15 with life satisfaction and .00 with rated happiness in a sample of 388 white Americans; the corresponding correlations in a group of 423 African Americans were −.06 and −.09, respectively. Finally, Lykken and Tellegen (1996) found that SES accounted for only 2–3% of the variance in well-being in their large U.S. twin sample. Clearly, high-status jobs are not associated with substantially greater happiness.

Another line of research has examined affect levels as a function of employment status, that is, whether or not one is working full or part time. To interpret these data properly, it is crucial that one distinguish between the voluntarily (e.g., full-time homemakers and those who are retired) and involuntarily (e.g., those who have been fired or laid off) unemployed. On the one hand, comparisons of the employed versus the voluntarily unemployed suggest that employment per se has little effect on well-being (e.g., Diener, 1984). For instance, Adelmann et al. (1989) investigated this issue in a sample of 684 middle-age women. They found that employment status (coded so that a higher score indicated that the respondent was employed outside of the home) correlated only −.08 with self-rated anxiety, −.10 with depression, and .18 with self-reported health. Similarly, retired people report relatively high levels of well-being (Argyle, 1987).

On the other hand, the evidence strongly indicates that the involuntarily unemployed report low levels of happiness and life satisfaction and elevated levels of depression and other psychological problems (Argyle, 1987; Diener, 1984; Weerasinghe & Tepperman, 1994). Campbell, Converse, and Rodgers (1976), for instance, found that unemployed individuals had the lowest levels of happiness, even after controlling for differences in income. Similarly, Weerasinghe and Tepperman (1994) reported that unemployment was associated with low levels of happiness and elevated rates of suicide.

The bulk of this evidence comes from cross-sectional designs. As noted earlier, such studies yield causally ambiguous results. This is particularly problematic in the current case, as there are data indicating that the unemployed tend to have somewhat poorer psychological health even *before* they lose their jobs. Thus, it could be argued that unhappiness causes unemployment, rather than vice versa (see Argyle, 1987). Fortunately, longitudinal data clearly confirm that unemployment has adverse effects on happiness and well-being. For instance, in an analysis of 954 men, Warr and Jackson (1984) found that unemployment led to increased levels of depression and anxiety. Similarly, Banks and Jackson (1982) followed a sample of British adolescents for nearly 2 years after they quit school. Interestingly, those who subsequently were successful in finding jobs reported *increased* levels of well-being after leaving school, whereas those who failed to find jobs reported *decreased* well-being.

With the notable exception of involuntary unemployment, we see little evidence that occupational and employment status have a major impact on well-being. Generally speaking, people in seemingly uninteresting, low-status jobs report levels of happiness and life satisfaction that are quite comparable to those of individuals in high-status occupations. Moreover, the employed and voluntarily unemployed report extremely similar levels of affect and well-being.

Marriage, Family, and Social Relations

Marriage and Family

Most people consider marriage and family life to be extremely important sources of happiness (Argyle, 1987). Are people who are married really that much happier than those who are not? An enormous research literature has examined this issue (Diener, 1984). Although the available data are not entirely consistent, the bulk of the evidence surprisingly suggests that marriage per se has relatively little effect on well-being. Most notably, a meta-analysis of 58 U.S. studies showed that marital status (coded such that a higher score indicated that the respondent was married) correlated only .14 with reported well-being (Haring-Hidore, Stock, Okun, & Witter, 1985). More recent studies have reported similar findings (e.g., Demo & Acock, 1996). For instance, Adelmann et al. (1989) obtained near-zero correlations between marital status and measures of anxiety, depression, and self-rated health in a large sample of middle-age women. Similarly, Lykken and Tellegen (1996) reported that marital status predicted less than 1% of the variance in their sample of nearly 4,000 adult twins.

Although marital status accounts for little overall variance in well-being, it nevertheless is true that married people tend to be disproportionately represented among the very happiest subgroup in the population. For instance, in an analysis of several large U.S. national surveys, Veroff et al. (1981) found that 35% of married men rated themselves as being very happy, compared with only 18.5% of single men (a difference of 16.5%). Women showed essentially the same pattern; specifically, 41.5% of married women described themselves as very happy, compared with only 25.5% of single women (a difference of 16.0%). In a subsequent analysis of data from the National Opinion Research Center, Lee, Seccombe, and Shehan (1991) obtained virtually identical results: Once again, married people were much more likely to describe themselves as very happy than were those who were single, and this "marriage gap" was quite similar for both men (17.6%) and women (15.9%).

These analyses of the "very happy" could be interpreted as suggesting that the intimacy and companionship of marriage may help people to achieve the highest levels of well-being. Unfortunately, these data all are cross-sectional and, therefore, are causally ambiguous. Indeed, it is noteworthy that happy, optimistic people are viewed as more attractive marriage partners and, therefore, are more likely to marry (Mastekaasa, 1992; Scott, 1992); conversely, depressed, unhappy people are perceived as unattractive and encounter increased social rejection (Joiner & Metalsky, 1995). Consequently—to some extent, at least—happiness causes marriage rather than vice versa (see Lykken & Tellegen, 1996; Myers & Diener, 1995).

As we have seen, marriage per se has little overall effect on rated happiness and satisfaction. Surprisingly, the evidence regarding parenthood is even more negative. In his review of the literature, Diener (1984) concluded that "most studies find either negligible or negative effects of having children" on well-being (p. 556). Argyle (1987) reached a similar conclusion, arguing that children both "provide great positive satisfaction" and "considerable costs" (p. 21). In terms of the latter, the data indicate that children can place a significant strain on the marital relationship, so that marital satisfaction tends to increase after they leave home (Argyle, 1987; Myers & Diener, 1995).

Social Behavior

Moving beyond family relationships, numerous studies have examined how well-being is more broadly related to individual differences in interpersonal activity and social behavior. These data indicate that objective indicators of social behavior (e.g., number of close friends and membership in organizations) are moderately positively correlated with measures of well-being (Argyle, 1987; Diener, 1984; Lewinsohn, Redner, & Seeley, 1991; Myers & Diener, 1995).

However, the strength of these relations varies systematically as a function of the type of well-being measure used. In light of the short-term mood data summarized in Chapter 3, it hardly is surprising that social activity correlates more strongly and consistently with Positive Affect than with Negative Affect (Watson & Clark, 1997a; Watson et al., 1992). For instance, several studies have shown that individual differences in Positive Affect—but not Negative Affect—are related to various indicators of social behavior, including frequency of contact with friends and relatives, making new acquaintances, and involvement in social organizations (Beiser, 1974; Bradburn, 1969; Phillips, 1967).

My colleagues and I have observed the same basic pattern in our own data (for a review, see Watson & Clark, 1997a). For example, I collected daily mood and activity questionnaires from 71 student participants over a 6- to 7-week period (M = 44.4 assessments per student; see Watson, 1988a). Each day, the students rated the number of hours they had spent socializing with friends; these ratings then were collapsed across all available days to yield an overall index of social activity. This index was significantly correlated with various measures of trait Positive Affect (r ranged from .25 to .34) but was unrelated to trait Negative Affect (r ranged from .01 to −.03).

These results subsequently were replicated in two studies reported in Watson et al. (1992). In Study 1, 85 students rated their mood and social activity once a week for 13 weeks (M = 12.2 assessments per person). At each assessment, the students rated how frequently they had engaged in each of 15 broad classes of social activity (e.g., going out for a meal, exercising or playing sports, and going to a movie or play); these ratings were averaged over all items and weeks to create a single overall index of social behavior. As expected, overall social activity correlated significantly (r =.35) with positive emotionality but was unrelated (r = .01) to negative emotionality. In Study 2, 120 students rated their mood and social activity once each day for several weeks (M = 42.9 ratings per person). The social activity questionnaire was quite similar to that used in Study 1, except that the students estimated the amount of time they had spent in each of 21 different social activities that day; these again were averaged across all items and days to yield a summary index of social activity. Once again, overall social behavior correlated significantly with individual differences in Positive Affect (r = .28) but not Negative Affect (r = .16).

Thus, social behavior is moderately correlated with individual differences in positive emotionality but not negative emotionality. As I discussed in Chapter 3, the evidence further suggests that the underlying causality is bidirectional, with social activity and trait Positive Affect mutually influencing each other. On the one hand, it seems reasonably clear that social interaction typically leads to increased positive emotionality; nevertheless, it also is true that feelings of joy and enthusiasm are associated with an enhanced desire for affiliation and an increased preference for interpersonal contact (see McIntyre et al., 1991; Watson, 1988a; Watson & Clark, 1997a; Watson et al., 1992). Thus, positive emotionality is both a cause and an effect of social behavior.

Religion and Spirituality

In contrast to most of the other variables I have reviewed, the evidence regarding religious faith and commitment generally is positive and suggests a moderate degree of association. People who describe themselves as spiritual or religious report higher levels of happiness and life satisfaction than those who do not, both in the United States and in Europe (Andrews & Withey, 1976; Argyle, 1987; Campbell et al., 1976; Diener, 1984; Myers & Diener, 1995; Okun & Stock, 1987). For instance, Gallup (1984) found that respondents who rated themselves as being high in spiritual commitment were twice as likely to rate themselves as very happy than were those low on this variable. Furthermore, the data indicate that well-being varies as a function of the strength of a person's faith and religious commitment. Specifically, well-being levels are particularly elevated among individuals who (1) report a strong, committed religious affiliation; (2) attend religious services regularly; and (3) espouse fairly traditional religious beliefs (Diener, 1984; Inglehart, 1990; Myers & Diener, 1995; Witter, Stock, Okun, & Haring, 1985). In addition, a strong religious faith has been shown to help people cope more effectively with catastrophic life events, such as bereavement, illness, and unemployment (Ellison, 1991; McIntosh, Silver, & Wortman, 1993). Finally, it is noteworthy that our own data show that religion and spirituality are significantly related to individual differences in Positive Affect but not Negative Affect (e.g., Watson & Clark, 1993).

Why do spiritual and religious people tend to be happier? Two basic explanations have been offered by researchers in this area (Argyle, 1987; Myers & Diener, 1995). First, religion may provide people with a profound sense of meaning and purpose in their lives. Put another way, religion can provide people with plausible answers to the basic existential questions of life ("Why am I here?" "What should I do with my life?" "What will happen to me after I die?"), thereby delivering them from existential angst and freeing them to enjoy their lives more fully. Second, religious activity simply may represent a particular variety of social behavior. In other words, membership in a religious denomination allows people to congregate together, espouse shared views, and form close supportive relationships. Consistent with this explanation, people who are religious rate themselves as being less lonely than those who are not (Argyle, 1987; Paloutzian & Ellison, 1982). Note that this view also offers a particularly plausible explanation for the finding that more frequent attendance at religious services is associated with greater levels of well-being.

Both of these explanations assume that religious activity (perhaps in conjunction with other variables, such as social behavior and support) generates elevated levels of well-being. As always, however, these cross-sectional correlational data are causally ambiguous and subject to various interpretations. In this regard, Waller, Kojetin, Lykken, Tellegen, and Bouchard (1990) showed that genetic factors accounted for roughly half of the variance in measures of religious interests, attitudes, and values; similarly, Beer, Arnold, and Loehlin (1998) found evidence of substantial heritability in a measure of religious orthodoxy. These genetic data raise the possibility that happiness and religiosity actually are linked through shared, underlying biological processes (e.g., both may reflect inherited individual differences in gregariousness and social engagement).

THE SUBJECTIVE NATURE OF HAPPINESS

Subjective versus Objective Influences on Happiness

This review has shown that happiness and well-being can be linked to a number of objective demographic factors. For instance, people in wealthy countries tend to be happier than those in poor countries. Moreover, the evidence clearly demonstrates that losing one's job leads to lower levels of well-being and elevated levels of depression. Finally, people who are socially active and religiously committed tend to be happier than those who are not. Objective factors such as these obviously must be included in any comprehensive model of human happiness (Argyle, 1987; Diener, 1996; Veenhoven, 1991, 1994).

Nevertheless, study after study has shown that objective factors—even when considered together—account for relatively little of the observed variance in happiness and well-being (Diener, 1996; Myers & Diener, 1995). For example, in a large national U.S. sample, Campbell et al. (1976) showed that the combined effect of several demographic variables (age, gender, income, education, and race) was quite small; Kammann (1983) obtained very similar results in New Zealand, concluding that "objective life circumstances have a negligible role to play in a theory of happiness" (p. 18).

Consequently, contemporary researchers have concluded that happiness is primarily a *subjective* phenomenon. That is, it is much more a function of subjective internal processes (e.g., attitudes, orientation toward life, and temperamental factors) than of objective external forces (e.g., income level and job quality) (see Csikszentmihalyi, 1991; Diener, 1996; Lykken & Tellegen, 1996; Myers & Diener, 1995). Consistent with this view, Diener and Diener (1996) recently summarized an enormous body of evidence indicating that most people—including those who are disadvantaged and those who are facing extreme hardships—report that they are at least relatively happy (see also Veenhoven, 1991). For example, persons with severe physical disabilities generally report that they are at least somewhat happy and satisfied with their lives. Hellmich (1995), for instance, studied individuals with severe quadriplegia; 93% of his respondents reported that they were glad to be alive, and 84% considered their quality of life to be average or above average. Similarly, Mehnert, Krauss, Nadler, and Boyd (1990) found that 68% of a sample of disabled adults rated themselves as being somewhat to very satisfied with their lives. In a related vein, even people with (1) extremely low levels of income (e.g., Andrews & Withey, 1976) and (2) chronic mental problems (e.g., Delespaul & deVries, 1987) tend to report positive levels of well-being.

These data closely parallel findings based on short-term affect that were discussed in Chapter 1. In Chapter 1, I showed that most people experience a pleasant, positive mood most of the time. Diener and Diener (1996) have extended this basic finding by demonstrating that it (1) also applies to long-term well-being and (2) holds true across a remarkable array of environmental conditions.

This basic pattern makes good evolutionary sense (see also Myers & Diener, 1995; Veenhoven, 1991). As I discussed in Chapter 1, positive mood states are part of a more general BFS that has evolved to ensure that organisms obtain the resources (e.g., food and water, warmth and shelter, and sexual partners) that are necessary for the survival of both the individual and the species. In general, these essential approach behaviors will be performed only when negative mood levels are relatively low and positive mood predominates. Consequently, individuals who failed to exhibit a predominance of positive mood would have shown poor adaptive fitness and would have been at a selective disadvantage in our distant evolutionary past. As Veenhoven (1991) put it, "Nature is unlikely to have burdened us with characteristic unhappiness, because evolution is unlikely to result in a species that does not fit its characteristic environment subjectively. Like 'health,' happiness would seem to be a normal condition" (p. 14).

Adaptation and the "Set Point"

Adaptation Level Theory

Several theoretical models have been developed to explain why objective events and circumstances account for little variance in happiness and life satisfaction. One prominent example is Adaptation Level Theory (Brickman & Campbell, 1971; Brickman, Coates, & Janoff-Bulman, 1978). According to this model, new events are evaluated against a standard that is based on the range of relevant stimuli that have been experienced in the past. Events that are better than this standard are viewed positively; those that fall below it are evaluated negatively, whereas those that are judged to be similar to the standard are perceived as neutral. Over time, even dramatic events and experiences gradually merge into this standard; they thereby become increasingly neutral and eventually lose their power to affect us. Thus, people gradually adapt to almost any event or circumstance, so that these experiences no longer affect them emotionally. In colloquial terms, we eventually "get used to things" and begin to "take them for granted."

Although Adaptation Level Theory has its limitations (see Argyle, 1987; Eysenck, 1990; Headey & Wearing, 1991), accumulating evidence establishes that it has considerable merit. Stone and Neale (1984), for instance, found that the mood-altering effects of severe, negative daily events tended to dissipate within a day. Similarly, Suh, Diener, and Fujita (1996) observed that only major life events occurring within the previous 3 months had a significant impact on rated well-being, indicating that people already had adapted to earlier experiences.

More striking support comes from studies of individuals who have experienced dramatic life changes. Brickman et al. (1978) found that although lottery winners initially were quite elated, they gradually adapted to their good fortune and eventually reported average levels of well-being. Similarly, Smith and Razzell (1975) studied 191 people who had won £160,000 or more in the British football pools; they found that even this sudden, dramatic increase in wealth had little long-term effect on overall happiness. Studies of catastrophic negative experiences yield comparable results. Brickman et al. (1978), for instance, observed that after an initial period of adjustment, quadriplegic patients eventually reported unremarkable levels of well-being. Along these same lines, Silver (1982) found that individuals with spinal cord injuries were extremely unhappy immediately following their trauma but within 3 weeks had rebounded and were reporting normal levels of happiness (see also Wortman & Silver, 1987).

Aspiration Level

A related theoretical model emphasizes the importance of *level of aspirations* in human happiness (Argyle, 1987; Diener, 1984; Michalos, 1985, 1991; Taylor, 1982). In brief, proponents of this view argue that happiness depends on the discrepancy between the actual conditions in a person's life and his or her aspirations: When the gap between conditions and aspirations is small, people tend to be happy and satisfied; however, they become increasingly dissatisfied as the gap widens.

The problem for human happiness is that objective improvements in life conditions tend to produce rising expectations and higher aspirations (Argyle, 1987; Taylor, 1982). In other words, the more we have, the more we want. In many instances, this might mean that even dramatic improvements may fail to reduce the gap between conditions and aspirations and, therefore, have little impact on happiness and well-being. In fact, if expectations increase faster than objective circumstances, improved conditions actually may lead to *lower* levels of satisfaction.

This model has received broad support in the recent literature (e.g., Michalos, 1985; Taylor, 1982). Moreover, it helps to explain some of the more puzzling findings that have emerged, such as instances in which people have reported greater dissatisfaction during periods of increasing affluence (Taylor, 1982). Data such as these strikingly indicate that "happiness is less a matter of getting what you want than wanting what you have" (Myers & Diener, 1995, p. 13).

The Emotional "Set Point"

These theoretical models—together with the empirical data they have generated—suggest that human affect is strongly inertial in character, and that few events or experiences are likely to have much long-term impact on levels of well-being. This, in turn, has led to the recent suggestion that human affect is characterized by a baseline or "set point" (Diener, 1996; Diener & Diener, 1996; Headey & Wearing, 1992). According to this view, each person has a characteristic baseline level of affect that represents his or her typical level of well-being. Positive and negative life events will deflect affect levels away from this set point, but eventually they drift back to the baseline and reestablish an emotional equilibrium.

Similar to earlier theories (e.g., Adaptation Level), this concept of the emotional set point emphasizes that (1) people eventually will adjust to almost anything and (2) even dramatic events and experiences gradually lose their power to influence us emotionally. Thus, even things that initially thrill us (such as winning the lottery) or terrify us (such as becoming disabled) gradually fail to move us. As Frijda (1988) put it, "Pleasure is always contingent upon change and disappears with continuous satisfaction" (p. 353). Interestingly, Freud (1961) reached virtually the same conclusion several decades earlier, noting that "We are so made that we can derive intense enjoyment only from a contrast and very little from a state of things" (p. 23).

At first glance, this seems to represent a highly unsatisfactory state of affairs. After all, wouldn't we all be happier if we really could "count our blessings" every day and take renewed pleasure in the positive events and experiences in our lives? What if we were able to reexperience positive events indefinitely, so that we still could derive substantial pleasure from the first kiss of adolescence, from an athletic triumph in high school, or from a promotion and raise that was received several years ago? Moreover, wouldn't it better if humans could learn to be satisfied with what they have rather than constantly raising their aspiration levels so that they always want more? Why are so many of us disinterested in—and dissatisfied with—the good things we already have, restlessly searching for new and better things (which we eventually will adapt to anyway)?

These are worthwhile questions to ponder, and they raise some important issues regarding the nature of human happiness. Certainly, it is difficult to argue that the key forces that have emerged in this literature (rising aspirations, set points, etc.) will maximize human happiness. Nevertheless, it must be emphasized that—regardless of any negative implications they might have for our subjective well-being—these processes are highly adaptive and play an extremely important role in our survival. As I have discussed previously, the basic dimensions of mood evolved as part of broader biobehavioral systems that regulate essential, survival-related activities. Negative moods are associated with the BIS, which is designed to keep organisms out of trouble—that is, it inhibits behavior that might lead to pain, punishment, or some other unpleasant consequence. Conversely, positive moods are part of the BFS, which has evolved to ensure that organisms obtain essential survival-related resources.

As such, it is crucially important that these mood systems be acutely sensitive to changing internal and external conditions rather than to static aspects of the environment. For instance, in the distant evolutionary past, would it have been adaptive for animals to be completely "satisfied" with the resources (food, water, shelter, etc.) they already had accumulated and consumed, so that they no longer perceived any need to acquire more? The answer must surely be "no": Natural selection generally should favor restless, acquisitive creatures that relentlessly seek new (and it is hoped better) resources. Similarly, would it ever have been adaptive for animals to stop "worrying" about potential threats and dangers in their environment? Again, the answer clearly is "no": An apprehensive vigilance is the necessary price one must pay to survive in a dangerous world. Thus, even though they may diminish our overall sense of well-being, feelings of restlessness, acquisitiveness, dissatisfaction, and apprehension are an essential part of our nature, irrespective of current environmental conditions.

Social Comparison

Models such as the Adaptation Level and Aspiration Level theories posit that people judge new events against some internal standard (e.g., their own relevant experiences in the past). In contrast, Social Comparison Theory argues that people judge new events against an *external* standard, namely, the experiences and circumstances of other people. This view is based on the seminal work of Festinger (1954), who proposed that people have a strong need to evaluate themselves accurately and, therefore, seek out others for comparison. Festinger further assumed that people are most likely to seek out *similar* others as a particularly salient basis for comparison; for instance, individuals of the same age, gender, and/or occupational status form a natural comparison group.

When applied to the well-being literature, Social Comparison Theory emphasizes that people judge their current life conditions largely in relative—rather than absolute—terms. If people perceive that their current circumstances are superior to those in their social comparison group, they will tend to be happy and satisfied regardless of the actual quality of these circumstances. Conversely, if people perceive that their current circumstances are inferior to those in their comparison group, they will become unhappy and dissatisfied, even if conditions are favorable in an absolute sense. Thus, an unskilled laborer who makes more money than other laborers at the same plant is likely to be relatively happy, whereas a highly paid executive who has a lower salary than other executives in the same corporation will be discontented. The great American cynic Ambrose Bierce perhaps had this model in mind when he defined happiness as "an agreeable sensation arising from contemplating the misery of another" (1958, p. 53).

Social comparison processes can be expected to build considerable inertia into human happiness. The reason is that significant changes in objective life conditions also tend to lead to the formation of an entirely new comparison group. For example, promotion within a corporation typically is associated with significant increases in both income and authority, which might be expected to generate elevated levels of well-being. The problem is that promotion also is likely to lead to a significant change in a person's comparison group, so that he or she now is using more powerful and affluent others as the standard for comparison. Note, moreover, that this theory is equally capable of explaining inertia following negative life events; for instance, the physically handicapped can maintain positive levels of well-being by comparing themselves to other individuals with disabilities rather than to the physically healthy (Veenhoven, 1991). Thus, it again seems that we may be fated to remain on an "hedonic treadmill" (Eysenck, 1990)—no matter how dramatically our life changes, we always fall back to the same familiar level of happiness.

Social Comparison Theory has received considerable support in the literature (see Argyle, 1987; Diener, 1984; Freedman, 1978). Several studies, for instance, have shown that life satisfaction varies more as a function of relative—rather than absolute—income levels. For example, in an analysis of U.S. data, Freedman (1978) reported that college-educated people at a given level of income (who can be expected to compare themselves to other college graduates) were less satisfied than nongraduates at the same income level (who should compare themselves to other nongraduates). Runciman (1966) obtained parallel results in a study of British workers. Finally, this model also offers perhaps the best existing explanation of an extremely curious phenomenon, namely, that many of the most highly paid members of our society (e.g., professional athletes and motion picture actors and actresses) often express great dissatisfaction with their enormous earnings. The explanation, of course, is that they compare themselves to their very highly paid colleagues rather than to more typical members of society.

THE BIOLOGICAL ORIGINS
OF INDIVIDUAL DIFFERENCES

Genetic Evidence

Models such as Adaptation Level Theory do an excellent job of explaining inertia in well-being and clarifying why changing life conditions tend to have little long-term impact on happiness and life satisfaction. Generally speaking, however, they are less adept at explaining why some people are happier than others. Why do some people tend to feel happy and enthusiastic about life, whereas others characteristically experience profound feelings of apprehension or gloom?

In recent years, it has become quite clear that innate biological processes play an important role in the emergence of these individual differences and so form an essential component in any comprehensive model of human happiness. Among other things, an enormous amount of evidence has clearly established that affect and well-being are strongly heritable and contain a substantial genetic component. For example, numerous studies have demonstrated that inherited factors are strongly implicated in the temperamental dimensions of Neuroticism and Extraversion, traits that (see Chapter 6) are strongly related to individual differences in Negative and Positive Affect, respectively (Eaves, Eysenck, & Martin, 1989; Heath, Cloninger, & Martin, 1994; Pedersen, Plomin, McClearn, & Friberg, 1988; Saudino, Pedersen, Lichtenstein, McClearn, & Plomin, 1997; Scarr, Webber, Weinberg, & Wittig, 1981; Viken et al., 1994).

Furthermore, in their meta-analysis of dozens of twin studies, McCartney, Harris, and Bernieri (1990) examined several traits related to affect and emotionality, including Anxiety, Emotionality, and Activity–Impulsivity. Each of these traits showed evidence of substantial heritability. In fact, using the traditional Falconer (1960) formula for calculating heritabilities in twin data (i.e., doubling the difference between the observed correlations for monozygotic and dizygotic twins), more than 50% of the variance in each of these traits could be attributed to genetic factors (see also Plomin & Daniels, 1987).

To date, the most directly relevant evidence has come from the Minnesota twin series; unlike most studies in this area, this series includes data from a large number of twins who were put up for adoption and, therefore, reared apart in different households. Tellegen et al. (1988) analyzed data from four different groups of twins—monozygotic (MZ) and dizygotic (DZ) twins reared both together and apart—across a wide range of scales included in the Multidimensional Personality Questionnaire (MPQ; Tellegen, in press). For our purposes, the two most interesting MPQ scales are Stress Reaction and Well-Being. The MPQ Stress Reaction scale is a strong, clear marker of trait Negative Affect; high scorers describe themselves as nervous, apprehensive, irritable, overly sensitive to minor frustrations, and emotionally labile. In contrast, the MPQ Well-Being scale is an excellent measure of trait Positive Affect; high scorers describe themselves as happy, enthusiastic, and optimistic and as leading an interesting and exciting life.

The results reported by Tellegen et al. (1988) clearly establish that genetic factors contribute substantially to individual differences in both Negative and Positive Affect. Specifically, 53% of the variance in Stress Reaction could be attributed to genetic factors. Consistent with the more general personality literature in this area (Loehlin, 1992; Plomin & Daniels, 1987), the shared familial environment had no discernible influence on this trait; rather, all the remaining variance could be attributed to the unshared environment. The results for Well-Being were virtually identical:

Once again, genes (48% of the variance) and the unshared environment (40% of the variance) both made enormous contributions to this trait, whereas the shared familial component was insignificant.

On the basis of these data—together with the larger body of evidence concerning Neuroticism, Extraversion, and other relevant measures—we can conclude that approximately half of the observed variance in both trait Negative Affect and trait Positive Affect is due to inherited factors. This striking genetic evidence confirms the wisdom of Meehl's (1975) conjecture that "some persons [are] born with more cerebral 'joy-juice' than others" (p. 299), as well as the old "Wild West" maxim (quoted by Meehl, 1975, p. 298) that "some men are just born three drinks behind."

Neurobiological Evidence

Frontal Brain Asymmetry

How do these innate genotypic differences manifest themselves as systematic phenotypic differences in affect and well-being? The accumulating data indicate that these phenotypic differences arise, in part, from substantial variations in central nervous system activity across different individuals. Davidson, Tomarken, and their colleagues have conducted an especially intriguing line of research that focuses on hemispheric asymmetry in the prefrontal cortex (for a review, see Tomarken & Keener, 1998). This research was stimulated by both experimental evidence and clinical reports (e.g., case studies of stroke patients and accident victims) suggesting that anterior asymmetry had profound emotional consequences. Specifically, unilateral lesions or sedation of the left frontal lobe were associated with a "depressive–catastrophic" reaction, whereas lesions or sedation of the right frontal area were associated with either a relatively neutral mood or heightened Positive Affect (Gainotti, Caltagirone, & Zoccolotti, 1993; Starkstein & Robinson, 1989; Tomarken & Keener, 1998). For instance, stroke patients with unilateral left frontal lesions show a significant increase in depressive symptoms, whereas those with right frontal lesions do not.

This evidence led Davidson, Tomarken, and their colleagues to explore the affective–temperamental implications of resting anterior asymmetry more systematically (see Davidson, 1992; Davidson & Tomarken, 1989; Larsen, Davidson, & Abercrombie, 1995; Tomarken, Davidson, Wheeler, & Doss, 1992; Tomarken & Keener, 1998). Their data consistently demonstrate that happy, euthymic individuals tend to show relatively greater resting activity in the left prefrontal cortex than in the right prefrontal area; conversely, dysphoric and dissatisfied individuals display relatively greater right anterior activity. For instance, Tomarken et al.

(1992) found that people with relatively greater left frontal activation reported higher trait Positive Affect and lower trait Negative Affect than those with relatively greater right frontal activity.

It has been difficult to isolate the specific effects of left versus right prefrontal activity in these studies. Some recent evidence, however, suggests that individual differences in trait Positive Affect primarily reflect the level of resting activity in the left prefrontal area, whereas trait Negative Affect is more strongly and systematically related to right frontal activation (see Bruder et al., 1997; Davidson, 1992; Larsen et al., 1995; Tomarken & Keener, 1998). Moreover, it is apparent that these effects are not state dependent but, rather, reflect stable individual differences in temperament. For instance, Henriques and Davidson (1990) reported that formerly depressed patients who were currently euthymic also showed relatively greater right prefrontal activity. In addition, the asymptomatic adolescent children of depressed mothers also exhibit this same pattern of anterior asymmetry (Tomarken & Keener, 1998).

On the basis of these accumulating data, Davidson, Tomarken, and their colleagues have linked frontal brain activity to individual differences in the general biobehavioral systems that I discussed earlier (see Davidson, 1992; Henriques & Davidson, 1991; Henriques, Glowacki, & Davidson, 1994; Tomarken & Keener, 1998). Specifically, they argue that resting levels of left prefrontal activation reflect individual differences in the approach-oriented BFS—which, in turn, is associated with the experience of Positive Affect. Tomarken and Keener (1998), for example, argue that "relative left frontal activation is associated with heightened appetitive or incentive motivation, heightened responsivity to rewards or other positive stimuli, and greater contact with those features of the external environment that are rewarding or engaging" (p. 395). Conversely, resting levels of right frontal activation reflect individual differences in the withdrawal-oriented BIS, which is related to the experience of Negative Affect. It therefore appears that the prefrontal cortex plays a critical role in determining whether one was born "three drinks behind" or "three drinks ahead."

Dopamine and Positive Affect

We can take this analysis a step further by asking: Why is prefrontal activity systematically related to individual differences in affectivity? One likely possibility is that anterior asymmetry reflects, at least in part, the operation of the major neurotransmitter systems. In this regard, each of the major ascending monoaminergic systems—norepinephrine, serotonin, and dopamine—has significant projections to the frontal cortex (Goldman-Rakic, Lidow, & Gallagher, 1990). Moreover, it is increasingly clear that the major dimensions of temperament are systematically related to these monoaminergic systems (Cloninger, 1987; Depue et al., 1994; Fowles, 1994; Siever & Davis, 1991).

To date, the clearest evidence concerns the dopaminergic system, which plays a key role in positive affective experience. The ascending dopamine system arises from cell groups located in the ventral tegmental area (VTA) of the midbrain and has projections throughout the cortex (Depue et al., 1994; Le Moal & Simon, 1991). It is noteworthy that these cortical projections tend to be concentrated in the left hemisphere, with a particularly strong asymmetry in the frontal region (Tucker & Williamson, 1984). Moreover, it is well established that the dopaminergic system mediates various approach-related behaviors, including heightened appetitive motivation, enhanced behavioral approach to incentive stimuli, and increased engagement with the environment (e.g., Depue et al., 1994; Depue & Iacono, 1989; Stellar & Stellar, 1985; Willner, 1985; Wise & Rompre, 1989). Taken together, these data suggest that the dopaminergic system plays a key role in left frontal activity and, therefore, in the experience of Positive Affect.

Depue et al. (1994) examined this idea by administering biological agents known to stimulate dopaminergic activity and then measuring the strength of the system's response. Consistent with their expectation, Depue et al. found that various measures of dopaminergic activity were strongly correlated with individual differences in trait Positive Affect but were unrelated to trait Negative Affect. Interestingly, Depue et al. (1994) noted further that "many of the behavioral and hormonal effects of dopamine activation are significantly influenced by genetic variation in dopamine cell number, including those dopamine cell groups in the VTA" (p. 486), implicating interindividual variation in the number of dopamine neurons as a possible source for the heritability of trait Positive Affect. In other words, variation in dopamine cell number in critical regions such as the VTA may cause some individuals to be born with more "cerebral joyjuice" than others.

Sensitivity to Punishment and Reward

Again, these intriguing data raise a further question: How do these variations in dopamine and other neurotransmitter systems give rise to observed individual differences in affect and well-being? A number of researchers in this area have argued that differential sensitivities to affect-eliciting stimuli may play a crucial role in the development of these observed individual differences (e.g., Cloninger, 1987; Larsen & Ketelaar, 1991; Tellegen, 1985; Tomarken & Keener, 1998; Zuckerman, 1987). Specifically, it is argued that Extraversion and trait Positive Affect reflect innate individual differences in sensitivity to pleasurable and rewarding stimuli. In other words, happy and enthusiastic individuals are more responsive to—and better able to derive pleasure from—rewarding stimuli. Conversely, Neuroticism and trait Negative Affect reflect innate differences in sensitivity to painful, punishing, and stressful stimuli. That is, distressed and dissatisfied individuals show stronger adverse reactions to noxious and threatening stimuli.

This "stimulus sensitivity" model has received some support in recent research (e.g., Berenbaum & Williams, 1995; Larsen & Ketelaar, 1991). The best, most direct evidence comes from two studies that assessed affect levels both before and after various mood inductions (Gross, Sutton, & Ketelaar, 1998; Rusting & Larsen, 1997). Consistent with the stimulus sensitivity model, Neuroticism scores predicted increases in negative mood following an unpleasant induction (e.g., watching a gruesome film) but were unrelated to changes in positive mood following the pleasant inductions (e.g., watching a funny film). Conversely, Extraversion scores predicted increases in positive mood following a pleasant mood induction but were unrelated to negative mood changes in the unpleasant conditions. Accordingly, it appears that Extraversion/Positive Affectivity and Neuroticism/Negative Affectivity do reflect individual differences in a person's sensitivity to pleasurable versus aversive stimuli, respectively.

TOWARD A GENERAL THEORY OF HAPPINESS

Happiness Is Not Highly Constrained by Objective Conditions

What lessons can be drawn from this enormous literature on happiness, well-being, and life satisfaction? First, the accumulating data clearly demonstrate that happiness is primarily a subjective phenomenon. To be sure, external conditions—such as poverty and unemployment—do show significant associations with happiness and life satisfaction. Nevertheless, most of the available evidence indicates that objective factors account for relatively little of the variance in measures of well-being (Campbell et al., 1976; Diener, 1984; Diener & Diener, 1996; Kammann, 1983; Myers & Diener, 1995).

One further implication of these data is that human happiness is not highly constrained by objective circumstances. The evidence clearly shows that people do not require all that much—in terms of material conditions, life circumstances, and so on—to be happy. For instance, it is obvious that one does not need to get married and have children, to obtain an advanced educational degree, or to find a glamorous, high-paying job in order to be happy. Rather, the data reveal that people can maintain reasonably good levels of satisfaction and well-being across a broad range of life conditions. Indeed, Diener and Diener (1996) demonstrated that most people—including the poor and the physically handicapped—describe themselves as being at least reasonably happy.

This further suggests that happiness is available to virtually everyone. One does not need to achieve a certain state of affairs—such as getting married or building a successful career—before happiness is possible. Rather, happiness rests primarily on the subjective internal processes (e.g., attitudes, aspirations, and outlook on life) of the individual. Csikszentmihalyi (1991) discusses this point at some length, arguing that happiness "is not something that money can buy or power command. It does not depend on outside events, but, rather, on how we interpret them" (p. 2).

Is Change Possible?

If happiness truly is available to anyone who has the right outlook on life, then an individual should be able to increase his or her level of well-being by adopting attitudes that promote satisfaction (e.g., by lowering aspiration levels). Csikszentmihalyi (1991) makes this point forcefully, asserting that "over the endless dark centuries of its evolution, the human nervous system has become so complex that it is now able to affect its own states, making it to a certain extent functionally independent of its genetic blueprint and of the objective environment. A person can make himself happy, or miserable, regardless of what is happening 'outside,' just by changing the contents of consciousness" (p. 24). In other words, rather than struggling to transform the material conditions of our lives, we can achieve happiness simply by changing *ourselves*.

At this point, we must confront a crucial issue: Is true, long-term change really possible? I have discussed several conceptual models—including Adaptation Level and Social Comparison Theory—that emphasize inertial forces in human happiness. Proponents of these views acknowledge that life events can produce significant short-term changes in well-being; nevertheless, they argue that people gradually adjust to these experiences and eventually drift back to their "emotional set point." Moreover, recent data establish that affect and well-being are strongly influenced by hereditary factors that apparently influence the structure and functioning of the central nervous system. Taken together, these converging lines of evidence suggest that although we may not be limited by external factors, we may well be constrained by internal forces that are strongly resistant to change.

It is increasingly apparent that these internal constraints exist, and that they must be acknowledged in any comprehensive model of happiness. In view of the twin data, it seems quite likely that hereditary factors do place certain restrictions on the experienced happiness of a given individual. In this regard, behavior geneticists have developed the concept of the "reaction range" to represent the phenotypic limits imposed by genes (see Gottesman, 1963, 1974; Gottesman & Goldsmith, 1994; Hall, 1987; Turkheimer & Gottesman, 1991; Weinberg, 1989). The reaction range concept includes two key principles. First, any given genotype is associated with a range of possible phenotypes across a specified range of environments. For instance, a person with "medium–tall" genes for height may be shorter than average if he or she grows up in relatively poor circumstances but may be taller than average if good nutrition is readily available. Second, the maximum and minimum phenotypic values that define the boundaries of this range will vary systematically across different genotypes. For instance, no matter how well fed, someone endowed with "short" genes will never be substantially taller than average; conversely, no matter how ill fed, someone endowed with "tall" genes will never be significantly shorter than average (Hall, 1987). When applied to well-being, this second principle implies that because of innate genotypic differences, some people are destined to be happier than others, regardless of past or present environmental conditions.

Nevertheless, it is easy to exaggerate the constraints imposed by genetic and biological factors by focusing solely on this second principle. Note that the first principle acknowledges that an enormous range of phenotypic values is possible for any given genotype. Returning to my earlier example, even though height is strongly heritable, the same individual may emerge as average, below average, or above average in height, depending on access to good nutrition and other qualities of the nurturing environment. In terms of human happiness, this first principle establishes that unless a person already has reached his or her maximum phenotypic level (a condition that should occur rarely, if at all), it should be possible to increase levels of satisfaction and well-being significantly, regardless of whether one was born "three drinks behind" or "three drinks ahead." Indeed, behavior geneticists repeatedly have attacked the overly simplistic view that evidence of heritability necessarily implies that change is impossible. As Weinberg (1989) put it, "There is a myth that if a behavior or characteristic is genetic, it cannot be changed. Genes do not fix behavior. Rather, they establish a range of possible reactions to the range of possible experiences that environments can provide" (p. 101).

This brings me to a crucial point that sometimes is forgotten in the contemporary literature: People do, in fact, show evidence of significant change in their overall levels of well-being. In Chapter 5, for instance, I presented data demonstrating that trait affect measures were moderately stable over periods of several years, with long-term stability coefficients typically falling in the .35-to-.55 range. Although these results establish an important continuity in affect levels, they also indicate that many respondents display substantial change over time (for related discussions, see Veenhoven, 1991, 1994). Along these same lines, Headey and Wearing (1991) reported that 25.1% of their respondents had life satisfaction scores that shifted by more than one standard deviation over a 6-year period; equivalent shifts in 31.1% and 27.3% of the respondents were observed on measures of Positive and Negative Affect, respectively.

Furthermore, there is suggestive evidence that changing circumstances can lead to broader cultural shifts over time. For example, the cross-cultural data reviewed earlier indicate that average levels of well-being vary considerably across nations, with respondents in richer countries reporting substantially higher levels of happiness and life satisfaction than those in poorer countries (Diener, 1996; Diener et al., 1995; Veenhoven, 1994). Diener et al. (1995), for instance, found that mean well-being in Denmark (which had the highest overall scores) and the Dominican Republic (which had the lowest scores) differed by 6.5 points on a 10-point scale (i.e., nearly two-thirds of the possible range). These data strongly suggest that improving the material conditions in a country may lead to marked increases in well-being. Conversely, other sociocultural changes may produce elevated levels of depression and dysphoria. Seligman (1991), for example, has argued that the growth of individualism in Western societies has led to an erosion of social support networks and, hence, to a rising epidemic of depression.

Consequently, the genetic and biological data should not induce a fatalistic resignation regarding the impossibility of change in human happiness. Although it is true that innate biological factors may place certain constraints on an individual's observed level of well-being, these constraints probably are more important theoretically than pragmatically. Because few of us ever reach the extreme upper bound of our "reaction range" of happiness, we ultimately are not constrained by our genetic endowment: We still are free to move around within our "range" and to increase our overall level of well-being.

Evolutionary Constraints on Happiness

Although true affective change is possible, ultimately there are important limits on the magnitude of the change that can reasonably be expected. Genetic factors may not seriously limit an individual's level of happiness, but evolutionary processes conspire to keep well-being within a certain restricted range. As I have discussed throughout this volume, the basic dimensions of mood evolved as part of broader biobehavioral systems that regulate essential, survival-related activities. Negative moods are associated with the BIS, which is designed to keep us out of trouble; whereas positive moods are part of the BFS, which has evolved to ensure that we obtain essential survival-related resources. Thus, these feeling states do not exist purely for their own sake; rather, they evolved to help motivate the occurrence of essential behaviors. In other words, mood systems have evolved through natural selection to maximize our *survival* rather than our happiness (see Nesse, 1991, for a similar analysis).

As I discussed previously, it is important that positive feelings predominate most of the time, so that we have the energy and confidence to emit necessary BFS-related behaviors (see also Diener & Diener, 1996). Nevertheless, as also noted earlier, feelings of restlessness, acquisitiveness, sadness, dissatisfaction, and apprehension also are essential to survival and an important part of our evolutionary heritage (Nesse, 1991). Thus, evolution has designed us to be happy—but not *too* happy. As Csikszentmihalyi (1991) put it, "Contrary to the myths mankind has developed to reassure itself, the universe was not created to answer our needs. Frustration is deeply woven into the fabric of life" (p. 7). Accordingly, we should not expect to achieve the transcendent bliss of pure happiness via money, sex, Prozac, or any other means.

The Importance of Goals

One particularly interesting implication of this literature is that people apparently devote much of their lives to striving after things—education, marriage, money, and so on—that ultimately have little effect on their happiness. At first glance, it may appear that this massive expenditure of time and energy is largely wasted in that it is devoted to the pursuit of things that really do not matter—at least in terms of our subjective well-being.

Are most of us, in fact, wasting away our lives in pursuit of things that ultimately do not matter? The answer clearly is "no." This is because it is the pursuit itself—the striving after important goals—that is crucial to maintaining psychological health and well-being (Csikszentmihalyi, 1991; Diener, 1984; Diener & Larsen, 1993; Emmons, 1986; Myers & Diener, 1995; Singer & Salovey, 1996). To appreciate the importance of goals, consider what would happen if people simply decided that things such as money, marriage, and family really did not matter in the long run and, therefore, were not worth pursuing after all. These feelings most likely would lead to a pervasive sense of hopelessness and despair; indeed, the perception that one is incapable of achieving positive outcomes is a hallmark of clinical depression (Abramson, Metalsky, & Alloy, 1989;

Alloy, Kelly, Mineka, & Clements, 1990; Beck, Rush, Shaw, & Emery, 1979). Consequently, happiness and well-being rest on the perception that (1) there are goals worth pursuing in life and (2) one is making significant progress toward those goals. Contemporary researchers therefore emphasize that it is the process of striving after goals—rather than goal attainment per se—that is crucial for human happiness. Myers and Diener (1995) express this point quite nicely, concluding that "Happiness grows less from the passive experience of desirable circumstances than from involvement in valued activities and progress toward one's goals" (p. 17). Similarly, Csikszentmihalyi (1991) argued that "The best moments usually occur when a person's body or mind is stretched to its limits in a voluntary effort to accomplish something difficult and worthwhile" (p. 3).

Thus, I conclude this survey by noting a curious paradox. As we have seen, most of the events and experiences in our lives ultimately are unimportant in terms of their long-term impact on our happiness. Nevertheless, it is extremely important that we *perceive* these things to be important and as representing goals that are well worth pursuing. In other words, although little of what we do really is important for our happiness, it is crucial that we do them, and that we *see* them as important.

8

AFFECT AND PSYCHOPATHOLOGY

Throughout this book, I have emphasized that our basic mood systems perform important adaptive functions: Negative moods help the organism to avoid painful and aversive stimuli, whereas positive moods facilitate the procurement of survival-related resources. Note, however, that although the basic *systems* themselves are highly adaptive, this by no means suggests that all our affective *responses* are functional and adaptive. Indeed, it is painfully obvious that each of us is capable of responding to situations and stimuli in dysfunctional and counterproductive ways. Of course, some people are much more prone to dysfunctional responses than are others; individuals who are particularly susceptible to these maladaptive states represent a major problem in our society. This chapter focuses on dysfunctional emotional responses, emphasizing in particular their relevance to major psychopathological syndromes.

What distinguishes an adaptive from a maladaptive affective response? To answer this question, I briefly note four ways in which affective responses may be dysfunctional (see also Clark & Watson, 1994). First, affective responses may be inappropriately *intense*. For instance, although it is adaptive to be concerned about how one is evaluated by others, the extreme nervousness and apprehension displayed by social phobics is dysfunctional and debilitating. The problem of intensity perhaps is best illustrated by the bipolar disorders, wherein the individual wildly fluctuates between the extremes of mania (i.e., feeling elated and euphoric and having tremendous energy, confidence, and optimism) and depression (i.e., feeling extremely sad, blue, tired, and disinterested); both these states represent exaggerated versions of adaptive responses that are too intense to be functional (Depue et al., 1987).

Second, affective responses may be too *prolonged* in duration. For instance, although it is evolutionarily adaptive to feel anxious or sad when one is initially separated from loved ones (Bowlby, 1980), extended feelings of depression serve no useful purpose and, indeed, may be highly counterproductive. Similarly, although it is understandable that one might feel irritated after being insulted by another, it clearly would be inappropriate to hold onto this feeling for several weeks. At the clinical level, this property is exemplified by posttraumatic stress disorder (PTSD), a syndrome in which the afflicted individual may continue to show striking symptoms of distress decades after the precipitating event (e.g., Barrett et al., 1996).

Third, affective responses may occur with unnecessary *frequency*. For instance, feelings of vigilance and apprehension are highly adaptive and can help organisms to avoid danger. However, the lives of individuals suffering from generalized anxiety disorder (GAD) become dominated by such feelings; in fact, to be diagnosed with this disorder, one has to experience excessive feelings of anxiety and worry "more days than not for at least 6 months" (American Psychiatric Association, 1994, p. 435). Clearly, the pervasive worry of these individuals no longer serves any useful purpose.

Fourth, affective responses may be *situationally inappropriate*. Situationally inappropriate responses are a common feature of many types of psychopathology. For instance, individuals suffering from schizophrenia may respond with silliness and laughter for no apparent reason (American Psychiatric Association, 1994). Similarly, persons afflicted with panic disorder experience sudden, debilitating panic attacks—that is, episodes of intense anxiety accompanied by hyperactivation of the sympathetic nervous system (American Psychiatric Association, 1994; Clark & Watson, 1994). This sympathetic arousal is highly adaptive when it occurs in response to threat or danger; in panic disorder, however, it occurs in the absence of threat and, therefore, is dysfunctional.

As these examples illustrate, dysfunctional affective responses are common, core features of many forms of psychopathology, particularly the anxiety and mood disorders. Indeed, "present distress" is listed as one of the defining features of mental disorder in the fourth edition of the *Diagnostic and Statistical Manual of Mental Disorders* (DSM-IV; American Psychiatric Association, 1994, p. xxi). In this chapter, I show how an examination of the basic negative and positive mood systems can clarify our understanding of psychopathology, focusing in particular on the mood disorders (e.g., depression, dysthymic disorder) and the anxiety disorders (e.g., panic disorder, simple phobia, social phobia, GAD, PTSD, and obsessive–compulsive disorder).

THE TWO-FACTOR AFFECTIVE MODEL OF ANXIETY AND DEPRESSION

The Relation between Anxiety and Depression

My interest in this area was stimulated by a problem that has vexed psychopathology researchers for years, namely, the strong overlap between anxiety and depression. Countless studies have shown that self-report measures of anxiety and depression are highly intercorrelated, with coefficients typically in the .50-to-.80 range (Clark & Watson, 1991b; Feldman, 1993; Mineka, Watson, & Clark, 1998; Watson, Weber, et al., 1995). This finding is highly robust and has been observed in college students (Gotlib, 1984; Joiner, 1996; Watson & Clark, 1992a; Watson, Weber, et al., 1995), children and adolescents (Brady & Kendall, 1992; Cole, Truglio, & Peeke, 1997; Wolfe et al., 1987) and community-dwelling adults (Orme, Reis, & Herz, 1986; Watson, Weber, et al., 1995). In a comprehensive review of the literature, Clark and I noted that somewhat better differentiation was obtained in psychiatric patient samples (Clark & Watson, 1991b); nevertheless, we concluded that even in patient samples, "self-ratings of anxiety and depression typically provide more information about the overall level of subjective distress than about the relative salience of depressive versus anxious symptomatology" (p. 326). This conclusion has been reinforced by several subsequent analyses demonstrating strong correlations between measures of depression and anxiety in clinical populations (Clark, Steer, & Beck, 1994; Jolly & Dykman, 1994; Lonigan, Carey, & Finch, 1994; Steer, Clark, Beck, & Ranieri, 1995).

Furthermore, this problem is not simply confined to self-report data. In fact, considerable overlap also is found in clinicians' ratings of depression and anxiety, although the level of differentiation in these data tends to be somewhat greater than in self-ratings (Clark & Watson, 1991b; Mineka et al., 1998). It currently is unclear, however, whether this improved differentiation represents (1) an increased sensitivity to subtle cues that patients themselves discount or are unaware of, which would imply that clinicians' ratings are more valid than self-ratings, or (2) rating biases on the part of clinicians, which would suggest that clinicians' ratings actually may be less valid than self-ratings (see Clark & Watson, 1991b; Mineka et al., 1998).

In this regard, it is noteworthy that clinicians', teachers', and parents' ratings of anxiety and depression in children show relatively little differentiation. Indeed, in their review of the literature, Brady and Kendall (1992) concluded that analyses of behavioral and observational ratings typically have yielded a single anxiety–depression factor in children (see also Cole et al., 1997). Again, however, it currently is unclear whether (1) these syndromes actually are less differentiated in children or (2) the scales used to assess child psychopathology are less adequate than those available for adults. Some evidence, however, suggests that child anxiety scales perform particularly poorly, and that ratings of anxiety differentiate less well between depressed and anxious children than do ratings of depression (Brady & Kendall, 1992).

Finally, substantial comorbidity has been observed at the diagnostic level (Clark, 1989; Maser & Cloninger, 1990; Mineka et al., 1998). For instance, in Clark's (1989) meta-analysis, 57% of those with major depression also met diagnostic criteria for one or more anxiety disorders. The National Comorbidity Survey (NCS) yielded remarkably similar data: Of those who met criteria for depression, 58% had one or more anxiety disorders during their lifetime, and 51.2% had an anxiety disorder during the preceding year (Kessler et al., 1996). Conversely, Clark's (1989) meta-analysis revealed that 56% of patients with an anxiety disorder also met diagnostic criteria for depression (see also Alloy, Kelly, Mineka, & Clements, 1990; Kessler et al., 1996; Mineka et al., 1998).

Development of the Two-Factor Affective Model

Why are depression and anxiety so difficult to distinguish empirically? My colleagues and I suspected that it would be helpful to consider the basic affective states that underlie these syndromes. Anxiety is an experience that is dominated by the emotion of fear (i.e., feelings of worry, apprehension, and dread), whereas depression centers on sadness (i.e., feelings of sorrow and gloom; see Izard, 1972, 1977; Watson & Kendall, 1989). As was discussed in detail in Chapter 2, ratings of fear, sadness, guilt, hostility, and other negative emotions all tend to be moderately to strongly interrelated because they all share a common component of general Negative Affect (see also Watson & Clark, 1992a). Extending this analysis to the clinical syndromes suggested that anxiety and depression are strongly intercorrelated because they both are centered around negative mood states and, therefore, share this common component of general Negative Affect. Put another way, general Negative Affect is a common feature of both depression and anxiety that accounts for the substantial overlap between them.

How, then, might anxiety and depression be differentiated? As I noted in Chapter 2, most types of negative mood (including fear) are essentially uncorrelated with positive affective experience. The one major exception is sadness, which tends to have moderate negative correlations with indicators of positive mood, particularly those reflecting joy and happiness. For instance, Table 2.4 reported correlations between the basic positive and negative mood scales of the PANAS-X. The PANAS-X Fear scale correlated only –.07 and –.02 with Joviality (i.e., feelings of happiness, enthusiasm, and energy) in moment and general ratings, respectively; in contrast, the corresponding correlations between Sadness and Joviality were –.34 and –.30, respectively. Extended to the clinical syndromes, data such as these strongly suggest that Positive Affect is much more relevant to depression than anxiety and, therefore, can serve to differentiate these syndromes.

Putting these considerations together, my colleagues and I proposed the following model: Anxiety is a state of high Negative Affect, and has no substantial connection to general Positive Affect; in contrast, depression is a mixed state that represents both high Negative Affect and low Positive Affect (Clark & Watson, 1991a; Clark et al., 1994; Watson, Clark, & Carey, 1988; Watson & Kendall, 1989). This affect-based model thus posits both a specific and a nonspecific factor. That is, Negative Affect is a nonspecific factor that is common to both depression and anxiety; as suggested earlier, the influence of this common factor helps to explain the strong associations between these syndromes. In contrast, (low) Positive Affect is relatively unique to depression. One important implication of this model is that the syndromes can be better differentiated by augmenting the assessment of the Positive Affect component—relative to the Negative Affect component—in measures of depression.

Evidence for the Two-Factor Affective Model

This two-factor model has received extensive support in the literature (Ahrens & Haaga, 1993; Dyck, Jolly, & Kramer, 1994; Joiner, 1996; Lonigan et al., 1994; Tellegen, 1985; Watson & Kendall, 1989). For instance, Blumberg and Izard (1986) used self-report emotion scales to predict anxiety and depression in children; consistent with the general pattern discussed earlier, anxiety and depression correlated .58 with one another. Multiple regression analyses indicated that fear was the best single predictor of anxiety, with various other negative affects (guilt, shame, sadness) also making lesser contributions. As expected, scales assessing positive emotions did not add significantly to the prediction of anxiety. In contrast, depression scores were best predicted by sadness; other negative affect scales (hostility, anger, fear) also made modest contributions. Most important—and consistent with our two-factor model—the two assessed Positive Affect scales (Joy and Interest) contributed significantly to the prediction of depression.

Similarly, Jolly, Dyck, Kramer and Wherry (1994) examined correlations between Negative and Positive Affect and symptoms of depression and anxiety in an outpatient sample. Consistent with our model, Negative Affect scores were strongly related to individual symptoms of both anxiety and depression, with mean correlations of .53 and .51, respectively. In contrast, Positive Affect scores were much more strongly associated with depression (mean $r = -.42$) than with anxiety (mean $r = -.27$). Moreover, after controlling for the influence of Negative Affect, the significant associations between Positive Affect and anxiety essentially vanished, leading the authors to conclude that "low positive affectivity (PA) was significantly related only to depressive symptoms" (p. 544).

Other support has come from factor-analytic investigations of anxiety and depression symptoms (Joiner, Catanzaro, & Laurent, 1996; Watson, Clark, et al., 1995). For example, Clark, Beck, and Beck (1994) subjected the items included in the Beck Anxiety Inventory (BAI; Beck, Epstein, Brown, & Steer, 1988) and BDI (Beck, Rush, Shaw, & Emery, 1979) to a principal factor analysis in a college student sample. They were able to extract well-defined factors representing anxiety and depression. Consistent with our two-factor model, a measure of trait Negative Affect was substantially correlated with both the anxiety ($r = .43$) and depression ($r = .47$) factors; importantly, these strong associations were maintained even after statistically controlling for trait Positive Affect (partial $r = .40$ and .37, respectively). In contrast—and as expected—trait Positive Affect was strongly correlated with depression ($r = -.47$) but not anxiety ($r = -.18$). Moreover, after statistically controlling for trait Negative Affect, its correlation with depression remained substantial ($r = -.36$), whereas its correlation with anxiety was weak and nonsignificant ($r = -.08$).

Thus far, I have considered only self-report symptoms; however, similar findings emerge when structured interview data are analyzed. Table 8.1 presents results from a sample of 150 psychiatric patients (previously reported in Watson, Clark, & Carey, 1988). Trait Negative and Positive Affect were assessed using the Negative and Positive Emotionality scales, respectively, of the MPQ (Tellegen, in press). Symptom and diagnostic data were obtained from each respondent using Version 3.0 of the Diagnostic Interview Schedule (DIS; Robins, Helzer, Croughan, & Ratcliff, 1981) according to DSM-III (American Psychiatric Association, 1980) criteria.

The upper portion of Table 8.1 reports correlations between trait Negative and Positive Affect and the number of clinically present symptoms in each of four areas—panic disorder, obsessive–compulsive disorder (OCD), phobias, and depression—whereas the lower section presents

TABLE 8.1. Correlations of Negative and Positive Emotionality with Symptoms and Diagnoses of Anxiety and Depression in a Psychiatric Patient Sample

Symptom/diagnostic index	Negative emotionality	Positive emotionality
Symptom indices		
No. of panic symptoms	.36**	−.15
No. of obsessive–compulsive symptoms	.37**	−.13
No. of phobias	.25**	−.11
No. of depressive symptoms	.57**	−.40**
Anxiety disorders		
Obsessive–compulsive disorder	.39**	−.12
Simple phobia	.16*	−.01
Social phobia	.20*	−.23*
Any anxiety diagnosis	.32**	−.12
Depressive disorders		
Major depression	.50**	−.41**
Dysthymic disorder	.39**	−.37**
Any depressive diagnosis	.51**	−.38**

Note. $N = 150$. Data adapted from Tables 1–3 of Watson, Clark, and Carey (1988). All diagnoses are scored dichotomously (0 = absent, 1 = present).
*$p < .05$, two-tailed; **$p < .01$, two-tailed.

corresponding coefficients with DIS-derived diagnoses (scored dichotomously, where 0 = absent and 1 = present). As expected, Negative Affect was broadly related to symptoms and diagnoses of both depression and anxiety, with correlations ranging from .16 to .57. Moreover, follow-up analyses indicated that it was significantly correlated with 18 of the 33 individual anxiety complaints (median $r = .22$) and with 19 of the 20 depression symptoms (median $r = .28$).

Consistent with our two-factor model, Positive Affect was moderately correlated with the number of depressive symptoms but was unrelated to all three anxiety symptom indices. Follow-up analyses indicated that it was significantly correlated with 11 of the 20 individual depression symptoms (median $r = −.25$) but with only 3 of 33 anxiety symptoms (median $r = −.10$). Positive Affect also correlated significantly with the diagnoses of both major depression and dysthymic disorder; among the anxiety disorders, however, it was significantly related only to social phobia. This significant connection with social phobia is not surprising in view of the strong links between Positive Affect and both Extraversion (Chapter 6) and social activity (Chapter 3). This is a robust finding that has emerged in several other studies as well (Amies, Gelder, & Shaw, 1983;

Brown, Chorpita, & Barlow, 1998; Trull & Sher, 1994); it has interesting implications for our model, which I explore subsequently.

THE TRIPARTITE MODEL OF ANXIETY AND DEPRESSION

Development of the Tripartite Model

Our two-factor model continues to show an impressive ability to explain key aspects of the mood and anxiety disorders. Nevertheless, my colleagues and I quickly became aware of its limitations. One notable limitation is that it fails to articulate a unique factor (paralleling the role of low Positive Affect in depression) that is specific to anxiety. Fortunately, Clark and I subsequently were able to identify a second specific factor that is relatively unique to anxiety: After reviewing a wide range of evidence, we concluded that symptoms of physiological hyperarousal are more strongly characteristic of anxiety than depression (Clark & Watson, 1991b).

This conclusion was based on three lines of evidence. First, content analyses indicated that anxiety scales with the best discriminant validity (i.e., having the lowest correlations with depression) tended to measure the somatic symptoms of anxiety rather than anxious mood per se. Second, autonomic manifestations of panic disorder (e.g., dizziness and racing heart) reliably differentiated anxious and depressed patient groups, whereas other types of anxiety symptoms did not. Third, factor-analytic investigations consistently identified three meaningful symptom dimensions. The three replicable dimensions consisted of (1) a general neurotic factor that included feelings of inferiority and rejection, oversensitivity to criticism, and anxious and depressed mood (i.e., general Negative Affect); (2) a specific depression factor that was defined by the loss of interest or pleasure (note that clinicians often use the term "anhedonia" to describe the pervasive loss of pleasure that frequently is manifested in depression), anorexia, crying spells, and suicidal ideation; and (3) a specific anxiety factor that was defined by items reflecting tension, shakiness, and panic (Clark & Watson, 1991b).

Putting all this evidence together, we proposed that a tripartite model best captures the underlying structure of depression and anxiety (Clark & Watson, 1991b). In this model, symptoms of anxiety and depression are grouped into three basic subtypes. First, many relevant symptoms are strong indicators of general Negative Affect. These symptoms are relatively nonspecific—that is, they are commonly experienced by both anxious and depressed individuals. This nonspecific group includes both anxious and depressed mood as well as other symptoms that are prevalent in both types of disorder, such as insomnia, restlessness, irritability, and poor concentration. In addition to these nonspecific symptoms, each syndrome is characterized further by a cluster of relatively unique symptoms: Somatic tension and hyperarousal (e.g., shortness of breath, dizziness and lightheadedness, and dry mouth) are relatively specific to anxiety, whereas manifestations of anhedonia and the absence of Positive Affect (e.g., loss of interest and feeling that nothing is interesting or enjoyable) are relatively specific to depression.

Subsequent Support for the Tripartite Model

Early Studies

The formulation of this tripartite model has stimulated a new wave of research into the structure of anxious and depressive symptoms (see Mineka et al., 1998). Several early studies—published within a few years of the formulation of the model in 1991—subjected existing psychometric instruments to exploratory factor analyses. Consistent with the tripartite model, these studies found clear evidence of three factors: a specific anxiety factor, a specific depression factor, and a general factor that contained symptoms relevant to both syndromes (Clark, Beck, & Stewart, 1990; Jolly & Dykman, 1994; Jolly & Kramer, 1994).

Unfortunately, these early studies were forced to rely on measures that were not explicitly designed to assess the major symptom groups of the tripartite model; most notably, most of these instruments were heavily laden with items assessing general Negative Affect but covered the two specific symptom groups (i.e., somatic hyperarousal and anhedonia/low Positive Affect) less satisfactorily. The paucity of good hyperarousal and/or anhedonia items (particularly the latter) made it difficult to identify specific dimensions that closely matched the predictions generated by the tripartite model. Nevertheless, several investigators managed to identify structures that strongly supported this model, finding evidence of (1) a general Negative Affect factor, (2) a specific anxiety factor that was primarily defined by symptoms of somatic arousal, and (3) a specific depression factor characterized by anhedonia and hopelessness (Clark et al., 1994; Steer et al., 1995; Steer, Clark, & Ranieri, 1994).

Analyses of the MASQ

Nevertheless, to address the measure-based limitations of these early studies, Clark and I created the 90-item Mood and Anxiety Symptom Questionnaire (MASQ; Watson & Clark, 1991a), which we used in two studies that examined key aspects of the tripartite model. In one of these

studies, Watson, Clark, et al. (1995) subjected the 90 MASQ items to separate principal factor analyses in each of five samples (three student, one
adult, one patient). Consistent with the tripartite model, the same three
dimensions could be identified in each data set: a nonspecific factor of
general Negative Affect, a bipolar dimension of positive mood versus
anhedonia, and a factor defined largely by somatic manifestations of anxiety. However, this specific anxiety factor was somewhat broader than expected and included several somatic symptoms that do not clearly reflect
sympathetic arousal (e.g., nausea and diarrhea). Consequently, this third
factor probably is better characterized as somatic anxiety rather than somatic hyperarousal per se.

In a second study, Watson, Weber, et al. (1995) tested the key prediction that symptoms of somatic arousal and anhedonia offer the best differentiation of anxiety and depression. Two pairs of anxiety and depression scales were created from the MASQ items. One set (the "specific"
scales) was composed of items assessing anhedonia/low Positive Affect
and somatic arousal—that is, items that are hypothesized to be relatively
unique to depression and anxiety, respectively, in the tripartite model.
The second pair (the "nonspecific" scales) was composed primarily of
symptoms reflecting depressed and anxious mood, as well as other symptoms predicted to be relatively nonspecific in the tripartite model. Clearly,
the tripartite model would predict that the correlation between the two
specific scales should be substantially lower than that between the two
nonspecific scales. This prediction was strongly confirmed in each of five
samples.

It is instructive to examine these MASQ scales in greater detail. The
90 MASQ items were culled from the symptom criteria for the anxiety
and mood disorders in DSM-III-R (American Psychiatric Association,
1987). The tripartite model then was used to group these items into five
scales, only four of which need concern us here. As noted earlier, one pair
of scales is composed of symptoms that—according to the tripartite
model—should be strongly related to general Negative Affect and, therefore, relatively nonspecific to depression and anxiety. Thus, the General
Distress: Anxious Symptoms scale (GD: Anxiety; 11 items) contains several indicators of anxious mood (e.g., felt nervous and felt afraid), as well
as other symptoms of anxiety disorder that were hypothesized to be relatively nondifferentiating (e.g., inability to relax and diarrhea). Conversely,
the General Distress: Depressive Symptoms scale (GD: Depression; 12
items) includes several items reflecting depressed mood (e.g., felt depressed, felt sad, felt discouraged), along with other relatively nonspecific
symptoms of mood disorder (e.g., feelings of disappointment and failure,
self-blame, and pessimism).

In contrast, the second pair is composed of symptoms that were hypothesized to be relatively specific to either anxiety or depression. Anxious Arousal (17 items) includes various symptoms of somatic tension and hyperarousal (e.g., feeling dizzy or lightheaded, shortness of breath, dry mouth, frequent urination, and shaking hands). Conversely, Anhedonic Depression (22 items) contains 8 items that directly assess the loss of interest and pleasure (e.g., felt bored, slowed down, felt that nothing was interesting or enjoyable, and felt withdrawn from other people), as well as 14 reverse-keyed items that assess positive emotional experiences (e.g., felt cheerful, optimistic, "up"; had a lot of energy; and looked forward to things with enjoyment). Preliminary analyses demonstrated that these two sets of Anhedonic Depression items were strongly intercorrelated, thereby justifying their combination in a single scale (see Watson, Weber, et al., 1995).

To date, correlational analyses of these MASQ scales are available in eight large samples, with a combined *N* of more than 3,600 respondents. Data from five of these samples (Student 1, Student 2, Student 3, Adult, Patient) were reported in the two MASQ-based studies noted previously (Watson, Clark, et al., 1995; Watson, Weber, et al., 1995). Data from an additional student sample (Student 4) were presented in Watson and Walker (1996); these respondents actually were former students at SMU, who were assessed on the MASQ following graduation. The seventh sample (Student 5) is based on an unpublished study that I conducted at the University of Iowa. Finally, findings from a large sample of University of Illinois undergraduates (Student 6) were reported in Nitschke, Heller, Imig, and Miller (1997).

The tripartite model clearly predicts that the correlation between the two nonspecific scales (i.e., GD: Anxiety and GD: Depression) should be substantially higher than that between the two specific scales (i.e., Anxious Arousal and Anhedonic Depression). Before examining these correlations, however, I first must consider the issue of *convergent validity*. One could plausibly argue that in the process of creating these specific scales, we lost the essence of the underlying syndromes; put another way, it is possible that these new scales no longer are clearly recognizable as measures of anxiety and depression.

The easiest way to test this idea is to correlate these specific scales with other, more traditional measures of the target syndromes. Accordingly, Table 8.2 presents correlations between the MASQ specific scales and their nonspecific counterparts in each of the eight samples. These data clearly establish that the two sets of measures converge quite well, with weighted mean correlations of .71 (anxiety) and .70 (depression) across the eight data sets. These findings indicate that convergent validity was not seriously compromised in the creation of the MASQ specific scales.

TABLE 8.2. Convergent Correlations between the MASQ Anxiety and
Depression Scales

Sample	N	GD: Anxiety vs. Anxious Arousal	GD: Depression vs. Anhedonic Depression
Student 1 (SMU)	516	.71	.68
Student 2 (SMU)	381	.71	.68
Student 3 (SMU)	516	.68	.71
Student 4 (SMU)	334	.72	.73
Student 5 (Iowa)	312	.81	.70
Student 6 (Illinois)	772	.62	.66
Adults	328	.69	.72
VA patients	470	.78	.72
Weighted mean r		.71	.70

Note. All correlations are significant at $p < .01$, two-tailed. MASQ, Mood and
Anxiety Symptom Questionnaire; GD, General Distress; SMU, Southern
Methodist University; VA, Veterans Administration.

Furthermore, respondents in three samples also were assessed on the
BAI and BDI. The Beck inventories are among the best validated and most
widely used instruments in the contemporary literature; they therefore offer particularly compelling evidence of convergent validity. Table 8.3 reports correlations between the Beck inventories and the MASQ scales. Not
surprisingly, the nonspecific scales display excellent convergent validity in
relation to the Beck inventories, with weighted mean correlations of .69
(BAI vs. GD: Anxiety) and .69 (BDI vs. GD: Depression). Note, however,
that the two specific scales demonstrate a similarly high level of convergent

TABLE 8.3. Convergent Correlations between the MASQ Anxiety and Depression Scales
and the Beck Inventories

Sample	N	BAI correlations		BDI correlations	
		GD: Anxiety	Anxious Arousal	GD: Depression	Anhedonic Depression
Student 3 (SMU)	516	.71	.72	.67	.60
Student 6 (Illinois)	772	.65	.72	.69	.60
Adults	328	.76	.79	.71	.68
Weighted mean r		.69	.74	.69	.62

Note. All correlations are significant at $p < .01$, two-tailed. MASQ, Mood and Anxiety
Symptom Questionnaire; GD, General Distress; SMU, Southern Methodist University.

validity, with weighted mean correlations of .74 (BAI vs. Anxious Arousal) and .62 (BDI vs. Anhedonic Depression). Thus, the MASQ specific scales clearly are recognizable as measures of anxiety and depression (for further discussion of this issue, see Watson, Weber, et al., 1995).

Turning now to discriminant validity, Table 8.4 presents the discriminant correlations among the MASQ anxiety and depression scales in each of the eight data sets, along with weighted mean correlations collapsed across all samples. As I have discussed, the tripartite model predicts that the GD: Anxiety and GD: Depression scales should be highly intercorrelated and display poor discriminant validity. This prediction has been strongly and consistently confirmed. Across the eight data sets, the discriminant correlations range from .61 to .78, with a weighted average of .69; this weighted mean coefficient indicates that these two scales share nearly half of their variance with one another.

The tripartite model further predicts that the syndromes will become better differentiated as the specific symptom clusters play an increasingly prominent role in their assessment. The data again strongly confirm this prediction. If we substitute Anxious Arousal for GD: Anxiety, the average discriminant correlation drops substantially from .69 to .52. We can achieve even better differentiation, however, by substituting Anhedonic Depression for GD: Depression; indeed, the weighted mean correlation between GD: Anxiety and Anhedonic Depression is only .42. Clearly, however, the best differentiation is obtained using both of the specific

TABLE 8.4. Discriminant Correlations among the MASQ Anxiety and Depression Scales

Sample	N	GD: Dep vs. GD: Anx	GD: Dep vs. AnxArous	GD: Anx vs. AnheDep	AnxArous vs. AnheDep
Student 1 (SMU)	516	.68[a]	.57[b]	.38[c]	.31[d]
Student 2 (SMU)	381	.67[a]	.47[b]	.41[b]	.28[c]
Student 3 (SMU)	516	.61[a]	.46[b]	.39[b]	.25[c]
Student 4 (SMU)	334	.69[a]	.52[b]	.42[b]	.32[c]
Student 5 (Iowa)	312	.75[a]	.66[b]	.47[c]	.41[c]
Student 6 (Illinois)	772	.64[a]	.43[b]	.32[c]	.20[d]
Adults	328	.69[a]	.49[b]	.41[b,c]	.38[c]
VA patients	470	.78[a]	.59[b]	.60[b]	.49[c]
Weighted mean r		.69[a]	.52[b]	.42[c]	.32[d]

Note. All correlations are significant at $p < .01$, two-tailed. Within a sample, correlations not sharing the same superscript differ significantly from one another at $p < .05$, two-tailed. MASQ, Mood and Anxiety Symptom Questionnaire; GD: Anx, General Distress: Anxiety; AnxArous, Anxious Arousal; GD: Dep, General Distress: Depression; AnheDep, Anhedonic Depression; SMU, Southern Methodist University; VA, Veterans Administration.

scales. In fact, the average correlation between Anxious Arousal and Anhedonic Depression is only .32. Overall, substituting the specific scales for the nonspecific scales reduces the overlapping variance between anxiety and depression from approximately 48% to only 10%. Thus, it is quite possible to distinguish depression from anxiety; the key is to focus assessment primarily on the unique symptoms that define each syndrome.

Other Support for the Tripartite Model

Several recent studies have broadened the empirical support for the tripartite model. For instance, Joiner et al. (1996) showed that the three hypothesized factors emerged in a sample of child and adolescent psychiatric inpatients, thereby extending the model to younger respondents. Joiner (1996) explicitly tested the viability of a three-factor model—consisting of general Negative Affect, anhedonia/low Positive Affect, and somatic arousal—in college students using confirmatory factor analysis. Supporting the tripartite model, Joiner found that it provided an excellent fit to the observed data, whereas one- and two-factor structures did not. Chorpita, Albano, and Barlow (1998) replicated and extended these results using confirmatory factor analysis in a clinical sample of children and adolescents, again finding that the hypothesized three-factor model best fit the data. It is noteworthy that whereas all previous studies relied solely on self-report data, Chorpita et al. (1998) based their analyses on both self- and parent ratings. Similarly, Brown et al. (1998) obtained evidence supporting the tripartite model in structural modeling analyses of both self-report and interview-based data.

Recent psychophysiological analyses offer further, indirect support for the tripartite model by demonstrating that the three hypothesized symptom groups reflect highly distinctive patterns of brain activity (Mineka et al., 1998). Specifically, individuals reporting elevated levels of general Negative Affect consistently show exaggerated startle reactions in response to negative stimuli (Cook, Hawk, Davis, & Stevenson, 1991; Lang, Bradley, & Cuthbert, 1992; Lang, Bradley, Cuthbert, & Patrick, 1993); this exaggerated startle response is thought to be mediated within the limbic system by the bed nucleus of the stria terminalis (Cuthbert et al., 1997). Other evidence has linked heightened levels of Negative Affect to increased activity in the right frontal cortex (see Chapter 7).

The two specific symptom clusters—anhedonia and anxious arousal—show markedly different patterns of psychophysiological activity. Anxious arousal consistently has been linked to *hyper*activation of the right parietotemporal region (Bruder et al., 1996, 1997; Heller, 1993; Heller, Etienne, & Miller, 1995). In sharp contrast, anhedonia and low Positive Affect are associated with *hypo*activation of this same region (Bruder et al., 1996, 1997; Heller, 1993; Heller et al., 1995), as well as hypoactivation of the left prefrontal area (Larsen et al., 1995; Tomarken & Keener, 1998). As I discussed in Chapter 7, it appears that this latter finding reflects stable individual differences in temperament.

In a related vein, recent evidence indicates that symptoms of anxious arousal are genetically distinct from other manifestations of anxiety and depression (Mineka et al., 1998). These data are worth considering in some detail. Beginning in the 1980s, numerous studies have examined the genetic links among the mood and anxiety disorders, primarily investigating whether a common genetic diathesis might render certain individuals vulnerable to multiple syndromes. The first major analysis was reported by Jardine, Martin, and Henderson (1984), who investigated anxious and depressive symptoms in a sample of Australian twins. Their data indicated that the observed phenotypic covariation between the two types of symptoms was largely due to a single common genetic factor (see also Kendler, Heath, Martin, & Eaves, 1987). Moreover, this same genetic factor was shared with Neuroticism, a trait that reflects individual differences in trait Negative Affect (see Chapter 6). Thus, their findings indicated that anxiety and depression could be linked to a single genetic diathesis that apparently represents an underlying vulnerability to experience Negative Affect. Put another way, these researchers had identified the apparent genetic basis of the general Negative Affect component of the tripartite model.

Subsequent analyses of these same data, however, revealed that panic-related symptoms of anxious arousal (e.g., "breathless or heart pounding") were associated with a specific genetic factor that differentiated them from other symptoms of depression and anxiety (Kendler et al., 1987) and from Neuroticism/trait Negative Affect (Martin, Jardine, Andrews, & Heath, 1988). Thus, these symptom-level data provided clear evidence of two distinct genetic factors, one broadly linked to general individual differences in Negative Affect (and, therefore, nonspecific to depression and anxiety) and the other more specifically focused on the somatic manifestations of panic.

This same basic pattern subsequently has been observed at the diagnostic level. Analyses consistently have found that major depression and GAD are genetically indistinguishable; that is, they reflect a single, common genetic diathesis (Kendler, 1996; Kendler, Neale, Kessler, Heath, & Eaves, 1992; Roy, Neale, Pedersen, Mathé, & Kendler, 1995). Moreover, replicating results at the symptom level, Kendler, Neale, Kessler, Heath, and Eaves (1993a) found that this common genetic diathesis also was strongly linked to individual differences in Neuroticism. On the basis of these data, Kendler and his colleagues have argued that this shared genetic factor represents a general tendency to respond poorly to stressful life experiences and, therefore, to experience frequent and intense episodes of Negative Affect (Kendler et al., 1992; Kendler et al., 1995).

Again, however, several studies have reported that panic disorder is genetically distinguishable from both GAD and major depression (Kendler, 1996; Kendler et al., 1995; Reich, 1993; Weissman, 1993; Woodman, 1993), thereby replicating the symptom-level results. For instance, Kendler et al. (1995) examined the genetic links among major depression, GAD, panic, and the phobias. They found evidence of two significant genetic factors. One factor was primarily defined by major depression and GAD, and clearly represented a nonspecific dimension of general distress/Negative Affect. In contrast, the second factor was primarily defined by panic disorder and the phobias.

Thus, consistent with the tripartite model, twin studies have identified two distinct genetic diatheses that represent (1) general Negative Affect and (2) the somatic manifestations of panic (i.e., anxious arousal). Regrettably, symptoms reflecting anhedonia and low Positive Affect were not examined in any of these studies.

AN INTEGRATIVE HIERARCHICAL MODEL OF ANXIETY AND DEPRESSION

The Heterogeneity of the Anxiety Disorders

Although these data offer strong support for several key aspects of the tripartite model, they also have exposed its limitations. As the evidence has accumulated, it has become painfully clear that the anxiety disorders are quite heterogeneous and subsume a diverse array of symptoms (Brown et al., 1998; Mineka et al., 1998; Zinbarg & Barlow, 1996). In light of this heterogeneity, it is apparent that a single specific factor—such as the anxious arousal component of the tripartite model—is insufficient to account fully for the enormous diversity of symptoms that define the anxiety disorders.

The heterogeneity of the anxiety disorders has been established at both the genotypic and phenotypic levels. At the genotypic level, I noted earlier that panic disorder is genetically distinguishable from GAD (as well as depression). Other evidence, however, indicates that OCD is genetically distinct from major depression, GAD, panic disorder, and the phobias (Pauls, Leckman, & Cohen, 1994); in fact, unlike these other disorders, OCD apparently has a strong genetic link to Tourette syndrome (Pauls, 1992; Pauls, Alsobrook, Goodman, Rasmussen, & Leckman, 1995). Moreover, the phobias (e.g., social phobia, situational phobia, and animal phobia) themselves are genetically heterogeneous and reflect multiple diatheses (Kendler, Neale, Kessler, Heath, & Eaves, 1993b). The genetic diversity of the anxiety disorders is further highlighted by their differential communalities with major depression: The available data indicate that depression is genetically indistinguishable from GAD, moderately related to panic, and more modestly related to the phobias (e.g., Kendler et al., 1995; Mineka et al., 1998). Thus, a simple dual-diathesis model (consisting of general Negative Affect and anxious arousal) cannot account for the genetic factors that give rise to the anxiety disorders.

Similar findings have been reported at the phenotypic level. For instance, recent structural analyses have shown that multiple specific factors are needed to capture the diversity of anxiety-related symptoms (Brown et al., 1998; Spence, 1997; Zinbarg & Barlow, 1996). Moreover, closely paralleling the genetic evidence, although depression is strongly related to symptoms of GAD, it shows more moderate associations with symptoms of the other anxiety disorders (Brown et al., 1998). Finally, the individual anxiety disorders are differentially related to one another. For example, Brown et al. (1998) found that GAD was strongly related to both panic disorder and OCD, but that the latter two disorders were only modestly associated with one another.

Barlow's Hierarchical Model of the Anxiety Disorders

Barlow and his colleagues recently proposed a hierarchical model that neatly addresses the heterogeneity of the anxiety disorders (Barlow, 1991; Barlow & DiNardo, 1991; Brown & Barlow, 1992; Zinbarg & Barlow, 1996). Barlow asserts that each of the individual anxiety disorders contains a shared component in a two-level hierarchical scheme. This higher-order factor originally was labeled "anxious apprehension" (Barlow, 1991, Brown & Barlow, 1992); in subsequent papers, however, Barlow has acknowledged that it essentially represents the general Negative Affect component of the tripartite model (Brown et al., 1998; Zinbarg & Barlow, 1996). Consequently, this higher-order factor not only is common across the anxiety disorders but also is shared with depression. Therefore, it primarily is responsible for the observed overlap both (1) among the individual anxiety disorders and (2) between depression and anxiety.

In addition, each of the anxiety disorders also contains a specific, unique component that distinguishes it from all of the others. Thus, each disorder can be decomposed into (1) a common component of general Negative Affect that is shared with all of the others, plus (2) a specific component that uniquely defines it. Spence (1997) recently proposed and tested a parallel model of the childhood anxiety disorders.

Several recent structural analyses have yielded strong support for this hierarchical organization of the anxiety disorders (Brown et al., 1998; Spence, 1997; Zinbarg & Barlow, 1996). The results of Brown et al. (1998) are particularly interesting in light of my lengthy consideration of the tripartite model. They found that anxious arousal was not broadly characteristic of the anxiety disorders; rather, it essentially represented the specific, unique component of panic disorder. Indeed, after eliminating the influence of general Negative Affect, anxious arousal was found to be largely unrelated to both OCD and social phobia and *negatively* related to GAD.

An Integrative, Hierarchical Model of Anxiety and Depression

After reviewing the recent literature, Mineka et al. (1998) proposed an expanded structural model that integrates key features of our tripartite model with Barlow's hierarchical organization of the anxiety disorders. In this integrative, hierarchical model, each individual syndrome can be viewed as containing both a common and a unique component. Following the original logic of the tripartite model, this shared component represents broad individual differences in Negative Affect; it is a pervasive higher-order factor that is (1) common to both the mood and anxiety disorders and (2) primarily responsible for the observed overlap among these disorders. In addition, however, each disorder also includes a unique component that differentiates it from all the others. For instance, anhedonia, disinterest, and the absence of Positive Affect comprise the core features of the specific component of depression.

Of course, these assertions are fully consistent with the original tripartite model. The major change is that anxious arousal no longer is viewed as broadly characteristic of all anxiety disorders; rather, it assumes a much more limited role as the specific component of panic disorder (Brown et al., 1998; Mineka et al., 1998). Each of the other anxiety disorders has its own unique component that is distinct from anxious arousal. One possible exception is GAD, which is strongly saturated with nonspecific Negative Affect and, therefore, may not have a well-defined specific component of its own (Barlow & DiNardo, 1991; Brown & Barlow, 1992; Brown et al., 1998).

FUTURE DIRECTIONS: CLARIFYING THE ROLE OF AFFECT IN PSYCHOPATHOLOGY

Clarifying the Relation between Negative Affect and Psychological Disorder

The Ubiquity of Negative Affect in Psychopathology

I believe that this integrative, hierarchical model offers an accurate representation of the existing data and, moreover, that it will provide a valuable heuristic guide for future work in this area. Nevertheless, it is clear that this model—similar to the others I have discussed—also has some important limitations and needs to be extended and clarified in future research. One notable problem with it—and with all other existing models in this area—is its somewhat sketchy and undeveloped characterization of the higher-order Negative Affect dimension.

The precision and scope of the model can be enhanced by careful consideration of two additional issues concerning the role of Negative Affect in psychopathology. First, all these affect-based models assume that Negative Affect is a general, nonspecific factor across the mood and anxiety disorders. This assumption is not wrong, but it does not go far enough. The available data clearly establish that this factor is not confined solely to the mood and anxiety disorders but is much more broadly related to psychopathology (Hinden, Compas, Howell, & Achenbach, 1997; Steer et al., 1994; Watson & Clark, 1984, 1995). Significant elevations in Negative Affect and Neuroticism have been reported in an enormous array of syndromes, including substance use disorders (Krueger, Caspi, Moffitt, Silva, & McGee, 1996; Sher & Trull, 1994; Trull & Sher, 1994), somatoform disorders (Kirmayer, Robbins, & Paris, 1994), eating disorders (Vitousek & Manke, 1994), personality and conduct disorders (Krueger et al., 1996; Widiger & Costa, 1994; Widiger & Trull, 1992), and schizophrenia (Berenbaum & Fujita, 1994).

Indeed, it has become increasingly apparent that most DSM syndromes can be linked to individual differences in Negative Affect. The pervasiveness of Negative Affect in psychopathology is unsurprising, given that subjective distress is one of the defining criteria of psychological disorder (American Psychiatric Association, 1994). Nevertheless, it has yet to be fully incorporated into major structural models of psychopathology, including those formulated by my colleagues and myself. Future investigators should expand the scope of this model by incorporating a much broader range of associated phenomena, such as the personality and somatoform disorders.

Quantifying the Size
of the Negative Affect Component

Second, it now is quite clear that the size of this general Negative Affect component differs markedly across various disorders, including the individual anxiety disorders. For example, both the genetic and the phenotypic data establish that depression and GAD are distress-based disorders containing an enormous amount of variance attributable to general Negative Affect. Indeed, as noted earlier, GAD may be so strongly saturated with this nonspecific variance that it essentially represents a disorder of elevated Negative Affect (Barlow & DiNardo, 1991; Brown & Barlow, 1992; Brown et al., 1998). Interestingly, several investigators have reached essentially the same conclusion regarding borderline personality disorder, arguing that it simply may represent "an extreme variant of Neuroticism" (Widiger & Trull, 1992, p. 369; see also Widiger & Costa, 1994; Wiggins & Pincus, 1989). In contrast, many of the anxiety disorders—including OCD, social phobia, and specific phobia—contain a more modest component of Negative Affect (Brown et al., 1998; Kendler, 1996; Kendler et al., 1995). Future research should move beyond the simple truism that each disorder is characterized by both a common and a unique component and instead seek to quantify the proportions of general and specific variance that characterize each syndrome.

Research along these lines can help to clarify three key issues: (1) comorbidity, (2) etiology, and (3) taxonomy. With regard to comorbidity, this shared component of general Negative Affect is primarily responsible for the observed overlap among the mood and anxiety disorders. Accordingly, evidence that establishes the size of the nonspecific component can be used to provide meaningful estimates of the phenotypic overlap between two disorders even before good comorbidity data actually become available. That is, all other things being equal, two disorders containing large Negative Affect components can be expected to be highly comorbid, whereas two syndromes with relatively small nonspecific components should be less comorbid. More generally, evidence regarding the relative salience of this nonspecific component can provide a useful organizing scheme for understanding comorbidity patterns across multiple syndromes.

Comorbidity data, in turn, can yield important insights into the underlying etiology of disorder. One striking aspect of the anxiety–depression data is the extent to which the phenotypic evidence has closely paralleled findings at the genotypic level. For instance, phenotypic analyses consistently have revealed that depression is differentially related to the individual anxiety disorders; generally speaking, depression shows the greatest overlap with GAD and its weakest associations with certain types of specific phobia (Brown et al., 1998; Clark, Beck, & Beck, 1994; Mineka et al., 1998). The genotypic data show a strikingly similar pattern, indicating that depression is genetically indistinguishable from GAD, more moderately related to panic, and only weakly related to the phobias (e.g., Kendler et al., 1995; Mineka et al., 1998). Thus, clarifying the nature of the phenotypic associations among disorders can be expected to produce parallel increases in our understanding of the underlying genetic diatheses.

Finally, these data have potentially important taxonomic implications. As I have discussed, depression and GAD are both distress-based disorders with large components of general Negative Affect. Not surprisingly, therefore, these disorders show a close affinity with one another. In fact, genetic, comorbidity, and structural modeling data all establish that GAD is more closely linked to major depression than to the other anxiety disorders (Brown, Antony, & Barlow, 1995; Brown et al., 1998; Kendler et al., 1995; Mineka et al., 1998). This, in turn, suggests that classification within the DSM might be improved by reorganizing the mood and anxiety disorders to place greater emphasis on the close affinity between these distress-based disorders.

For instance, the mood and anxiety disorders could be combined into a superordinate class of *distress disorders* (Clark et al., 1994). One possibility would be to define this new category quite broadly to include all the current mood and anxiety disorders. Alternatively, it might make more sense to restrict it to those disorders with a strong general distress component. This more restrictive conceptualization certainly would subsume GAD and major depression; it also might include other disorders (e.g., borderline personality disorder, and dysthymic disorder) that have been strongly linked to individual differences in Negative Affectivity. It is noteworthy that most of the candidate syndromes for this proposed new class reflect chronic, long-term dysfunction and clearly have a strong characterological component. This, of course, is entirely consistent with the evidence indicating that depression, GAD, and Neuroticism all reflect a single genetic diathesis (Kendler et al., 1993a). Thus, these distress-based disorders appear to arise from a genetically inherited predisposition to experience frequent and intense episodes of Negative Affect (Kendler et al., 1992, 1995).

Another taxonomic approach would be to recognize formally that anxious and depressed mood are strongly intercorrelated and, therefore, that many patients essentially report elevated levels of nonspecific Negative Affect (Clark & Watson, 1991b; Clark, Watson, & Mineka, 1994). That is, rather than arbitrarily labeling distress as "anxious" or "depressed," it might be preferable to assign a nonspecific affective diagnosis, such as generalized affective disorder (Clark & Watson, 1991b) or mixed anxiety–depression (Katon & Roy-Byrne, 1991; Roy-Byrne, 1996; Zinbarg & Barlow, 1991; Zinbarg et al., 1994). Diagnosticians recently have made some important progress toward implementing this approach. Most notably, the nonspecific diagnosis of "mixed anxiety and depressive disorder" has been included in the 10th revision of the *International Classification of Diseases* (ICD-10; World Health Organization, 1992; see Sartorius, Üstün, Korten, Cooper, & van Drimmelen, 1995); furthermore, a provisional diagnosis of "mixed anxiety–depressive disorder" was examined in a DSM-IV field trial (Zinbarg et al., 1994) and has been included in the DSM-IV appendix for proposed diagnostic categories that merit further study (American Psychiatric Association, 1994).

Clarifying the Relation between Positive Affect and Psychological Disorder

Further Consideration of the Specificity of Positive Affect

In the integrative, hierarchical model, low Positive Affect is hypothesized to represent the core of the specific, unique component of depression. In support of this prediction, the data clearly demonstrate that measures of low Positive Affect (1) are substantially correlated with indicators of depression and (2) help to distinguish depression from other types of psychopathology. Nevertheless, the accumulating evidence also has established that low levels of Positive Affect are not confined solely to depressed individuals. For instance, I already have shown that social phobia consistently has been linked to low Positive Affect. In addition, low levels of Positive Affect have been observed in individuals diagnosed with agoraphobia and PTSD (Trull & Sher, 1994), eating disorder (Vitousek & Manke, 1994), substance disorders (Trull & Sher, 1994), and schizophrenia (Berenbaum & Fujita, 1994). Thus, although Positive Affect clearly shows much greater specificity than Negative Affect, low scores on this dimension are not uniquely characteristic of depression.

Clarifying the Links between Positive Affect and the Mood Disorders

Other evidence, however, suggests that low Positive Affect plays a particularly salient role in—and has an especially strong affinity with—the mood disorders. One striking aspect of these disorders is their cyclical, episodic course over time. This systematic temporal sequencing is an unusual component of the symptom picture, one that is not nearly as salient in most other disorders. For instance, the intensity of phobic fear does not vary systematically as a function of the hour of the day or the season of the year. Similarly, the compulsive rituals of individuals with OCD do not occur in well-defined episodes, with periods of extreme disturbance alternating with intervals of relative normalcy.

In sharp contrast, most of the mood disorders are characterized by well-defined cycles and episodes. The cyclicity of the mood disorders is most apparent in the bipolar disorders, in which the individual fluctuates between well-defined episodes of mania (or hypomania) and depression. The temporal patterning of unipolar depression is less dramatic, but it still is the case that this disorder tends to occur in episodes that may spontaneously remit over time (American Psychiatric Association, 1994). Moreover, the melancholic subtype—which is characterized by a "loss of pleasure in all, or almost all, activities" and/or a "lack of reactivity to usually pleasurable stimuli" (American Psychiatric Association, 1994,

p. 384)—frequently shows a marked diurnal pattern in which the symptoms are worst in the morning and then lessen in strength over the course of the day. Finally, both unipolar depression and bipolar disorder can show a marked seasonal pattern; in most cases, the onset of the depressive episode is in the fall or winter, with remission in the spring (American Psychiatric Association, 1994; Bauer & Dunner, 1993; Booker & Helleckson, 1992; see also Chapter 4).

Thus, symptoms of mood disorder tend to ebb and flow systematically over time, exhibiting recurring circadian and seasonal trends. As I discussed in Chapter 4, Positive Affect also shows these same basic cyclical patterns. These parallel cyclical patterns surely are not coincidental; indeed, the evidence strongly suggests that melancholic depression and bipolar disorder represent marked perturbations in the positive mood system (see Clark et al., 1994; Depue & Iacono, 1989; Depue et al., 1987). That is, mania and hypomania typically are episodes of extremely elevated Positive Affect (i.e., the individual feels elated and euphoric; he or she has also tremendous energy, confidence, and enthusiasm), whereas melancholic depression is characterized by a profound anhedonia and an almost total inability to experience pleasure (i.e., extremely low Positive Affect).

As I discussed in Chapter 4, cyclical rhythms are an endogenous, preprogrammed feature of positive moods and of the more general BFS. Cyclicity likely evolved to promote the efficient use of energy and bodily resources. Because the approach behaviors mediated by this system represent high-activation states, they should be emitted only when reward is relatively likely and the risk of danger is low; when the probability of reward is relatively low (e.g., because food is scarce), sluggish inactivity—which conserves precious energy—is more adaptive. Furthermore, for most species, the relative availability of resources—and the risk of harm—is a probabilistic function of time. For instance, in many of the world's ecosystems, food is much more plentiful in the spring and summer than during the dead of winter. Similarly, animals with poor night vision may have little hope of reward after dark. Accordingly, the function of these endogenous biological cycles is to maximize the probability that organisms will be active, alert, and energetic at those times that food and other resources are easily obtainable and the risk of harm is low; conversely, when these environmental conditions are not met, animals are preprogrammed to be sluggish and inactive.

Thus, preprogrammed periods of sluggishness and inactivity are an inherent feature of positive moods and the BFS; note, moreover, that mechanisms must have evolved to induce these recurring periods of quiescence. The sleep–wake cycle represents the most obvious example of such a mechanism. As discussed in Chapter 4, sleep has evolved as a highly efficient means of energy conservation. During periods of sleep (especially slow-wave sleep) the metabolic rate falls, so that animals burn fewer calories and require less food to survive (e.g., Berger & Phillips, 1995; Walker et al., 1979; Webb, 1979). The energy conservation function of sleep is most clearly seen in the case of hibernation, which essentially represents a prolonged episode of slow-wave sleep (Mrosovsky, 1988; Walker et al., 1979). Hibernation is associated with a marked reduction in the metabolic rate, thereby promoting survival during periods of food scarcity.

Various lines of evidence link depression to the sleep–wake cycle (e.g., Kupfer, 1976; 1995; Vogel, Neill, Hagler, & Kors, 1990; Wu & Bunney, 1990). For instance, the fall/winter depression observed in SAD appears to represent a hibernation-like state (Kasper & Rosenthal, 1989; Mrosovsky, 1988). Moreover, disordered sleep is one of the most prominent symptoms of depression (e.g., Kupfer, 1976, 1995). Sleep in depressed individuals (particularly those with melancholic depression) tends to be relatively shallow, with increased Stage 1 and reduced amounts of slow-wave sleep. In addition, insomnia is a common symptom in all forms of depression, with early morning awakening being particularly prominent in the melancholic subtype (American Psychiatric Association, 1994). Furthermore, the architecture of REM sleep is seriously disturbed in depressed individuals: REM episodes occur (1) unusually early in the NREM/REM cycle and (2) with unusual frequency during the early hours of sleep (e.g., Kupfer, 1976; Vogel, Vogel, McAbee, & Thurmond, 1980). Finally, sleep deprivation is one of the most effective short-term treatments for depression (e.g., Vogel, Buffenstein, Minter, & Hennesey, 1990; Wu & Bunney, 1990).

These considerations suggest that the depressive episodes seen in melancholic depression and bipolar disorder may have evolved as part of this energy conservation system (Beck, 1987; Clark & Watson, 1994; Nesse, 1991). Clearly, however, something has gone terribly wrong in these disorders, so that this normally adaptive system now is operating in a highly dysfunctional manner. What might account for this dysfunction? In the case of the bipolar disorders, it appears that faulty regulatory systems are at least partly responsible. As I discussed in Chapter 5, control mechanisms must have evolved to regulate the preprogrammed cyclicity of the BFS and to ensure that it is kept within reasonable bounds (Depue et al., 1987). It appears that the bipolar disorders reflect a pathological breakdown of these regulatory control mechanisms; this regulatory malfunction permits the system to vary in wildly exaggerated cycles, fluctuating between the extraordinary heights of mania and the profound depths of depression. The fall/winter depression seen in SAD undoubtedly involves some additional factors; for instance, Reme, Terman, and

Wirz-Justice (1990) have argued that it may arise from a deficiency in retinal photoreceptor mechanisms.

How, then, can we account for the profound anhedonia and other symptoms of melancholic depression? Three intriguing possibilities are suggested by the recent evidence in this area. The first two explanations arise from the enormous literature linking depression to sleep. First, melancholic depression may reflect a dysregulation of the normally adaptive circadian rhythms (Healy & Williams, 1988; Stroebel, 1985; Wehr & Wirz-Justice, 1982). As discussed in Chapter 4, circadian rhythms appear to be regulated by two biological control systems, the "strong oscillator" (which regulates body temperature and REM sleep) and the "weak oscillator" (which more strongly influences the general sleep–wake cycle). Both of these systems have been linked to variations in Positive Affect: Generally speaking, our positive mood levels are elevated when our body temperature is high and when we are the farthest removed from sleep.

The two oscillators normally work in close synchrony, which promotes adaptive functioning. That is, the synchrony of the two systems ensures that our body temperature will be relatively high (and, therefore, that we will feel alert, energetic, and enthusiastic) while we are awake and relatively low (thereby promoting restfulness and deep, slow-wave sleep) when we are asleep. Under certain circumstances, however, these two systems may become desynchronous, which clearly would have devastating consequences for the afflicted individual (Healy & Williams, 1988). Most notably, desynchrony could lead to a situation in which the body temperature was relatively low (with concomitant feelings of sluggishness, disinterest, and inattentiveness) during the waking hours and relatively high (producing restlessness and fitful, light sleep) at night. This desychrony model nicely explains both the (1) anhedonia and low Positive Affect and (2) insomnia and sleep disturbance experienced by many depressed individuals.

Second, Wu, and Bunney (1990) argue that a depressogenic substance is produced during sleep; this substance may play a key role in inducing the restfulness and relaxation of deep, slow-wave sleep. Wu and Bunney posit that this depressogenic substance gradually is metabolized during wakefulness, which would explain why levels of positive mood increase systematically during the first few hours following sleep (see Chapter 4). To test their model, Wu and Bunney (1990) examined extensive evidence regarding the association between sleep and depression, based on a meta-analysis of 61 studies. Across all these studies, Wu and Bunney found that 59% of depressed patients showed a marked decrease in depressive symptomatology following a night of total sleep deprivation; the improvement rate was even greater among those with melancholic depression. The patients who improved showed an interesting temporal course. Specifically, their initial depression gradually improved over the course of the first day and continued to improve throughout their sleepless night and the second day. After they were allowed to sleep during the second night, however, their depression returned in full force the following day. Furthermore, other evidence indicated that a relapse into depression could occur after naps as short as 90 seconds. Although these data are not conclusive, they are quite consistent with Wu and Bunney's (1990) model.

Wu and Bunney's (1990) model offers a parsimonious explanation for why (1) Positive Affect levels initially are low on awakening but then rise steadily during the morning and (2) symptoms of depression can be alleviated by sleep deprivation. It is less clear, however, why the release of this depressogenic substance should lead to a profound anhedonia only in certain afflicted individuals. The most likely possibility is that it stems from the more general disturbance in the sleep–wake cycle that is observed in depression. The regulatory mechanisms that control the release of this depressogenic substance likely respond to feedback concerning the depth, quality, and amount of sleep; once it is determined that sufficient sleep has been induced, these mechanisms would inhibit any further release of the substance (Wu & Bunney, 1990). Because depressed individuals tend to have light and fitful sleep, however, these regulatory mechanisms might fail to receive signals of sleep satiety and, therefore, would continue to stimulate the release of the substance over an abnormally extended period. This, in turn, would mean that depressed individuals would have an abnormally large quantity of the substance that would take unusually long to metabolize on awakening. This account also would explain why melancholic depression typically shows a marked diurnal pattern in which the symptoms are worst in the morning and then lessen in strength over the course of the day.

Third, melancholic depression may reflect a malfunction in the ascending dopamine system. As discussed in Chapter 7, the dopaminergic system mediates various approach-related behaviors (Depue et al., 1994; Depue & Iacono, 1989; Fibiger & Phillips, 1986; Wise & Rompre, 1989). Moreover, individual differences in Positive Affect have been linked to the strength of the system's response (Depue et al., 1994). It therefore appears that this system plays a key role in regulating the subjectively experienced "reward" that reinforces such goal-directed behaviors as eating and drinking.

Melancholic depression is characterized by "loss of pleasure in all, or almost all, activities" and/or "lack of reactivity to usually pleasurable stimuli" (American Psychiatric Association, 1994, p. 384). It therefore seems likely that it reflects a dysfunctional dopaminergic system, one that fails to deliver sufficient pleasure or reward following approach behaviors. Not surprisingly, the individual loses interest in pursuing these goal-directed activities and begins to show a marked reduction in motivated behavior. This "shutdown" response of reduced behavior is quite adaptive from an evolutionary viewpoint. As I have emphasized throughout this book, high-activation states (such as approach behaviors) should only be emitted when they are likely to lead to reward. In the general absence of reward, the best strategy is to reduce behavior and conserve energy for a later (and it is hoped more hedonically advantageous) time. Thus, melancholic depression may represent another example of how energy conservation mechanisms powerfully shape our subjective experience of Positive Affect. In this case, the problem is that the afflicted individual repeatedly fails to receive sufficient signals of reward, thereby producing an abnormally prolonged episode of anhedonia and inactivity.

CONCLUSION

Negative Affect is very broadly related to psychopathology; indeed, elevated Negative Affect seems to characterize most of the major DSM syndromes. Consequently, Negative Affect is a highly nonspecific dimension that is common to many types of psychopathology and, therefore, is primarily responsible for the observed comorbidities among many of the major clinical syndromes. In addition, certain disorders (such as GAD and borderline personality disorder) contain an extremely large general distress component and appear to reflect a genetically inherited predisposition to experience frequent and intense episodes of Negative Affect.

Positive Affect shows far greater specificity when related to psychological disorder. Although low levels of positive emotionality have been identified in other disorders (e.g., social phobia), anhedonia and low Positive Affect seem to play a particularly important role in the mood disorders, especially the melancholic subtype of depression. On the basis of both theoretical and empirical evidence, it appears that the mood disorders reflect—at least in part—malfunctions in the energy-conserving mechanisms that regulate the ongoing cycles of Positive Affect and the BFS.

9

AFFECT, PERSONALITY, AND HEALTH

In this concluding chapter, I examine the complex and somewhat puzzling links between affective experience and physical health. Paralleling the material covered in Chapter 8, this survey again focuses primarily on how evolutionarily adaptive mechanisms may become problematic and dysfunctional under certain circumstances. This focus on maladaptive emotional responses does not simply reflect a bias on my part; rather, it represents the primary thrust of this literature as it has developed during the 20th century. That is, although some investigators recently have explored how positive emotional reactions may promote survival (e.g., Cousins, 1989; Taylor, 1989), the bulk of the research has focused on how negative emotional responses may lead to illness and death.

THE PSYCHOSOMATIC HYPOTHESIS

Stress and the "Flight or Fight" Response

This negativistic focus reflects the broader development of emotion theory during this century. Indeed, it essentially represents a straightforward extension of a basic principle that I have emphasized throughout this book, namely, that high-activation states (e.g., fear and anger) are accompanied by an elevated expenditure of energy and, therefore, may put an added strain on the bodily resources of the individual.

The pioneering work in this area was conducted in the early 20th century by the great U.S. physiologist Walter Cannon (1927, 1929). Cannon observed that states of fear, anger, pain, and hunger all were associated with a generalized physiological reaction, which he termed the "flight or fight" response. As part of this response, epinephrine (adrenaline) and norepinephrine (noradrenaline) are poured into the bloodstream. Moreover, the sympathetic nervous system (SNS) is activated and initiates a series of changes that are designed to (1) promote the efficient mobilization of bodily resources and (2) permit a high level of sustained physical activity. Thus, the SNS increases the heart rate, systolic blood pressure, and blood sugar level, thereby augmenting the amount of oxygen available to the skeletal muscles; in a related vein, breathing becomes deeper and more rapid, which elevates the level of oxygen in the blood. The production of glucose is stimulated to increase the available stores of energy, and the pupils of the eyes dilate to let in more light. Furthermore, the sweat glands increase their level of activity in order to dissipate the extra body heat that is being generated. Finally, nonessential functions are temporarily shut down, so that digestion is inhibited and the salivary glands stop working.

Cannon recognized that this flight-or-fight response is tremendously adaptive, at least under normal circumstances. Its obvious function is to permit animals to respond to crises with quick, decisive—even extraordinary—activity. Suppose, for instance, that a predator suddenly appears and threatens the safety of a large prey animal. This emergency clearly calls for quick and decisive action—indeed, a sluggish response in this instance likely would cause the animal's death. Fortunately, massive SNS activation can be expected to initiate a classic "flight" response in which the animal bolts quickly and flees its dangerous adversary at maximum possible speed.

Although this flight-or-fight response clearly is highly adaptive during a short-term crisis, it is easy to see why it could become dysfunctional over time. The problem, of course, is that the animal is expending energy—and bodily resources—at an alarming rate. If this pattern of SNS activation were prolonged over an extended period, essential bodily resources could be depleted, which eventually might cause illness or death. This potential problem ordinarily is circumvented by the parasympathetic nervous system, which works to conserve energy by decreasing the heart rate, lowering the blood sugar, and so on, thereby returning the animal to a stable, homeostatic—and more restful—state.

However, this neat homeostatic model breaks down under certain circumstances. Selye (1936, 1976) was the first researcher to explore these circumstances systematically. Selye articulated the concept of "stress" to help characterize the types of environmental conditions that give rise to prolonged, dysfunctional emotional responses. Moreover, he developed the concept of the general adaptation syndrome (GAS) to clarify the over-all sequence of events that precede—and follow—these problematic responses. The GAS commences with the occurrence of a noxious environmental stimulus (the "stressor"), which generates an *alarm reaction* in the organism. During this stage, the animal prepares to resist the stressor through the pattern of SNS activation described earlier. When these SNS-initiated changes have fully prepared the animal to respond, it enters the stage of *resistance*, wherein it uses various coping strategies in an attempt to counteract the threat. Selye acknowledged that in most cases these coping behaviors should lead to successful adaptation and the elimination of the stressor. In those instances in which adaptation is unsuccessful, how-ever, the prolonged SNS activation eventually leads to *exhaustion*, the fi-nal stage of the GAS. At this point, physiological reserves are depleted and diseases of adaptation—such as cardiovascular or kidney dysfunc-tion—become increasingly likely. Sapolsky (1996) recently extended this model by demonstrating that sustained stress also has adverse effects on the brain, particularly in the hippocampus.

The Psychosomatic Hypothesis

The pioneering work of Cannon and Selye has important implications for our understanding of how emotional responses may be linked to physical health. Most notably, this research leads to the rather straightforward pre-diction that individuals who are chronically prone to high activation emotional states—especially those states associated with the classic flight-or-fight response, such as fear and anger—eventually should expe-rience increased rates of illness and generally poorer health. This is the classic *psychosomatic hypothesis*, which has had an enormous influence in health psychology (Alexander, 1950; Watson & Pennebaker, 1989).

Numerous variations on this basic theme have been proposed and investigated by health researchers, but all the models share the common assumption that chronically elevated levels of negative emotion eventu-ally will lead to significant health problems. Indeed, anxiety, depression, anger, hostility, and other negative affects have been causally implicated in a wide array of both minor (e.g., headaches, nausea, and acne) and more serious (e.g., ulcers, coronary heart disease, arthritis, asthma, and diabetes) health problems (e.g., Alexander, 1950; Anderson, Bradley, Young, McDaniel, & Wise, 1985; Diamond, 1982; Friedman & Booth-Kewley, 1987; Harrell, 1980). Most psychosomatic models have focused on the health effects of negative emotional responses that are overtly expressed and consciously experienced; in some cases, however, investigators have instead emphasized the effects of suppressed emotional reactions (e.g., Brown et al., 1996; Harrell, 1980; Spiro, Aldwin, Ward, & Mroczek, 1995).

TESTING THE PSYCHOSOMATIC HYPOTHESIS

Subjective versus Objective Measures of Health

Do chronically elevated levels of negative emotionality cause significant health problems? To answer this question, it is important to distinguish carefully between *subjective* and *objective* measures of health (Costa & McCrae, 1985a, 1987; Smith & Williams, 1992; Watson & Pennebaker, 1989, 1991). Subjective health measures reflect—at least in part—the respondents' perceptions of, and interpretations about, their ongoing physical condition. The most widely used subjective measures are self-report health complaint scales that ask respondents to assess how frequently or intensely they have experienced various physical symptoms and problems, such as headaches, back pain, nausea, sinus congestion, and so on. I should add that although subjectivity often is viewed as a problem that is confined strictly to self-ratings, this is not necessarily the case; indeed, non–self-report measures also may contain a significant subjective component. For instance, physicians may base their ratings of the extent of recovery following surgery—at least in part—on their patients' verbal reports of pain and discomfort.

In contrast, objective health measures are not based on respondents' subjective perceptions of their health. Examples of objective health indicators include health-related behaviors (e.g., number of sick days lost to illness, number of physician visits for illness during the past year, and frequency of pain medication use), biological markers (e.g., blood pressure levels, serum risk factors, immune system functioning, and objective evidence of dysfunction) and health outcomes (e.g., diagnosis of disease and mortality rates). These types of health measures can yield results that are quite different from those obtained using physical symptom scales.

In highlighting this distinction between subjective and objective measures, I am not arguing that self-report scales are invalid. Indeed, self-report scales have been extensively validated against hard, objective evidence of dysfunction, and it is clear that they assess a certain amount of true, health-related variance. For instance, physical symptom scales correlate significantly with external measures of health status, such as medical records, documented health visits, and objective indexes of illness severity (e.g., Cohen et al., 1995; LaRue, Bank, Jarvik, & Hetland, 1979; Linn & Linn, 1980; Pennebaker, 1982). Furthermore, prospective studies have shown that self-report health measures are significant predictors of mortality from ischemic heart disease and other causes (e.g., Kaplan & Camacho, 1983; Kaplan & Kotler, 1985). In light of such evidence, it would be a mistake simply to dismiss self-report health measures as invalid.

On the other hand, the correlations between somatic complaints and other types of health measures typically are only low to moderate in magnitude (e.g., Cohen et al., 1995). Consequently, it appears that health complaint scales subsume at least two distinct sources of variance, one that is clearly health relevant and another that is more subjective and psychological (Costa & McCrae, 1987; Mechanic, 1979, 1980; Watson & Pennebaker, 1989, 1991). Note, moreover, that the relative strength of these two components can be expected to vary systematically as a function of several assessment-related conditions. For instance, self-report data collected in samples containing a relatively large proportion of somatizers—that is, individuals who tend to focus on, and magnify the extent of, their physical problems (Kirmayer, Robbins, & Paris, 1994)—likely will contain a disproportionately large subjective component. Conversely, it appears that the subjective component in symptom measures can be attenuated by having respondents make on-line judgments of current symptoms rather than retrospective ratings of problems experienced in the past (Brown & Moskowitz, 1997; Larsen, 1992).

Affect and Symptom Reporting

I begin my evaluation of the psychosomatic hypothesis by examining relations between affect and subjective health complaints. The bulk of this evidence has been collected in traditional between-subject designs in which large groups of respondents rate both (1) their levels of trait and/ or state affect and (2) the frequency or intensity of their physical problems. Consequently, these data indicate whether individuals who experience elevated levels of various affects also tend to report more health complaints.

Watson and Pennebaker (1989) provided a comprehensive analysis of the relation between affect and symptom reporting. The data they presented were remarkably robust across different samples and a diverse array of affect and health measures. The most noteworthy finding was that—consistent with the psychosomatic hypothesis—measures of trait Negative Affect were reliably correlated with physical complaint scores, with the bulk of the coefficients falling in the .30-to-.50 range.

For instance, Watson and Pennebaker (1989) analyzed data from seven samples (with a combined N of 854) who were assessed on the Pennebaker Inventory of Limbic Languidness (PILL; Pennebaker, 1982). The PILL consists of 54 common physical symptoms and complaints (e.g., racing heart, chest pain, and diarrhea); respondents rate how frequently they have experienced each of these problems during the past year. Across these seven samples, correlations between the PILL and trait Negative Affect ranged from .27 to .47, with a weighted mean value of .40. Similar results were obtained using other popular health complaint measures, including the Somatization scale of the Hopkins Symptom Checklist (HSCL; Derogatis, Lipman, Rickels, Uhlenhuth, & Covi, 1974) and the Physical subscale of the Cornell Medical Index (CMI; Brodman, Erdmann, & Wolff, 1949). Furthermore, Watson and Pennebaker (1989) found that state measures of Negative Affect also were consistently related to symptom reports. In general, these correlations were not quite as high as those found with trait Negative Affect; still, most of the coefficients were in the .20-to-.40 range, with a median value of .30. These results have been replicated by several subsequent investigators (e.g., Cohen et al., 1995; Larsen, 1992; Leventhal, Hansell, Diefenbach, Leventhal, & Glass, 1996; Robbins, Spence, & Clark, 1991). Finally, negative mood inductions in controlled laboratory settings lead to increased reports of aches and pains (Salovey & Birnbaum, 1989).

In stark contrast, measures of state and trait Positive Affect essentially are unrelated to physical symptom reporting. For instance, across six samples with a combined N of 612, Watson and Pennebaker (1989) obtained a weighted mean correlation of only −.07 between trait Positive Affect and scores on the PILL. Moreover, across 3 samples with a combined N of 372, trait Positive Affect had a mean correlation of −.15 with the HSCL Somatization scale. Similarly, correlations between state measures of Positive Affect and symptom reporting in various samples clustered around zero (see Watson & Pennebaker, 1989). In other words—and somewhat surprisingly—it is entirely possible to lead a full, happy, and interesting life (i.e., experience elevated levels of Positive Affect) while reporting a large number of physical symptoms and problems.

Most of the data reviewed by Watson and Pennebaker (1989) were obtained from single assessments in which respondents rated their symptoms only once. However, similar results are obtained using longitudinal designs in which respondents report their physical symptoms on multiple occasions (e.g., Brown & Moskowitz, 1997; Larsen, 1992). For instance, Watson (1988a) studied daily mood and symptom reporting in 71 undergraduates. Prior to the daily rating period, the students were assessed on the Positive Emotionality and Negative Emotionality scales of the MPQ (Tellegen, in press). They then completed a daily mood and symptom questionnaire over a period of 7 weeks (M = 44.4 assessments per person).

Each day, the students rated their (1) Negative Affect, (2) Positive Affect, and (3) physical symptoms (summed across 18 PILL items). These daily assessments later were averaged across all available days to yield mean daily scores on all three variables. Finally, approximately 1 month after the end of the daily rating period, the participants completed the PILL, as well as a trait mood questionnaire in which they were asked to rate the extent to which they "generally" experienced various types of affect.

Consequently, this design yielded two measures of symptom reporting (the PILL and mean daily physical complaints), as well as three indexes of both trait Negative Affect (MPQ Negative Emotionality, mean daily Negative Affect, general Negative Affect) and trait Positive Affect (MPQ Positive Emotionality, mean daily Positive Affect, general Positive Affect). Table 9.1 reports correlations between the symptom and affect scores. Consistent with the findings reported by Watson and Pennebaker (1989), both symptom indices were moderately correlated with trait negative affect; the individual coefficients ranged from .20 to .41, with a median value of .35. In sharp contrast, symptom reporting was entirely unrelated to individual differences in Positive Affect; the individual coefficients ranged from only −.10 to .06, with a median value of .00.

Taken together, these data clearly establish that individuals who experience chronically elevated levels of Negative Affect also report more somatic problems. One potentially serious problem in interpreting these data, however, is that many "physical symptom" measures contain items that actually may assess distress, negative emotionality, and psychopathology rather than physical health problems per se. For instance, Leventhal et al. (1996) used a "physical symptom checklist" that contained sev-

TABLE 9.1. Correlations between General Positive and Negative Affectivity and Health Complaints

Affect measure	PILL	Mean daily physical complaints
Negative Affectivity		
MPQ Negative Emotionality	.39*	.20
General Negative Affect	.41*	.34*
Mean Daily Negative Affect	.36*	.31*
Positive Affectivity		
MPQ Positive Emotionality	.06	.04
General Positive Affect	−.08	.05
Mean Daily Positive Affect	−.10	−.04

Note. N = 71. PILL, Pennebaker Inventory of Limbic Languidness; MPQ, Multidimensional Personality Questionnaire. Data adapted from Watson (1988a, Table 3).
*p < .05, two-tailed.

eral items assessing common symptoms of depression (e.g., fatigue, energy loss, and sleep disturbance) and anxiety (dizziness). Similarly, the PILL contains a great many items (e.g., racing heart, dizziness, faintness, chills, hot flashes, numbness and tingling, and trembling or shaky hands) that are classic symptoms of panic disorder; in fact, many of these items are virtually identical to those included in the Anxious Arousal scale of the MASQ (see Chapter 8).

As discussed in Chapter 8, anxiety and depression are distressed-based syndromes that contain a large component of general Negative Affect. Given the presence of such items in physical symptom scales, one could argue that the observed correlations between Negative Affect and health complaints are spurious. That is, these correlations simply may demonstrate that one type of distress (i.e., a trait Negative Affect scale) is related to another (i.e., a measure containing symptoms of depression and anxiety). If this were so, then the data I reviewed earlier are irrelevant to the psychosomatic hypothesis.

I agree that the inclusion of anxiety and depression symptoms in "physical symptom scales" is problematic, and that it would be highly desirable to bypass this problem entirely in the future. However, I also must emphasize that measures of trait Negative Affect do not simply correlate with symptoms of depression and anxiety; rather, the association between trait Negative Affect and somatic complaints is quite general. For instance, Costa and McCrae (1980b) found that individuals who were high in trait Negative Affect scored significantly higher on all 12 somatic sections of the CMI. Similarly, Watson and Pennebaker (1991) computed correlations between trait Negative Affect and the individual PILL items in each of four samples (with N ranging from 192 to 568). Of the 54 PILL items, 27 (50%) were significantly correlated with trait Negative Affect in all four samples. Moreover, an additional 24 items were significantly correlated with trait Negative Affect in at least one of the data sets. Thus, only 3 of the 54 PILL items (hemorrhoids, boils, and nonfacial acne) had nonsignificant coefficients in all four samples. In other words, trait Negative Affect was significantly related to numerous symptoms (e.g., running nose, swollen ankles, and toothaches) that are not common manifestations of depression or anxiety. These data demonstrate that trait Negative Affect has a broad and nonspecific association with physical symptom reporting; furthermore, they establish that the observed correlations do not simply reflect the presence of anxiety/depression symptoms.

Another important issue concerns the generality of this relation across different types of negative emotionality: Is the relation nonspecific, or is it instead limited to particular negative affects? This issue has direct relevance to the psychosomatic hypothesis, at least as it was initially formulated. As I discussed earlier, this hypothesis is based on the idea that prolonged SNS activation will lead to the depletion of vital bodily resources and, eventually, to exhaustion and illness. In this regard, certain types of negative affect are reliably associated with greater SNS activation than are others (e.g., Ekman et al., 1983; Levenson et al., 1990). Accordingly, one might expect that those negative affects associated with the greatest SNS arousal (e.g., fear and anger, the classic flight-or-fight emotions) would show particularly strong associations with health complaints.

To investigate this issue, Clark and I analyzed data from a large (N = 387) sample of undergraduates at SMU who were assessed twice over a 2-month interval (Watson & Clark, 1992a). At each assessment, the respondents completed (1) the PILL and (2) a general, trait version of the PANAS-X. We computed correlations between the total PILL score and the four basic negative emotion scales (Fear, Sadness, Guilt, Hostility) of the PANAS-X at each assessment. Table 9.2 presents these data—along with parallel correlations with general Negative and Positive Affect (which were not reported in the original article). As expected, somatic complaints were more strongly correlated with general Negative Affect than with Positive Affect at both assessments. In terms of the present discussion, however, the most noteworthy finding was that with the single exception of Hostility at Time 1, all the correlations with the basic Negative Affect scales were moderate and quite similar in magnitude, ranging from .34 to .46.

The striking similarity of these correlations across different types of negative emotionality suggests that the relation is largely nonspecific and essentially reflects the influence of the general Negative Affect dimen-

TABLE 9.2. Correlations between General and Specific Measures of Trait Affect and Health Complaints (Assessed Using the PILL)

Affect measure	Time 1	Time 2
General affect scales		
Positive Affect	−.15	−.21
Negative Affect	.44	.51
Specific negative affects		
Fear	.42	.46
Sadness	.38	.45
Guilt	.34	.43
Hostility	.24	.40

Note. N = 387. PILL, Pennebaker Inventory of Limbic Languidness. All correlations are significant at $p < .01$, two-tailed. The correlations with the specific negative affect scales are adapted from Watson and Clark (1992a, Table 9). Copyright 1992 by the American Psychological Association. Adapted by permission.

sion. To test this possibility, Watson and Clark (1992a) computed partial correlations between the specific negative affects and the PILL, controlling for individual differences in general Negative Affect. These partial correlations were invariably low, ranging from only –.12 to .14 at Time 1, and from –.08 to .08 at Time 2. Parallel analyses of the individual PILL items yielded very similar findings. On the basis of these results, it appears that somatic complaints are nonspecifically related to general Negative Affect (see also Leventhal et al., 1996; Robbins et al., 1991).

As we have seen, between-subject analyses consistently show that somatic complaints are moderately correlated with individual differences in Negative Affect but not Positive Affect. In contrast, the available evidence (which, unfortunately, is rather sparse) suggests that within-subject fluctuations in health complaints are more broadly associated with both greater Negative Affect and lower Positive Affect. I reported the most extensive analysis of this issue in a study in which I computed within-subject correlations between daily mood and physical complaints in each of 80 participants (Watson, 1988a). Contrary to my expectation, the average within-subject correlations for Negative Affect ($r = .14$) and Positive Affect ($r = -.18$) did not differ in magnitude (for a related discussion, see Brown & Moskowitz, 1997). Nevertheless, aggregated between-subject analyses of these same data yielded the typical pattern: Health complaints were associated with individual differences in Negative Affect but not Positive Affect (see Table 9.1). We currently lack a good explanation for this curious discrepancy between these two analytic approaches; this clearly is an important issue for future research.

General Explanations for the Link between Negative Affect and Symptom Reporting

One obvious interpretation of these results is that—consistent with the psychosomatic hypothesis—chronically elevated levels of Negative Affect eventually produce significant health problems, which then are manifested as higher scores on physical symptom scales. This is not the only plausible interpretation, however. Another possibility is that causality runs in the opposite direction, that is, that health problems generate higher levels of negative emotionality. Watson and Pennebaker (1989) labeled this alternative explanation the *disability hypothesis*. The underlying logic of this model is that significant health problems can generate substantial stress through a number of pathways, including chronic pain and discomfort, worries about the future, physical disability, and social and/ or occupational impairment. Under these adverse circumstances, it is easy to see why health problems might heighten feelings of distress and dissatisfaction.

The psychosomatic and disability hypotheses both assume that the health complaints of distressed individuals are real—put another way, they both seek to explain why individual differences in trait Negative Affect are associated with greater health problems. In contrast, a third explanation—which Watson and Pennebaker (1989) termed the "symptom perception hypothesis"—does not necessarily assume that individual differences in negative emotionality are significantly related to actual, objective indicators of health. According to this view, individuals differ in how they perceive, respond to, recall, and/or complain about bodily sensations. Stated in its strongest possible form, the symptom perception hypothesis posits that the observed association between Negative Affect and self-rated health is illusory and simply reflects the fact that elevated levels of negative emotionality are associated with an increased tendency to attend to, remember, and/or complain about internal physical sensations. A weaker form of this general model would posit that perceptual/ attentional processes magnify or exaggerate any true affect-related differences in actual, objective health status. In essence, therefore, the symptom perception hypothesis argues that individuals who are high in trait Negative Affect tend to be somatizers who are prone to overreport physical problems (Costa & McCrae, 1985a, 1987; Salovey, O'Leary, Stretton, Fishkin, & Drake, 1991; Watson & Pennebaker, 1989, 1991).

It must be emphasized that these three explanations are not incompatible or mutually exclusive. It is entirely possible, for example, that elevated negative emotionality produces significant physical problems in some individuals but is a consequence of health difficulties in others. It also is possible that individuals who are high in trait Negative Affect actually suffer from poorer health in some objective sense, but they nevertheless exaggerate or overreact to these legitimate health concerns. Indeed, as I show shortly, at least some evidence can be mustered in support of all three hypotheses, so that we eventually need to integrate them to arrive at some larger truth.

I first consider evidence related to the psychosomatic hypothesis and its central prediction that chronically elevated Negative Affect causes health problems. I begin by examining two major foci of behavioral medicine research—(1) cardiac health and illness and (2) cancer and the immune system—and then consider trait affect in relation to a broader array of health indicators.

Cardiac Health and Illness

In examining this literature, it again is necessary to distinguish between subjective health complaints and objective indicators of cardiac pathology. I already have shown that individual differences in Negative Affect are broadly correlated with somatic symptoms. Coronary symptoms are no exception to this general rule: Trait Negative Affect is significantly correlated with self-reported complaints that often are associated with heart disease, such as chest pain and angina pectoris (i.e., persistent attacks of severe chest pain) (e.g., Costa, Fleg, McCrae, & Lakatta, 1982; Shekelle, Vernon, & Ostfeld, 1991).

It appears, however, that although trait Negative Affect is moderately correlated with angina and chest pain—and angina, in turn, is a significant predictor of heart disease—that negative emotionality is largely unrelated to objective indices of cardiac health, including risk factors for heart disease, coronary artery stenosis and other evidence of cardiac pathology, and heart-related mortality (Costa et al., 1982; Shekelle et al., 1991; Watson & Pennebaker, 1989). I consider this objective evidence in more detail.

Blood Pressure and Hypertension

Hypertension is a well-known risk factor for heart disease: High premorbid levels of both systolic blood pressure (SBP) and diastolic blood pressure (DBP) are significant predictors of later cardiac pathology (Aberg, Lithell, Selinus, & Hedstrand, 1985; Newman et al., 1986; Steinberg, 1985). Watson and Pennebaker (1989) presented extensive evidence relating each of these variables to individual differences in both positive and negative emotionality. Generally speaking, trait affect measures were not consistently related to any indices of either SBP or DBP, including both (1) mean levels and (2) variability. Moreover, the few significant findings that did emerge tended to run counter to the psychosomatic hypothesis. That is, individuals who described themselves as euthymic (i.e., high Positive Affect, low Negative Affect) had slightly *higher* blood pressure.

Findings from other studies have been inconsistent. For example, Kidson (1973) found that trait Negative Affect was unrelated to either SBP or DBP in a normal healthy sample. Similarly, Almada, Zonderman, Shekelle, and Dyer (1991) reported that negative emotionality was unrelated to SBP in a large sample ($N = 1,871$) of adult men. In contrast, Davies (1970) divided participants into three groups on the basis of their mean DBP levels; contrary to the psychosomatic hypothesis, the high-DBP group had trait Negative Affect scores that were significantly *lower* than those of the lowest-DBP group. Finally, in a study of high school students, Ewart and Kolodner (1994) found that negative emotionality was significantly associated with higher SBP and DBP but only among white boys. Among girls and black boys, only 1 of 12 correlations was statistically significant, and the median coefficient was only .06. Consistent with the results reported by Watson and Pennebaker (1989), the most reasonable conclusion is that trait Negative Affect has no clear, replicable association with either SBP or DBP.

The conclusion is similar when affect is related to hypertension. Watson and Pennebaker (1989) compared the negative emotionality scores of normotensives versus hypertensives in two samples. Contrary to the psychosomatic hypothesis, the hypertensives had *lower* trait Negative Affect scores than did the normotensives in both cases, although this difference was significant in only one of the samples. The evidence from other studies is inconsistent. Some researchers have reported that hypertensives have higher Negative Affect scores (Davies, 1970; Kidson, 1973; Sainsbury, 1964), whereas others have found no differences between hypertensives and normotensives (Cochrane, 1969, 1973; Costa, McCrae, Andres, & Tobin, 1980; Robinson, 1962).

Two large-scale prospective studies have explored the affective precursors of hypertension. First, Markovitz, Matthews, Kannel, Cobb, and D'Agostino (1993) studied a large cohort of adult men (N = 497) and women (N = 626). The members of this cohort—all of whom were healthy and asymptomatic at the beginning of the study—were followed up for 18 to 20 years; at the end of this period, they were classified as either normotensive or hypertensive. Premorbid anxiety levels were significantly related to the development of hypertension among middle-age men, thereby offering some support for the psychosomatic hypothesis. Among older men, however, baseline anxiety levels failed to predict the development of hypertension; moreover, within this latter group, hypertensives had significantly *lower* levels of premorbid anger. Finally, anxiety and anger both were completely unrelated to hypertensive status in both middle-age and older women. Overall, these results offer weak, qualified support for the psychosomatic hypothesis.

Second, Spiro et al. (1995), followed a large sample (N = 838) of adult men—all of whom were normotensive at the initial assessment—over an average interval of 17.3 years. During this intervening period, 39% of the sample developed hypertension. Spiro et al. (1995) then compared the hypertensive and normotensive groups on a broad range of personality traits. The only difference to emerge was that the hypertensives showed a slight, marginally significant ($p < .06$) tendency to report higher levels of trait anxiety, which again provides some support for the psychosomatic hypothesis.

Serum Risk Factors

High serum cholesterol—particularly low-density lipoprotein (LDL) cholesterol—is a well-known predictor of heart disease (Aberg et al., 1985; Steinberg, 1985). Premorbid serum triglyceride and uric acid levels also are strongly predictive of later heart disease, although their independent contributions to cardiac pathology (after controlling for other known risk factors, such as obesity and cholesterol) have not been established (Aberg et al., 1985; Brand, McGee, Kannel, Stokes, & Castelli, 1985). Serum uric acid is an especially interesting cardiovascular marker because it is highly responsive to transient stress (e.g., Kasl, Cobb, & Brooks, 1968).

Watson and Pennebaker (1989) correlated four serum risk variables (uric acid, triglycerides, LDL, and total cholesterol) with negative and positive emotionality in two adult samples. In general, the affect scores were unrelated to coronary risk (see also Almada et al., 1991, who reported similar, nonsignificant findings). The single exception was that trait Negative Affect was *negatively* correlated with uric acid levels in both samples. Because high uric acid levels predict later coronary disease (e.g., Brand et al., 1985), these results again run counter to the psychosomatic hypothesis.

Coronary Heart Disease

The data concerning actual coronary disease are inconsistent. Individual studies generally have found that trait Negative Affect is unrelated to objective indicators of cardiac pathology. Several major prospective studies, with follow-up periods ranging from 4 to 20 years, have reported that premorbid Negative Affect does not predict the subsequent occurrence of coronary heart disease (Brozek, Keys, & Blackburn, 1966; Costa et al., 1982), myocardial infarction (Ostfeld, Lebovits, Shekelle, & Paul, 1964), or heart-related mortality (Almada et al., 1991; Keehn, Goldberg, & Beebe, 1974; Shekelle et al., 1981). Particularly noteworthy are the results of Shekelle et al. (1991), who followed a large ($N = 2,003$) cohort of middle-age men over a period of 10 years. They found that trait Negative Affect was significantly correlated with the incidence of uncomplicated angina pectoris; nevertheless, baseline Negative Affect levels failed to predict the incidence of either myocardial infarction or coronary death over the follow-up period.

Although individual studies generally have failed to support the psychosomatic hypothesis, Booth-Kewley and Friedman's (1987) meta-analytic examination of the literature suggests that individual differences in Negative Affect may be modestly related to the subsequent development of heart disease. Specifically, their meta-analysis of the relevant prospective studies yielded low but significant correlations between heart disease and individual differences in anxiety ($r = .14$), depression ($r = .17$), and hostility ($r = .07$). These results suggest that there is a systematic link between Negative Affect and the subsequent incidence of coronary disease—although this link clearly is substantially weaker than the association between negative emotionality and subjective indicators of cardiac pathology (such as angina). One problem in interpreting these data, however, is that Booth-Kewley and Friedman included an extremely heterogeneous array of affect measures in their meta-analysis. Some of these scales clearly assessed trait affect, whereas others measured state affect; in other instances (e.g., various projective tests), unfortunately, the constructs being assessed were unclear. Thus, it is impossible to isolate the specific effects of trait and state affect in these data.

Other evidence suggests that current distress levels are a significant predictor of subsequent disease course following a myocardial infarction. Specifically, several studies have established that current symptoms of depression (Frasure-Smith, Lespérance, & Talajic, 1993, 1995) and anxiety (Follick et al., 1988; Frasure-Smith, 1991) are important risk factors for (1) subsequent cardiac events and (2) mortality following an initial heart attack. For instance, Frasure-Smith et al. (1995) followed 222 patients—each of whom had suffered a recent myocardial infarction—over a 12-month period. It is noteworthy that whereas current levels of depression and anxiety predicted the occurrence of subsequent cardiac events, various measures of trait anger did not. Thus, it appears that although trait affect is not a strong predictor of initial cardiac disease, current state affect can have a powerful influence on prognosis following a major cardiac event.

In summary, although trait Negative Affect is moderately associated with subjective complaints of angina and chest pain, it is inconsistently related to objective indicators of cardiac pathology. Indeed, various studies have shown that negative affectivity is (1) positively related, (2) negatively related, and (3) completely unrelated to objective measures of coronary disease. Despite these inconsistencies, there is sufficient positive evidence to suggest that the psychosomatic hypothesis has merit, and that the links between Negative Affect and heart disease warrant further scrutiny. Nevertheless, it also is clear that negative emotionality is more strongly associated with subjective manifestations of cardiac pathology than with objective measures of coronary disease. Therefore, these data still are entirely compatible with a weak form of the symptom perception hypothesis.

Cancer and the Immune System

Cancer

A few studies have examined the association between premorbid Negative Affect and the subsequent development of cancer. Kaplan and Reynolds (1988) investigated the relation between various measures of subjective well-being and cancer in a prospective study spanning 17 years; they found that premorbid well-being scores were unrelated to cancer incidence and mortality in both men and women. Similarly, other large-scale prospective studies also have found that premorbid levels of trait Negative Affect are unrelated to cancer-related mortality over periods of 17 (Shekelle et al., 1981) and 24 (Keehn et al., 1974) years. In view of these null findings, perhaps the safest conclusion is that baseline levels of Negative Affect are unrelated to the development of cancer.

Other data, however, suggest that *low* levels of trait Negative Affect may increase one's vulnerability to cancer, at least among individuals who tend to suppress or deny their negative feelings. Indeed, after reviewing the evidence, Eysenck (1994) argued for the existence of a "cancer-prone personality" that is characterized by (1) an inability to cope with stress effectively and (2) a tendency to suppress negative emotions such as anxiety and anger. Eysenck's hypothesis generally has received good support from cross-sectional data: That is, although a few studies have reported no differences between cancer patients and normal controls (e.g., Bond & Pearson, 1969), several others have found that cancer patients had significantly lower levels of trait Negative Affect than did controls (Kissen, 1964; Kissen & Eysenck, 1962; Wistow, 1990).

Prospective data also provide some suggestive support for Eysenck's hypothesis. Dattore, Shontz, and Coyne (1980) compared 75 cancer patients to 125 controls with various diagnoses, including benign neoplasms, schizophrenia, and hypertension. All the respondents completed the Minnesota Multiphasic Personality Inventory (MMPI) at least 1 year prior to receiving any of these diagnoses. Dattore et al. found that the cancer patients reported significantly lower premorbid levels of trait Negative Affect than did the controls. Unfortunately, because of the heterogeneous composition of the control group, it is impossible to determine whether (1) the cancer patients were unusually low in Negative Affect premorbidly or (2) the controls reported elevated levels of baseline Negative Affect. Dattore et al. (1980) preferred the former interpretation and suggested that individuals who tend to suppress negative emotions are more vulnerable to cancer.

Researchers also have investigated how Negative Affect influences survival in patients who already are diagnosed with cancer; the results of these studies offer further support for Eysenck's model. Derogatis, Abeloff, and Melisaratos (1979) found that long-term survivors of breast cancer had significantly higher levels of hostility, guilt, and general negative emotionality; Rogentine et al. (1979) reported similar findings for patients with melanoma. On the basis of these data, Derogatis et al. (1979) suggested that the overt expression of negative emotionality promotes survival, at least among cancer patients.

Thus, low levels of Negative Affect may have deleterious health consequences, at least with regard to cancer; consistent with Eysenck's model, these findings may reflect the fact that many individuals who report low levels of negative emotionality also tend to suppress their negative feelings. A related line of research has examined this issue directly by examining the health implications of the "repressive" coping style. Repressors typically are defined as individuals who (1) report low levels of trait Negative Affect (as indexed by low scores on scales such as the Taylor Manifest Anxiety Scale [TMAS]; Taylor, 1953) and (2) tend to respond in an excessively socially desirable manner (as indexed by high scores on the Marlowe-Crowne [MC] Social Desirability Scale; Crowne & Marlowe, 1964). These repressors then are compared to groups of high-anxious (i.e., high TMAS, low MC) and low-anxious (i.e., low TMAS, low MC) individuals.

Corroborating Eysenck's model, repressors have a higher rate of cancer-related mortality than do both the high-anxious and low-anxious groups (Jensen, 1984). Moreover, repressors show greater autonomic activity (Weinberger, Schwartz, & Davidson, 1979), as well as elevated blood pressure (King, Taylor, Albright, & Haskell, 1990), cholesterol (Weinberger, 1990), and cortisol (Brown et al., 1996). It is noteworthy that the high- and low-anxious groups tended to have similar scores on these variables. These data therefore suggest that Negative Affect per se may be unrelated to the development of cancer; rather, it may be the tendency to suppress or deny negative emotions that is the crucial factor in increasing an individual's vulnerability.

In summary, high levels of trait Negative Affect do not play a significant role in the eventual development of cancer. If anything, the data suggest that *low* Negative Affect (perhaps because of a repressive coping style) may increase one's vulnerability to this disease. Thus, this literature offers no support for the psychosomatic hypothesis.

Immune Function

The immune system forms an important part of the body's natural defense against cancer and infectious disease. Natural killer cells, for instance, play a crucial role in arresting the spread of tumor cells and in halting the progression of cancer (Herberman, 1982; Herberman & Ortaldo, 1981). Therefore, on the basis of the cancer data, one might expect that Negative Affect was largely unrelated—or perhaps even positively related—to the quality of immune system functioning.

Contrary to this expectation, however, high levels of state Negative Affect generally are associated with poorer immune system functioning (see Cohen & Williamson, 1991; Herbert & Cohen, 1993). That is, although some studies have failed to find significant effects (e.g., Levy, Herberman,

Maluish Schlien, & Lippman, 1985), most investigators have reported that transient negative moods are associated with a significant decrease in immune function. Moreover, these significant findings have been obtained using both correlational (Herbert & Cohen, 1993; Stone, Cox, Valdimarsdottir, Jandorf, & Neale, 1987) and experimental (Futterman, Kemeny, Shapiro, Polonsky, & Fahay, 1992; Knapp et al., 1992) designs. For example, Cohen, Tyrrell, and Smith (1993) studied 394 healthy volunteers who were exposed to one of five different viruses and then quarantined for a week. Immediately prior to their exposure to the virus, all respondents rated their negative mood level during the previous week. Individuals with elevated Negative Affect showed a higher rate of clinical infection (88.2%) than did those reporting low levels of negative mood (76.9%). Interestingly, however, negative mood levels failed to predict the actual development of colds (the rates were 45.4% and 45.8% in the high and low Negative Affect groups, respectively).

Cohen et al. (1995) exposed 86 healthy individuals to either of two respiratory viruses. Of these participants, 70 subsequently developed a clinically significant illness. On the day they were exposed to the virus, the participants all completed measures of both trait and state Negative Affect; the state scale assessed their feelings over the previous 24 hours. State Negative Affect was a significant predictor of both subjective complaints following exposure (e.g., reports of congestion, running nose, sore throat, and headache; $r = .33$), as well as an objective indicator of illness severity (i.e., the overall weight of mucus discharge; $r = .26$). In contrast, although trait Negative Affect also was moderately associated with postexposure complaints ($r = .27$), it was entirely unrelated to the objective index of illness severity ($r = -.02$).

On the basis of these data, it appears that high levels of state—but not trait—Negative Affect are associated with poorer immune system functioning and an increased vulnerability to infectious disease. Furthermore, the findings of Cohen et al. (1995) again indicate that trait Negative Affect scores are much better predictors of subjective complaints than of objective indicators of disease. Consequently, although the findings in this area clearly indicate that transient negative moods may have significant short-term health consequences, they ultimately offer little support for the psychosomatic hypothesis.

General Health Correlates of Negative Emotionality

Mortality

I already have shown that premorbid Negative Affect is unrelated to mortality rates due to either coronary disease or cancer (e.g., Keehn et al.,

1974; Shekelle et al., 1981). Is it associated with overall mortality rates? Good data are scarce, but the available evidence suggests that negative emotionality is, at best, weakly related to mortality. Shekelle et al. (1981) found no association between premorbid Negative Affect levels and deaths from any cause across a 17-year follow-up period. Similarly, Costa and McCrae (1987) reported that negative emotionality was unrelated to overall mortality (assessed 7 to 26 years after the initial personality testing) in a large sample of adult males. In contrast, Kaplan and Reynolds (1988) found that high premorbid depression scores predicted non–cancer-related deaths in a 17-year follow-up. An inspection of the item content of this scale (see Kaplan & Reynolds, 1988, Table 1), however, indicates that it included prototypical markers of both Positive Affect (low) and Negative Affect (high); accordingly, it is unclear whether high Negative Affect, low Positive Affect, or some combination of the two contributed to this significant effect.

Keehn et al. (1974) compared normal versus neurotic individuals (this latter group can be expected to be high in negative emotionality; see Chapter 8) over a 24-year follow-up and found a significantly higher mortality rate among the latter. However, the bulk of this effect was due to an increased incidence of suicide, homicide, and alcoholism among the neurotics. Furthermore, the discrepancy between the groups declined sharply after the first few years and eventually vanished altogether. Commenting on their results, Keehn et al. (1974) concluded: "We see little evidence that the anxiety and emotional conflicts noted at hospitalization . . . have led to chronic disturbance of physiological function and so to organic disease later in life" (p. 44).

Analyses of the Terman Life-Cycle Study provide particularly compelling results in light of the large sample size (more than 1,100 participants) and the long follow-up intervals (ranging from 40 to 65 years across various published studies). Friedman et al. (1993) examined an array of personality measures that were collected in 1921, when the participants were, on average, approximately 11 years old. The final follow-up assessment occurred in 1986, allowing Friedman et al. to analyze these personality data in relation to deaths occurring between 1930 to 1986 (16 participants who had died prior to 1930 were excluded because they already might have been seriously ill at the initial assessment). A measure of low neuroticism/negative emotionality ("High Self-Confidence") essentially was unrelated to mortality, leading Friedman et al. (1993) to conclude that "simple models that propose that a neurotic constitution is a major factor in adult health are probably inadequate" (p. 181). An additional—and quite surprising—finding was that premorbid levels of Cheerfulness/Humor (defined as "sense of humor and cheerfulness-optimism"; Friedman et al., 1993, p. 178) were *positively* associated with subsequent mortality. The mechanisms underlying this effect are unclear, although Friedman et al. suggested that cheerful and optimistic people may "underestimate the danger of certain risks to their health and thereby fail to take precautions or to follow medical advice" (p. 181).

In a subsequent analysis of this same sample, Martin et al. (1995) investigated the health consequences of a trichotomous index of mental health that was constructed in 1950. This index classified all the participants into one of three categories: (1) satisfactory adjustment (i.e., "those who were able to cope normally with everyday problems and who were judged to be essentially typical in terms of their emotional makeup"), (2) some maladjustment (i.e., "those who, although experiencing excessive feelings of inferiority or inadequacy, anxiety, or emotional conflicts, were nonetheless able to function"), or (3) serious maladjustment ("individuals who had shown marked symptoms of anxiety, depression, personality maladjustment, psychopathic personality, or had suffered a nervous breakdown"; see Martin et al., p. 382). This index—which clearly contains a strong component of general negative emotionality—then was related to deaths occurring from 1950 to 1991; it was a significant predictor of mortality in men but not women, thereby offering some weak support for the psychosomatic hypothesis.

Health-Relevant Behaviors

Another way of evaluating the health consequences of negative emotionality is to examine how it correlates with various health-related behaviors. Watson and Pennebaker (1989) examined this issue by correlating measures of both negative and positive emotionality with (1) number of physician or health-center visits, (2) days hospitalized during the past year, and (3) days of work or school missed because of illness during the past year. Across five different samples, trait Negative Affect scores were completely unrelated to all three behavioral variables, with correlations ranging from −.17 to .19. Positive emotionality also was largely unrelated to health behaviors, although it was significantly negatively correlated with both health visits ($r = -.25$) and health-related absences ($r = -.25$) in one of the samples.

One significant limitation of the Watson and Pennebaker (1989) data, however, is that these health behaviors were based on the respondents' self-reports, which may not have been entirely accurate. I therefore attempted to replicate these findings using documented health visits—collected over an entire academic year—from the archival records of the SMU Student Health Center. As part of its electronic data base, the health center coded visits due to physical problems into one of five categories: (1) general illness, (2) headaches, (3) gastrointestinal and stomach problems, (4) upper respiratory problems, and (5) injuries. I subsequently combined the first four categories into an overall index of illness-related visits. Because injuries might be related to a somewhat different set of trait dimensions (e.g., recklessness or impulsivity), they were retained as a separate category.

I then correlated these health-visit scores with trait affect and personality measures collected from two different SMU student samples. Sample 1 consisted of 354 students who rated themselves on the NEO-FFI (Costa & McCrae, 1992) and the GTS (Clark & Watson, 1990) at the start of the Fall 1991 semester. Accordingly, this battery contained two measures of both negative emotionality (i.e., NEO-FFI Neuroticism and GTS Negative Temperament) and positive emotionality/extraversion (i.e., NEO-FFI Extraversion and GTS Positive Temperament). Sample 2 consisted of 185 students who were assessed at the beginning of the Spring 1992 semester; these respondents completed an alternative measure of the Big Five—the Big Five Inventory (John, Donahue, & Kentle, 1991)—as well as the Neuroticism and Openness scales from the NEO-FFI. Thus, this battery contained two measures of negative emotionality (i.e., NEO-FFI Neuroticism and BFI Neuroticism) and one index of positive emotionality (i.e., BFI Extraversion). I should note that the students in Sample 1 made an average of 1.84 visits for illness and 0.23 visits for injury; in Sample 2, the corresponding means were 1.69 and 0.19, respectively.

Table 9.3 presents correlations between both types of visits and all the assessed personality variables (the students' sex also is included for comparison purposes). The most noteworthy finding is that—contrary to the psychosomatic hypothesis but replicating the results reported by Watson & Pennebaker (1989)—trait Negative Affect scores were completely unrelated to both types of visits, with correlations ranging from only –.08 to .07. Somewhat surprisingly, individuals who reported high levels of positive emotionality made *more* illness-related visits in both samples and also had more injury-related visits in Sample 1. The only other replicable effect was that women made more illness-related visits than did men in both samples.

Other investigators have examined the association between negative emotionality and health visits. Schroeder (1972) also found that trait Negative Affect scores were unrelated to the number of visits to a student health center. Tessler, Mechanic, and Dimond (1976) obtained a significant but low ($r = .15$) correlation between negative emotionality and visits made to a health maintenance organization. Similarly, Mechanic (1980) reported significant but low correlations between trait Negative Affect and both physician visits ($r = .13$) and sick days ($r = .20$). Byrne, Steinberg, and Schwartz (1968) found that Negative Affect scores were significantly related to health-center visits in men but not in women. Finally, Gayton,

TABLE 9.3. Correlations between Personality Scores and Health Center Visits

Personality scale	Illness visits	Injury visits
	Sample 1	
Negative emotionality		
GTS Negative Temperament	.03	−.08
NEO-FFI Neuroticism	.01	−.07
Positive emotionality		
GTS Positive Temperament	.15**	.12*
NEO-FFI Extraversion	.17**	.17**
Other measures		
GTS Disinhibition	.04	.14**
NEO-FFI Conscientiousness	.01	.00
NEO-FFI Agreeableness	−.06	−.08
NEO-FFI Openness	.07	.05
Sex	.12*	−.09
	Sample 2	
Negative emotionality		
NEO-FFI Neuroticism	.00	.07
BFI Neuroticism	.04	.03
Positive emotionality		
BFI Extraversion	.15*	.00
Other measures		
BFI Conscientiousness	−.14*	−.15*
BFI Agreeableness	−.12	−.01
BFI Openness	.01	−.04
NEO-FFI Openness	.10	.16*
Sex	.25**	−.04

Note. N = 354 (Sample 1), 185 (Sample 2). GTS, General Temperament Survey; NEO-FFI, NEO Five-Factor Inventory; BFI, Big Five Inventory.
*$p < .05$, two-tailed; **$p < .01$, two-tailed.

Bassett, Tavormina, and Ozmon (1978) reported that prisoners who were high in Negative Affect made more sick-call visits (both medically justified and unjustified) than did those lower on the trait. Putting all these data together, it appears that trait Negative Affect is, at best, weakly related to health visits.

In a related vein, Watson (1988a) correlated negative emotionality with reported sick days. Recall that the participants in this study completed a daily mood and symptom questionnaire every day for 6 to 7 weeks. At the bottom of the rating form, the students noted whether they had been sick that day. Colds or flu were listed as the cause of almost all sick days (an average of 6.9 days per participant). Negative emotionality ($r = .00$) and positive emotionality ($r = -.06$) both were completely unrelated to the number of reported sick days. Overall, the data exhibited a familiar pattern:

1. Individuals who were high in Negative Affect reported more physical complaints (see Table 9.1); and
2. Health complaints, in turn, were associated with more frequent sick days; but
3. Negative Affect was unrelated to reported sick days.

Thus, we again find that negative emotionality is more highly correlated with subjective complaints than with objective health measures.

Fitness and Lifestyle Variables

Finally, Watson and Pennebaker (1989) related trait affectivity to a number of indicators of general fitness and health-related lifestyle, including weight, obesity, frequency of exercise, sleep (average number of hours per night), smoking, alcohol, coffee and total caffeine consumption, and the use of aspirin or other painkillers. Across five samples (three adult, two student), neither negative nor positive emotionality was strongly or consistently correlated with any of these variables.

Overall Status of the Psychosomatic Hypothesis

What overall conclusions can be drawn regarding the validity of the psychosomatic hypothesis? With regard to heart disease, the evidence is quite inconsistent, but there is enough positive evidence to suggest that chronically elevated levels of negative mood may play a modest role in the development of cardiac pathology. In contrast, although the evidence regarding cancer again is inconsistent, the data seem to suggest that *low* Negative Affect may represent the more salient vulnerability factor in the development of neoplasms; however, this effect may primarily be attributable to "repressors" who tend to suppress their negative feelings. Finally, negative emotionality is, at best, a weak predictor of overall mortality and health-related behaviors (doctor visits, sick days, etc.).

It seems unlikely that the psychosomatic hypothesis simply is wrong. Put another way, this hypothesis has received enough positive empirical support over the years to suggest that its basic proposition—namely, that chronically elevated Negative Affect has deleterious health effects—is not without merit. At the same time, however, the enormous inconsistencies in the literature strongly suggest that the original proposition was much too simplistic, and that future research should systematically explore additional factors (such as gender, race, age, emotional suppression vs. expression, and nonlinear effects) that may moderate the association between negative emotionality and health.

Finally, it must be emphasized that even when positive findings have been reported, the observed effects invariably are quite weak, typically reflecting correlations in the .10-to-.20 range. Thus, the available data clearly establish that negative emotionality is more strongly and consistently associated with subjective health complaints than with objective indicators of disease and dysfunction. Therefore, the psychosomatic hypothesis cannot completely account for the symptom correlations discussed earlier. Indeed, the data strongly suggest that individuals who report chronically high levels of Negative Affect tend to overreport physical problems, which is consistent with at least a weak form of the symptom perception hypothesis.

THE DISABILITY HYPOTHESIS

As noted earlier, the disability hypothesis proposes that health problems lead to distress and dissatisfaction and, ultimately, to elevated levels of negative emotionality. The preceding evidence already exposes some important limitations of this model as a general explanation for the symptom data. Similar to the psychosomatic hypothesis, the disability model assumes that trait Negative Affect is associated with actual health problems. To the extent this basic proposition is true, both explanations receive some preliminary support. To the extent it is *not* true, however, both explanations run into immediate problems. As we have seen, negative emotionality is only weakly related to objective indicators of disease and dysfunction, at least in general adult and student populations. Nevertheless, trait Negative Affect scores are strongly correlated with somatic complaints in these same populations. It follows, therefore, that *major* health problems (such as cancer or heart disease) are not a significant cause of elevated Negative Affect in these samples.

One still could argue, however, that *minor* health problems—the sorts of problems that are assessed in most of the widely used physical symptom scales—produce heightened negative emotionality in these respondents. For instance, it may be that people who experience frequent headaches, indigestion, diarrhea, and so on become distressed as a result of their chronic discomfort. This hypothesis is virtually impossible to test empirically because most minor physical complaints are inherently subjective, offering little opportunity for objective verification. Even in the absence of demonstrable pathology, who can disprove an individual's complaint of headache or stomach pain?

Nevertheless, the available data present one significant problem for this model. As discussed earlier, within-subject analyses indicate that ongoing physical problems are associated with a diffuse, unpleasant mood that is characterized by both elevated Negative Affect and lowered Positive Affect. For example, Watson (1988a) reported that Negative and Positive Affect had similar mean within-subject correlations with daily health problems (r = .14 and –.18, respectively). Similarly, Clark and Watson (1988) found that respondents experienced both heightened Negative Affect and lowered Positive Affect on days with reported health problems. Finally, Watson (1988a) found that sick days (i.e., days on which respondents reported suffering from a cold or flu) were associated with low Positive Affect but not elevated Negative Affect.

Thus, if trait affect scores reflect accumulated pain and discomfort—as the disability model proposes—then one would expect that negative and positive emotionality both would be substantially correlated with overall symptom levels in these data. As Table 9.1 indicates, however, this was not the case: Consistent with the typical pattern, Watson (1988a) found that trait Negative Affect was significantly correlated with the average physical complaint score, whereas trait Positive Affect was not. These findings indicate that trait Negative Affect levels do not simply reflect accumulated aches and pains, and that additional dispositional forces must be at work.

Thus, there is little evidence to suggest that persistent health problems cause elevated negative emotionality in nonpatient samples. We can view this issue somewhat differently, however, by asking whether serious health problems lead to higher Negative Affect in patient populations. In other words, do medical patients report consistently higher levels of Negative Affect? In their review of the literature, Watson and Pennebaker (1989) noted three important trends. First, patient groups do not have consistently elevated Negative Affect—they may be higher, lower, or no different from nonmedical controls (e.g., Cassileth et al., 1984; Sainsbury, 1964). Second Negative Affect scores seem to be largely unrelated to the severity of the medical condition. Most notably, patients with severe, life-threatening health problems are not necessarily high in negative emotionality. I already have shown, for instance, that cancer patients do not report elevated levels of Negative Affect (e.g., Wistow, 1990). More generally, Sainsbury (1964) compared various patient groups with a healthy control sample. Negative Affect scores were elevated among patients with various minor ailments (e.g., acne) but were normal among many groups with more serious problems, such as peptic ulcers and coronary disease (see also Cassileth et al., 1984). Third, specific illness groups often show inconsistent patterns. For example, as discussed earlier, when hypertensives are compared with normotensives, they may report higher (e.g., Davies, 1970; Kidson, 1973), lower (Watson & Pennebaker, 1989), or unremarkable (e.g., Costa et al., 1980) levels of Negative Affect.

Moreover, even when significant group differences are found, they are difficult to interpret for two reasons. First, patients who are high in Negative Affect may be overdiagnosed for certain disorders because of their tendency to complain about physical symptoms (Costa et al., 1982; Costa & McCrae, 1985a). Second, negative emotionality scores may be spuriously inflated in medical samples because many of the commonly used measures of trait Negative Affect contain health-related items (Watson & Kendall, 1983).

The picture here is quite similar to that seen with the psychosomatic hypothesis, and it leads to parallel conclusions. First, the disability hypothesis cannot simply be dismissed as invalid. The literature contains enough positive findings to establish that health problems can produce elevated levels of distress under certain circumstances. Again, however, it also is clear that additional considerations must be involved. For instance, patients with the most severe, life-threatening health problems do not report especially high levels of Negative Affect. It therefore would be helpful if future investigators could begin to specify which types of health problems are associated with the greatest elevations in negative emotionality. Finally, in view of the relatively weak support that the disability hypothesis has received, it seems unlikely that it can provide an acceptable general explanation for the robust link between trait Negative Affect and symptom reporting.

THE SYMPTOM PERCEPTION HYPOTHESIS

Negative Affectivity and Hypochondriasis

Neither the psychosomatic nor the disability hypothesis can fully explain the observed correlations between trait Negative Affect and physical symptoms. The problem is that negative emotionality is more strongly and consistently related to subjective health complaints than to objective indicators of health status. One must conclude, therefore, that subjective complaint scales significantly overestimate the true association between negative emotionality and health. Thus, the data support at least a weak form of the symptom-perception hypothesis, which posits that individuals who are high in Negative Affect are more likely to perceive, recall, overreact to, and/or complain about minor physical problems and sensations. This leads to a further question: Why exactly do those high in Negative Affect overreport physical problems?

One possible explanation is that these individuals simply are hypochondriacs with a persistent pattern of exaggerated somatic concern. This view has some merit and likely offers a partial explanation for the observed links between trait Negative Affect and symptom reporting. In this regard, it is well established that patients with somatoform disorders (e.g., hypochondriasis and somatization disorder) generally report elevated levels of negative emotionality (Kirmayer et al., 1994). It therefore seems likely that somatizing and an exaggerated somatic concern play a significant role in the observed associations between negative emotionality and health complaints.

One might even go further and argue that a few somatizing hypochondriacs are largely responsible for these observed correlations. This extreme view is implausible for two reasons. First, the association between Negative Affect and health complaints is strongly linear. At any level, higher negative emotionality is associated with an increasing number of physical complaints; for instance, individuals who experience moderate levels of Negative Affect report more health complaints than do those who are low on the trait. Moreover, the correlation between negative emotionality and somatic complaints remains significant even after respondents with the highest Negative Affect and/or physical complaint levels are removed from the analysis (Costa & McCrae, 1985a).

Second, individuals with elevated negative emotionality do not exhibit the "doctor shopping" characteristic of the classic hypochondriac (American Psychiatric Association, 1994, p. 463). Indeed, despite their myriad physical complaints, they are not unusually likely to visit a physician or health center (see Table 9.3). More generally, although it is true that most hypochondriacs report high levels of Negative Affect, most people who are high in negative emotionality are not hypochondriacs.

Possible Mechanisms for Symptom Overreporting

Pain Sensitivity

What specific mechanisms might account for symptom overreporting among individuals high in negative emotionality? One possible explanation is that these individuals are more sensitive to pain. In this regard, studies have shown that respondents experience painful stimuli more intensely when they are anxious (Barsky & Klerman, 1983; Sternbach, 1978). Because individuals who are high in negative emotionality are prone to episodes of anxiety, they may tend to respond more strongly to sensations of pain and discomfort.

Unfortunately, the data directly relating trait Negative Affect to pain sensitivity are inconsistent and difficult to interpret. Some studies have found that high scorers on this dimension report greater pain in response to the same standardized stimuli; however, these same studies also found evidence suggesting that positive emotionality is just as strongly related to pain sensitivity (Lynn & Eysenck, 1961; Morgan & Horstman, 1978). Given these results, it is difficult to explain why somatic complaints correlate with individual differences in negative emotionality but not positive emotionality. Furthermore, others have found that trait Negative Affect scores are unrelated to pain threshold and tolerance (Davidson & Bobey, 1970; Jamner & Schwartz, 1986). Consequently, although the pain-sensitivity notion may have some merit, other processes must be involved as well.

Vigilance and Scanning

As I have noted throughout this book, Negative Affect is associated with the BIS, a biobehavioral system that seeks to inhibit behavior that might lead to pain, punishment, or some other unpleasant consequence. Gray (1981, 1982, 1985) has argued that individuals who are high in negative emotionality have an overactive BIS, one that identifies all incoming environmental stimuli as potentially important and as requiring careful checking. As a result of this BIS activity, these individuals will be hypervigilant, constantly scanning the world for signs of impending trouble. In a related vein, Tellegen (1985) has proposed that trait Negative Affect is related to an unsettled and future-oriented cognitive mode in which the individual scans the environment with uncertainty and apprehension.

This hypervigilance may lead to symptom overreporting in two ways. First, high trait scorers simply may be more likely to notice and attend to normal bodily sensations and minor aches and pains. Second, because their scanning is fraught with anxiety and uncertainty, those who are high in negative emotionality may interpret normal, benign sensations as painful or pathological (Barsky & Klerman, 1983; Costa & McCrae, 1985a). Indeed, high trait Negative Affect individuals generally interpret ambiguous stimuli in a negative or threatening manner (Watson & Clark, 1984).

Introspection and Internal Self-Focus

Individuals who report elevated levels of Negative Affect tend to be introspective and ruminative (Watson & Clark, 1984). This suggests the possibility that these individuals report more physical problems, in part because they are more internally focused (see Salovey & Birnbaum, 1989; Salovey et al., 1991; Watson & Pennebaker, 1989). In support of this notion, several studies have demonstrated that an internal orientation increases physical symptom reporting. This line of research is based on a model of physical symptom reporting that originally was proposed by Pennebaker (1982; Pennebaker & Lightner, 1980).

Based on the assumption that the capacity of human information processing is limited, Pennebaker (1982) proposed that physical complaints will vary as a function of the relative availability of external stimuli. As the number and salience of external cues increase, attention to internal stimuli necessarily will decrease, and vice versa. In other words, internal sensory stimuli and external environmental cues compete for attention. When attention is focused internally, individuals are more likely to report a variety of physical symptoms and sensations. This model predicts, for example, that people will report more symptoms (e.g., headaches) in a boring environment than in an interesting one.

Several studies have supported this model. Pennebaker and Lightner (1980), for instance, found that joggers ran faster and reported less fatigue when their exercise environment was interesting (a wooded cross-country trail) than when it was boring (a track). Other studies demonstrated that people coughed more (Pennebaker, 1980) and reported greater fatigue (Pennebaker & Brittingham, 1982) when their environment was lacking in stimulation. Fillingim and Fine (1986) found that joggers reported more physical problems when they focused internally (attending to their own heart and breathing rate) rather than externally (listening to verbal stimuli). Finally, manipulations forcing heightened self-attention through the use of a mirror also lead to increased physical symptom reporting (Wegner & Vallacher, 1980; Wicklund, 1975).

Biased Recall and Retrieval

Thus far, I have examined processes that may influence how physical sensations are experienced, perceived, and interpreted. All these mechanisms involve the differential *encoding* of physical sensations. Recent evidence also demonstrates, however, that trait Negative Affect is significantly linked with the biased recall and *retrieval* of physical symptoms. Larsen (1992) first demonstrated this point in an influential study in which physical symptoms were assessed both concurrently and retrospectively. Specifically, participants rated their current physical problems (e.g., headache and dizziness) three times a day over a period of 8 weeks; they subsequently completed a retrospective assessment in which they rated how often they had suffered from each of these same problems during this 2-month period. Larsen found that negative emotionality was significantly related to both (1) the concurrent reporting of physical problems and (2) a biased retrieval process that exaggerated the nature of this link in the retrospective ratings. Larsen's basic findings subsequently were replicated by Brown and Moskowitz (1997).

Why is negative emotionality related to the biased retrieval of physical symptoms? Larsen (1992) suggests that trait Negative Affect is broadly associated with the selective processing of negative information about the self, such that individuals who are high in negative emotionality preferentially process various types of negative self-relevant information. The rapid accumulation of this negative self-relevant information helps to create a pervasively negative self-concept. This negative self-concept, in turn, plays a crucial role in the retrieval process. This is because recall is a selective and reconstructive process in which people fill in gaps in their memories by using preexisting beliefs and expectations to make inferences about past events and experiences. Because of their negative self-concept, individuals who are high in trait Negative Affect retrospectively assume that they *must* have experienced a multitude of physical problems in the past. In other words, individuals high in negative emotionality generally see themselves as suffering from various types of problems; they therefore tend to "remember" experiencing these problems in the past to a greater extent than is justified. This explanation therefore predicts that negative emotionality is not simply related to the biased retrieval of physical symptoms but is more broadly associated with negative self-relevant information.

Larsen (1992) further suggests that biased retrieval may also reflect mood-congruent memory processes. Some evidence indicates that current mood states can promote the recall of affectively congruent experiences from memory; for instance, inducing sad moods in research participants can lead to the increased retrieval of sad experiences (Bower, 1981; Salovey & Birnbaum, 1989). At any given point of time, individuals who are high in trait Negative Affect are more likely to be in a negative mood state than are those low on this trait. Consequently, these distressed individuals may be prone to recall affectively congruent memories involving physical pain and discomfort (and, hence, to overreport somatic problems retrospectively).

CONCLUSION

The data clearly establish a strong and robust link between negative emotionality and health complaints. I examined three competing (but not mutually exclusive) explanations for this finding. First, the psychosomatic hypothesis posits that chronic Negative Affect produces significant health problems. Conversely, the disability hypothesis argues that chronic health problems lead to distress and discomfort and, eventually, to elevated negative emotionality. Finally, the symptom-perception hypothesis proposes that trait Negative Affect is associated with individual differences in how people encode and retrieve bodily sensations; unlike the other explanations, this last model does not assume that negative emotionality is related to actual, objective indicators of health.

The data are complex and inconsistent. It is noteworthy, however, that all three models have received some support in the literature. It is clear, therefore, that none of these models—by itself—is able to offer a complete explanation for the findings in this area. Future investigators must strive to integrate them into a more comprehensive scheme that better captures the complex links between negative emotionality and health.

REFERENCES

Aberg, H., Lithell, H., Selinus, I., & Hedstrand, H. (1985). Serum triglycerides are a risk factor for myocardial infarction but not for angina pectoris: Results from a 10-year follow-up of Uppsala Primary Preventive Study. *Atherosclerosis, 54*, 89–97.

Abramson, L. Y., Metalsky, G. I., & Alloy, L. B. (1989). Hopelessness depression: A theory-based subtype of depression. *Psychological Review, 96*, 358–372.

Abramson, L. Y., Seligman, M. E. P., & Teasdale, J. D. (1978). Learned helplessness in humans: Critique and reformulation. *Journal of Abnormal Psychology, 87*, 49–74.

Adams, R. G. (1988). Which comes first: Poor psychological well-being or decreased friendship activity? *Activities, Adaptation and Aging, 12*, 27–41.

Adelmann, P. K., Antonucci, T. C., Crohan, S. F., & Coleman, L. M. (1989). Empty nest, cohort, and employment in the well-being of midlife women. *Sex Roles, 20*, 173–189.

Aganoff, A., & Boyle, G. J. (1994). Aerobic exercise, mood states and menstrual cycle symptoms. *Journal of Psychosomatic Research, 38*, 183–192.

Agho, A. O., Price, J. L., & Mueller, C. W. (1992). Discriminant validity of measures of job satisfaction, positive affectivity and negative affectivity. *Journal of Occupational and Organizational Psychology, 65*, 185–196.

Ahrens, A. H., & Haaga, D. A. F. (1993). The specificity of attributional style and expectations to positive and negative affectivity, depression and anxiety. *Cognitive Therapy and Research, 17*, 83–98.

Alexander, F. (1950). *Psychosomatic medicine: Its principles and applications.* New York: Norton.

293

Allik, J., & Realo, A. (1997). Emotional experience and its relation to the five-factor model in Estonian. *Journal of Personality, 65,* 625–647.

Allison, T., & van Twyver, H. (1970). The evolution of sleep. *Natural History, 79,* 56–65.

Alloy, L. B., Kelly, K. A., Mineka, S., & Clements, C. M. (1990). Comorbidity of anxiety and depressive disorders: A helplessness-hopelessness perspective. In J. Maser & R. C. Cloninger (Eds.), *Comorbidity of mood and anxiety disorders* (pp. 499–543). Washington, DC: American Psychiatric Press.

Allport, G. W., & Odbert, H. S. (1936). Trait-names: A psycholexical study. *Psychological Monographs, 47*(1, Whole No. 211).

Almada, S. J., Zonderman, A. B., Shekelle, R. B., & Dyer, A. R. (1991). Neuroticism and cynicism and risk of death in middle-aged men: The Western Electric study. *Psychosomatic Medicine, 53,* 165–175.

Almagor, M., & Ben-Porath, Y. S. (1991). Mood changes during the menstrual cycle and their relation to the use of oral contraceptive. *Journal of Psychosomatic Research, 6,* 721–728.

American Psychiatric Association. (1980). *Diagnostic and statistical manual of mental disorders* (3rd ed.). Washington, DC: Author.

American Psychiatric Association. (1987). *Diagnostic and statistical manual of mental disorders* (3rd ed., rev.). Washington, DC: Author.

American Psychiatric Association. (1994). *Diagnostic and statistical manual of mental disorders* (4th ed.). Washington, DC: Author.

Amies, P. L., Gelder, M. G., & Shaw, P. M. (1983). Social phobia: A comparative clinical study. *British Journal of Psychiatry, 142,* 174–179.

Anderson, K. O., Bradley, L. A., Young, L. D., McDaniel, L. K., & Wise, C. M. (1985). Rheumatoid arthritis: Review of psychological factors related to etiology, effects, and treatment. *Psychological Bulletin, 98,* 358–387.

Andrews, F. M., & Withey, S. B. (1976). *Social indicators of well-being: America's perception of life quality.* New York: Plenum.

Argyle, M. (1987). *The psychology of happiness.* New York: Methuen.

Argyle, M., & Martin, M. (1991). The psychological causes of happiness. In F. Strack, M. Argyle, & N. Schwarz (Eds.), *Subjective well-being: An interdisciplinary perspective* (pp. 77–100). New York: Pergamon Press.

Arvey, R. D., Bouchard, T. J., Jr., Segal, N. L., & Abraham, L. M. (1989). Job satisfaction: Environmental and genetic determinants. *Journal of Applied Psychology, 74,* 187–192.

Aschoff, J., Giedke, H., Poppel, E., & Wever, R. (1972). The influence of sleep-interrruption and of sleep-deprivation on circadian rhythms in human performance. In W. P. Colquhuon (Ed.), *Aspects of human efficiency: Diurnal rhythm and loss of sleep* (pp. 135–150). London: English Universities Press.

Assenheimer, J. S., & Watson, D. (1991). [Self- and partner-ratings of trait affect: Convergent and discriminant validity and correlations with relationship satisfaction.] Unpublished raw data.

Auerbach, S. M. (1973a). Effects of orienting instructions, feedback-information, and trait-anxiety level on state-anxiety. *Psychological Reports, 33,* 779–786.

Auerbach, S. M. (1973b). Trait–state anxiety and adjustment to surgery. *Journal of Consulting and Clinical Psychology, 40,* 264–271.

Averill, J. R. (1994). In the eyes of the beholder. In P. Ekman & R. J. Davidson (Eds.), *The nature of emotion: Fundamental questions* (pp. 7–14). New York: Oxford University Press.

Banks, M. H., & Jackson, P. R. (1982). Unemployment and risk of minor psychiatric disorder in young people: Cross sectional and longitudinal evidence. *Psychological Medicine, 12,* 789–798.

Barlow, D. H. (1991). The nature of anxiety: Anxiety, depression, and emotional disorders. In R. M. Rapee & D. H. Barlow (Eds.), *Chronic anxiety: Generalized anxiety disorder and mixed anxiety–depression* (pp. 1–28). New York: Guilford Press.

Barlow, D. H., & DiNardo, P. A. (1991). The diagnosis of generalized anxiety disorder: Development, current status, and future directions. In R. M. Rapee & D. H. Barlow (Eds.), *Chronic anxiety: Generalized anxiety disorder and mixed anxiety–depression* (pp. 95–118). New York: Guilford Press.

Barrett, D. H., Resnick, H. S., Foy, D. W., Dansky, B. S., Flanders, W. D., & Stroup, N. E. (1996). Combat exposure and adult psychosocial adjustment among U.S. army veterans serving in Vietnam, 1965–1971. *Journal of Abnormal Psychology, 105,* 575–581.

Barsky, A. J., & Klerman, G. L. (1983). Overview: Hypochondriasis, bodily complaints, and somatic styles. *American Journal of Psychiatry, 140,* 273–283.

Bauer, M. S., & Dunner, D. L. (1993). Validity of seasonal pattern as a modifier for recurrent mood disorders for DSM-IV. *Comprehensive Psychiatry, 34,* 159–170.

Beck, A. T. (1976). *Cognitive therapy and the emotional disorders.* New York: New American Library.

Beck, A. T. (1987). Cognitive models of depression. *Journal of Cognitive Psychotherapy, An International Quarterly, 1,* 5–37.

Beck, A. T. (1991). Cognitive therapy: A 30-year retrospective. *American Psychologist, 46,* 368–375.

Beck, A. T., Epstein, N., Brown, G., & Steer, R. A. (1988). An inventory for measuring clinical anxiety: Psychometric properties. *Journal of Consulting and Clinical Psychology, 56,* 343–352.

Beck, A. T., Rush, A. J., Shaw, B. F., & Emery, G. (1979). *Cognitive therapy of depression.* New York: Guilford Press.

Beck, A. T., Ward, C. H., Mendelson, M., Mock, J., & Erbaugh, J. (1961). An inventory for measuring depression. *Archives of General Psychiatry, 4,* 561–571.

Beer, J. M., Arnold, R. D., & Loehlin, J. C. (1998). Genetic and environmental influences on MMPI factor scales: Joint model fitting to twin and adoption data. *Journal of Personality and Social Psychology, 74,* 818–827.

Beiser, M. (1974). Components and correlates of mental well-being. *Journal of Health and Social Behavior, 15,* 320–327.

Bentler, P. M. (1969). Semantic space is (approximately) bipolar. *Journal of Psychology, 71,* 33–40.

Berenbaum, H., & Fujita, F. (1994). Schizophrenia and personality: Exploring the boundaries and connections between vulnerability and outcome. *Journal of Abnormal Psychology, 103,* 148–158.

Berenbaum, H., Fujita, F., & Pfennig, J. (1995). Consistency, specificity, and correlates of negative emotions. *Journal of Personality and Social Psychology, 68,* 342–352.

Berenbaum, H., & Williams, M. (1995). Personality and emotional reactivity. *Journal of Research in Personality, 29,* 24–34.

Berger, B. G., Owen, D. R., & Man, F. (1993). A brief review of literature and examination of acute mood benefits of exercise in Czechoslovakian and United States swimmers. *International Journal of Sport Psychology, 24,* 130–150.

Berger, R. J., & Phillips, N. H. (1995). Energy conservation and sleep. *Behavioral Brain Research, 69,* 65–73.

Berry, D. S., & Hansen, J. S. (1996). Positive affect, negative affect, and social interaction. *Journal of Personality and Social Psychology, 71,* 796–809.

Bierce, A. (1958). *The devil's dictionary.* New York: Dover. (Original work published 1911)

Blake, M. J. F. (1967). Relationship between circadian rhythm of body temperature and introversion–extraversion. *Nature, 215,* 896–897.

Block, J. (1995). A contrarian view of the five-factor approach to personality description. *Psychological Bulletin, 117,* 187–215.

Blood, M. R. (1969). Work values and satisfaction. *Journal of Applied Psychology, 53,* 456–459.

Blumberg, S. H., & Izard, C. E. (1986). Discriminating patterns of emotions in 10- and 11-year-old children's anxiety and depression. *Journal of Personality and Social Psychology, 51,* 852–857.

Bond, M. R., & Pearson, I. B. (1969). Psychological aspects of pain in women with advanced cancer of the cervix. *Journal of Psychosomatic Research, 13,* 13–19.

Booker, J. M., & Helleckson, C. J. (1992). Prevalence of seasonal affective disorder in Alaska. *American Journal of Psychiatry, 149,* 1176–1182.

Booth-Kewley, S., & Friedman, H. S. (1987). Psychological predictors of heart disease: A quantitative review. *Psychological Bulletin, 101,* 343–362.

Borgatta, E. F. (1964). The structure of personality characteristics. *Behavioral Science, 9,* 8–17.

Bosscher, R. J. (1993). Running and mixed physical exercises with depressed psychiatric inpatients. *International Journal of Sport Psychology, 24,* 170–184.

Botwin, M. D., & Foley, P. J. (1988, August). *Replication of the NEO-PI and its relationship to the EPQ.* Paper presented at the 96th annual convention of the American Psychological Association, Atlanta, GA.

Bower, G. H. (1981). Mood and memory. *American Psychologist, 36,* 129–148.

Bowlby, J. (1980). *Attachment and Loss: Vol. 3: Loss.* New York: Basic Books.

Boyle, G. J., & Grant, A. F. (1992). Prospective versus retrospective assessment of menstrual cycle symptoms and moods: Role of attitudes and beliefs. *Journal of Psychopathology and Behavioral Assessment, 14,* 307–321.

Bradburn, N. M. (1969). *The structure of psychological well-being.* Chicago: Aldine.

Brady, E. U., & Kendall, P. C. (1992). Comorbidity of anxiety and depression in children and adolescents. *Journal of Consulting and Clinical Psychology, 111,* 244–255.

Brand, F. N., McGee, D. L., Kannel, W. B., Stokes, J., III, & Castelli, W. P. (1985). Hyperuricemia as a risk factor of coronary heart disease: The Framingham study. *American Journal of Epidemiology, 121,* 11–18.

Brickman, P., & Campbell, D. T. (1971). Hedonic relativism and planning the good society. In M. H. Appley (Ed.), *Adaptation level theory: A symposium* (pp. 287–302). New York: Academic Press.

Brickman, P., Coates, D., & Janoff-Bulman, R. (1978). Lottery winners and accident victims: Is happiness relative? *Journal of Personality and Social Psychology, 36,* 917–927.

Brief, A. P., Burke, M. J., George, J. M., Robinson, B. S., & Webster, J. (1988). Should negative affectivity remain an unmeasured variable in the study of job stress? *Journal of Applied Psychology, 73,* 193–198.

Brief, A. P., Butcher, A. H., George, J. M., & Link, K. E. (1993). Integrating bottom-up and top-down theories of subjective well-being: The case of health. *Journal of Personality and Social Psychology, 64,* 646–653.

Brief, A. P., Butcher, A. H., & Roberson, L. (1995). Cookies, disposition, and job attitudes: The effects of positive mood inducing events and negative affectivity on job satisfaction in a field experiment. *Organizational Behavior and Human Decision Processes, 62,* 55–62.

Briggs, S. R. (1989). The optimal level of measurement for personality constructs. In D. M. Buss & N. Cantor (Eds.), *Personality psychology: Recent trends and emerging directions* (pp. 246–260). New York: Springer.

Brodman, K., Erdmann, A. J., & Wolff, H. G. (1949). *Cornell Medical Index—Health Questionnaire.* New York: Cornell University Medical College.

Brown, K. W., & Moskowitz, D. S. (1997). Does unhappiness make you sick? The role of affect and neuroticism in the experience of common physical symptoms. *Journal of Personality and Social Psychology, 72,* 907–917.

Brown, L. L., Tomarken, A. J., Orth, D. N., Loosen, P. T., Kalin, N. H., & Davidson, R. J. (1996). Individual differences in repressive-defensiveness predict basal salivary cortisol levels. *Journal of Personality and Social Psychology, 70,* 362–371.

Brown, T. A., Antony, M. M., & Barlow, D. H. (1995). Diagnostic comorbidity in panic disorder: Effect on treatment outcome and course of comorbid diagnoses following treatment. *Journal of Consulting and Clinical Psychology, 63,* 408–418.

Brown, T. A., & Barlow, D. H. (1992). Comorbidity among anxiety disorders: Implications for treatment and DSM-IV. *Journal of Consulting and Clinical Psychology, 60,* 835–844.

Brown, T. A., Chorpita, B. F., & Barlow, D. H. (1998). Structural relationships among dimensions of the DSM-IV anxiety and mood disorders and dimensions of negative affect, positive affect, and autonomic arousal. *Journal of Abnormal Psychology, 107,* 179–192.

Brozek, J., Keys, A., Blackburn, H. (1966). Personality differences between potential coronary and non-coronary subjects. *Annals of the New York Academy of Sciences, 134,* 1057–1064.

Bruder, G. E., Fong, R., Tenke, C. E., Leite, P., Towey, J. P., Stewart, J. E., McGrath, P. J., & Quitkin, F. M. (1997). Regional brain asymmetries in major depression with and without an anxiety disorder: A quantitative EEG study. *Biological Psychiatry, 41,* 939–948.

Bruder, G. E., Tenke, C., Towey, J., Leite, P., Fong, R., Stewart, J., & Quitkin, F.

(1996). Topographic analyses of brain potentials in depressed patients. *Biological Psychiatry, 39,* 566.

Burke, M. J., Brief, A. P., & George, J. M. (1993). The role of negative affectivity in understanding relations between self-reports of stressors and strains: A comment on the applied psychology literature. *Journal of Applied Psychology, 78,* 402–412.

Burke, M. J., Brief, A. P., George, J. M., Roberson, L., & Webster, J. (1989). Measuring affect at work: Confirmatory factor analyses of competing mood structures with conceptual linkage to cortical regulatory systems. *Journal of Personality and Social Psychology, 57,* 1091–1102.

Bushman, B. J., Cooper, H. M., & Lemke, K. M. (1991). Meta-analysis of factor analyses: An illustration using the Buss–Durkee Hostility Inventory. *Personality and Social Psychology Bulletin, 17,* 344–349.

Buss, A., & Plomin, R. (1984). *Temperament: Early developing personality traits.* Hillsdale, NJ: Erlbaum.

Byrne, A., & Byrne, D. G. (1993). The effect of exercise on depression, anxiety and other mood states: A review. *Journal of Psychosomatic Research, 37,* 565–574.

Byrne, D., Steinberg, M. A., & Schwartz, M. S. (1968). Relationship between Repression-Sensitization and physical illness. *Journal of Abnormal Psychology, 73,* 154–155.

Cacioppo, J. T., & Berntson, G. G. (1994). Relationship between attitudes and evaluative space: A critical review, with emphasis on the separability of positive and negative substrates. *Psychological Bulletin, 115,* 401–423.

Caminada, H., & de Bruijn, F. (1992). Diurnal variation, morningness–eveningness, and momentary affect. *European Journal of Personality, 6,* 43–69.

Campbell, A. (1981). *The sense of well-being in America.* New York: McGraw-Hill.

Campbell, A., Converse, P. E., & Rodgers, W. L. (1976). *The quality of American life: Perceptions, evaluations, and satisfactions.* New York: Russell Sage.

Campbell, J. (1986). *Winston Churchill's afternoon nap: A wide-awake inquiry into the human nature of time.* New York: Simon & Schuster.

Cannon, W. B. (1927). The James–Lange theory of emotions: A critical examination and an alternative. *American Journal of Psychology, 39,* 106–124.

Cannon, W. B. (1929). *Bodily changes in pain, hunger, fear and rage.* Boston: Branford.

Cantril, H. (1965). *The pattern of human concerns.* New Brunswick, NJ: Rutgers University Press.

Carp, F. M. (1985). Relevance of personality traits to adjustment in group living situations. *Journal of Gerontology, 40,* 544–551.

Cassileth, B. R., Lusk, E. J., Strouse, T. B., Miller, D. S., Brown, L., Cross, P. A., & Tenaglia, A. N. (1984). Psychosocial status in chronic illness: A comparative analysis of six diagnostic groups. *New England Journal of Medicine, 311,* 506–511.

Cattell, R. B. (1945). The principal trait clusters for describing personality. *Psychological Bulletin, 42,* 129–161.

Cattell, R. B. (1946). *The description and measurement of personality.* Yonkers-on-Hudson, NY: World Book.

Cattell, R. B., & Scheier, I. H. (1961). *The meaning and measurement of neuroticism and anxiety.* New York: Ronald Press.

Chapman, L. J. (1967). Illusory correlation in observational report. *Journal of Verbal Learning and Verbal Behavior, 6,* 151–155.

Chapman, L. J., & Chapman, J. P. (1969). Illusory correlation as an obstacle to the use of valid psychodiagnostic signs. *Journal of Abnormal Psychology, 74,* 271–280.

Charry, J. M., & Hawkinshire, F. B. W. (1981). Effects of atmospheric electricity on some substrates of disordered social behavior. *Journal of Personality and Social Psychology, 41,* 185–197.

Chen, P. Y., & Spector, P. E. (1991). Negative affectivity as the underlying cause of correlations between stressors and strains. *Journal of Applied Psychology, 76,* 398–407.

Chorpita, B. F., Albano, A. M., & Barlow, D. H. (1998). The structure of negative emotions in a clinical sample of children and adolescents. *Journal of Abnormal Psychology, 107,* 74–85.

Christie, M., & Venables, P. (1973). Mood changes in relation to age, EPI scores, time and day. *British Journal of Social and Clinical Psychology, 12,* 61–72.

Clark, D. A., Beck, A. T., & Beck, J. S. (1994). Symptom differences in major depression, dysthymia, panic disorder, and generalized anxiety disorder. *American Journal of Psychiatry, 151,* 205–209.

Clark, D. A., Beck, A. T., & Stewart, B. (1990). Cognitive specificity and positive–negative affectivity: Complementary or contradictory views on anxiety and depression? *Journal of Abnormal Psychology, 99,* 148–155.

Clark, D. A., Steer, R. A., & Beck, A. T. (1994). Common and specific dimensions of self-reported anxiety and depression: Implications for the cognitive and tripartite models. *Journal of Abnormal Psychology, 103,* 645–654.

Clark, L. A. (1989). The anxiety and depressive disorders: Descriptive psychopathology and differential diagnosis. In P. C. Kendall & D. Watson (Eds.), *Anxiety and depression: Distinctive and overlapping features* (pp. 83–129). San Diego, CA: Academic Press.

Clark, L. A., Ingersoll, K. S., Soutter, C., Hook, P., & Watson, D. (1989). *Exercise and its relation to Positive and Negative Affect.* Unpublished manuscript.

Clark, L. A., & Watson, D. (1988). Mood and the mundane: Relations between daily life events and self-reported mood. *Journal of Personality and Social Psychology, 54,* 296–308.

Clark, L. A., & Watson, D. (1990). *The General Temperament Survey.* Unpublished manuscript, University of Iowa, Iowa City.

Clark, L. A., & Watson, D. (1991a). Theoretical and empirical issues in differentiating anxiety from depression. In J. Becker & A. Kleinman (Eds.), *Psychosocial aspects of mood disorders* (pp. 39–65). Hillsdale, NJ: Erlbaum.

Clark, L. A., & Watson, D. (1991b). Tripartite model of anxiety and depression: Psychometric evidence and taxonomic implications. *Journal of Abnormal Psychology, 100,* 316–336.

Clark, L. A., & Watson, D. (1994). Distinguishing functional from dysfunctional affective responses. In P. Ekman & R. J. Davidson (Eds.), *The nature of emotion: Fundamental questions* (pp. 131–136). New York: Oxford University Press.

Clark, L. A., Watson, D., & Leeka, J. (1989). Diurnal variation in the positive affects. *Motivation and Emotion, 13,* 205–234.

Clark, L. A., Watson, D., & Mineka, S. (1994). Temperament, personality, and the mood and anxiety disorders. *Journal of Abnormal Psychology, 103,* 103–116.

Clements, P. R., Hafer, M. D., & Vermillion, M. E. (1976). Psychometric, diurnal, and electrophysiological correlates of activation. *Journal of Personality and Social Psychology, 33,* 387–394.

Cloninger, C. R. (1987). A systematic method for clinical description and classification of personality variants. *Archives of General Psychiatry, 44,* 573–588.

Clore, G. L., Ortony, A., & Foss, M. A. (1987). The psychological foundations of the affective lexicon. *Journal of Personality and Social Psychology, 53,* 751–766.

Cochrane, R. (1969). Neuroticism and the discovery of high blood pressure. *Journal of Psychosomatic Research, 13,* 21–25.

Cochrane, R. (1973). Hostility and neuroticism among unselected essential hypertensives. *Journal of Psychosomatic Research, 17,* 215–218.

Cohen, S., Doyle, W. J., Skoner, D. P., Fireman, P., Gwaltney, J. M., Jr., & Newsom, J. T. (1995). State and trait negative affect as predictors of objective and subjective symptoms of respiratory viral infections. *Journal of Personality and Social Psychology, 68,* 159–169.

Cohen, S., Tyrrell, D. A. J., & Smith, A. P. (1993). Negative life events, perceived stress, negative affect, and susceptibility to the common cold. *Journal of Personality and Social Psychology, 64,* 131–140.

Cohen, S., & Williamson, G. (1991). Stress and infectious disease in humans. *Psychological Bulletin, 109,* 5–24.

Cole, D. A., Truglio, R., & Peeke, L. (1997). Relation between symptoms of anxiety and depression in children: A multitrait-multimethod-multigroup assessment. *Journal of Consulting and Clinical Psychology, 65,* 110–119.

Coleman, R. M. (1986). *Wide awake at 3 a.m.: By choice or by chance?* New York: Freeman.

Cook, E. W., III, Hawk, L. W., Jr., Davis, T. L., & Stevenson, V. E. (1991). Affective individual differences and startle reflex modulation. *Journal of Abnormal Psychology, 100,* 5–13.

Cook, W. W., & Medley, D. M. (1954). Proposed Hostility and Pharisaic-Virtue scales for the MMPI. *Journal of Applied Psychology, 38,* 414–418.

Coppen, A., & Kessel, N. (1963). Menstruation and personality. *British Journal of Psychiatry, 109,* 711.

Costa, P. T., Jr., Fleg, J. L., McCrae, R. R., & Lakatta, E. G. (1982). Neuroticism, coronary artery disease, and chest pain complaints: Cross-sectional and longitudinal studies. *Experimental Aging Research, 8,* 37–44.

Costa, P. T., Jr., & McCrae, R. R. (1980a). Influence of extraversion and neuroticism on subjective well-being: Happy and unhappy people. *Journal of Personality and Social Psychology, 38,* 668–678.

Costa, P. T., Jr., & McCrae, R. R. (1980b). Somatic complaints in males as a function of age and neuroticism: A longitudinal analysis. *Journal of Behavioral Medicine, 3,* 245–257.

Costa, P. T., Jr., & McCrae, R. R. (1984). Personality as a life-long determinant of well-being. In C. Z. Malatesta & C. E. Izard (Eds.), *Emotion in adult development* (pp. 141–157). Beverly Hills, CA: Sage.

Costa, P. T., Jr., & McCrae, R. R. (1985a). Hypochondriasis, neuroticism, and aging: When are somatic complaints unfounded? *American Psychologist, 40,* 19–28.

Costa, P. T., Jr., & McCrae, R. R. (1985b). *The NEO Personality Inventory Manual.* Odessa, FL: Psychological Assessment Resources.

Costa, P. T., Jr., & McCrae, R. R. (1987). Neuroticism, somatic complaints, and disease: Is the bark worse than the bite? *Journal of Personality, 55,* 299–316.

Costa, P. T., Jr., & McCrae, R. R. (1988a). From catalog to classification: Murray's needs and the five-factor model. *Journal of Personality and Social Psychology, 55,* 258–265.

Costa, P. T., Jr., & McCrae, R. R. (1988b). Personality in adulthood: A six-year longitudinal study of self-reports and spouse ratings on the NEO Personality Inventory. *Journal of Personality and Social Psychology, 54,* 853–863.

Costa, P. T., Jr., & McCrae, R. R. (1992). *Revised NEO Personality Inventory (NEO-PI-R) and NEO Five-Factor Inventory (NEO-FFI) professional manual.* Odessa, FL: Psychological Assessment Resources.

Costa, P. T., Jr., & McCrae, R. R. (1994). Stability and change in personality from adolescence through adulthood. In C. F. Halverson, G. A. Kohnstamm, & R. P. Martin (Eds.), *The developing structure of temperament and personality from infancy to adulthood* (pp. 139–150). Hillsdale, NJ: Erlbaum.

Costa, P. T., Jr., McCrae, R. R., Andres, R., & Tobin, J. D. (1980). Hypertension, somatic complaints, and personality. In M. F. Elias & D. Streeten (Eds.), *Hypertension and cognitive processes* (pp. 95–110). Mt. Desert, ME: Beech-Hill.

Costa, P. T., Jr., McCrae, R. R., & Dembroski, T. M. (1989). Agreeableness vs. antagonism: Explication of a potential risk factor for CHD. In A. W. Siegman & T. M. Dembroski (Eds.), *In search of coronary-prone behavior* (pp. 41–63). Hillsdale, NJ: Erlbaum.

Costa, P. T., Jr., McCrae, R. R., & Zonderman, A. B. (1987). Environmental and dispositional influences on well-being: Longitudinal follow-up of an American national sample. *British Journal of Psychology, 78,* 299–306.

Cousins, N. (1989). *Head first: The biology of hope.* New York: Dutton.

Crohan, S. E., Antonucci, T. C., Adelmann, P. K., & Coleman, L. M. (1989). Job characteristics and well-being at midlife: Ethnic and gender comparisons. *Psychology of Women Quarterly, 13,* 223–235.

Cronbach, L. J., & Meehl, P. E. (1955). Construct validity in psychological tests. *Psychological Bulletin, 52,* 281–302.

Crowne, D. P., & Marlowe, D. (1964). *The approval motive: Studies in evaluative dependence.* New York: Wiley.

Csikszentmihalyi, M. (1991). *Flow: The psychology of optimal experience.* New York: Harper Perennial.

Cunningham, M. R. (1979). Weather, mood, and helping behavior: Quasi-experiments with the sunshine samaritan. *Journal of Personality and Social Psychology, 37,* 1947–1956.

Cunningham, M. R. (1988a). Does happiness mean friendliness? Induced mood and heterosexual self-disclosure. *Personality and Social Psychology Bulletin, 14,* 283–297.

Cunningham, M. R. (1988b). What do you do when you're happy or blue? Mood, expectancies, and behavioral interest. *Motivation and Emotion, 12,* 309–331.

Curtis, G. C., Fogel, M. L., McEvoy, D., & Zarate, C. (1966). The effect of sustained affect on the diurnal rhythm of adrenal cortical activity. *Psychosomatic Medicine, 28,* 696–713.

Cuthbert, B. N., Strauss, C., Drobes, D., Patrick, C., Bradley, M. M., & Lang, P. J. (1997). *Startle and the anxiety disorders.* Unpublished manuscript, University of Florida, Gainesville, FL.

Dark, J., & Zucker, I. (1985). Seasonal cycles in energy balance: Regulation by light. *Annals of the New York Academy of Sciences, 453,* 170–181.

Dattore, P. J., Shontz, F. C., & Coyne, L. (1980). Premorbid personality differentiation of cancer and noncancer groups: A test of the hypothesis of cancer proneness. *Journal of Consulting and Clinical Psychology, 48,* 388–394.

Davidson, J. T. R., Giller, E. L., Zisook, S., & Overall, J. E. (1988). An efficacy study of isocarboxazid in depression and its relationship to depressive nosology. *Archives of General Psychiatry, 45,* 120–128.

Davidson, P. O., & Bobey, M. J. (1970). Repressor–sensitizer differences on repeated exposure to pain. *Perceptual and Motor Skills, 31,* 711–714.

Davidson, R. J. (1992). Anterior asymmetry and the nature of emotion. *Brain and Cognition, 20,* 125–151.

Davidson, R. J., & Tomarken, A. J. (1989). Laterality and emotion: An electrophysiological approach. In F. Boller & J. Grafman (Eds.), *Handbook of neuropsychology* (pp. 419–441). Amsterdam: Elsevier.

Davies, M. (1970). Blood pressure and personality. *Journal of Psychosomatic Research, 14,* 89–104.

Davis-Blake, A., & Pfeffer, J. (1989). Just a mirage: The search for dispositional effects in organizational research. *Academy of Management Review, 14,* 385–400.

Delespaul, P. A. E. G., & deVries, M. W. (1987). The daily life of ambulatory chronic mental patients. *Journal of Nervous and Mental Disease, 175,* 537–544.

DeLongis, A., Folkman, S., & Lazarus, R. S. (1988). The impact of daily stress on health and mood: Psychological and social resources as mediators. *Journal of Personality and Social Psychology, 54,* 486–495.

Dembroski, T. M., MacDougall, J. M., Costa, P. T., Jr., & Grandits, G. A. (1989). Components of hostility as predictors of sudden death and myocardial infarction in the Multiple Risk Factor Intervention Trial. *Psychosomatic Medicine, 51,* 514–522.

Demo, D. H., & Acock, A. C. (1996). Singlehood, marriage, and remarriage: The effects of family structure and family relationships on mothers' well-being. *Journal of Family Issues, 17,* 388–407.

Depue, R. A., & Iacono, W. G. (1989). Neurobehavioral aspects of affective disorders. *Annual Review of Psychology, 40,* 457–492.

Depue, R. A., Krauss, S., & Spoont, M. R. (1987). A two-dimensional threshold model of seasonal bipolar affective disorder. In D. Magnusson & A. Ohman (Eds.), *Psychopathology: An interactional perspective* (pp. 95–123). San Diego, CA: Academic Press.

Depue, R. A., Luciana, M., Arbisi, P., Collins, P., & Leon, A. (1994). Dopamine and the structure of personality: Relation of agonist-induced dopamine activity to positive emotionality. *Journal of Personality and Social Psychology, 67,* 485–498.

Derogatis, L. R., Abeloff, M., & Melisaratos, N. (1979). Psychological coping mechanisms and survival time in metastatic breast cancer. *Journal of the American Medical Association, 242,* 1504–1508.

Derogatis, L. R., Lipman, R. S., Rickels, K., Uhlenhuth, E. H., & Covi, L. (1974). The Hopkins Symptom Checklist (HSCL): A self-report symptom inventory. *Behavioral Science, 19,* 1–15.

Diamond, E. L. (1982). The role of anger and hostility in essential hypertension and coronary heart disease. *Psychological Bulletin, 92,* 410–433.

Diener, E. (1984). Subjective well-being. *Psychological Bulletin, 95,* 542–575.

Diener, E. (1996). Traits can be powerful, but are not enough: Lessons from subjective well-being. *Journal of Research in Personality, 30,* 389–399.

Diener, E., & Diener, C. (1996). Most people are happy. *Psychological Science, 7,* 181–185.

Diener, E., Diener, C., & Diener, M. (1995). Factors predicting the subjective well-being of nations. *Journal of Personality and Social Psychology, 69,* 851–864.

Diener, E., Fugita, F., & Sandvik, E. (1994). What subjective well-being researchers can tell emotion researchers about affect. In N. Frijda (Ed.), *Proceedings of the 8th meeting of the International Society for Research on Emotion,* Cambridge, England.

Diener, E., Horwitz, J., & Emmons, R. A. (1985). Happiness of the very wealthy. *Social Indicators, 16,* 263–274.

Diener, E., & Iran-Nejad, A. (1986). The relationship in experience between various types of affect. *Journal of Personality and Social Psychology, 50,* 1031–1038.

Diener, E., & Larsen, R. J. (1984). Temporal stability and cross-situational consistency of affective, behavioral, and cognitive responses. *Journal of Personality and Social Psychology, 47,* 871–883.

Diener, E., & Larsen, R. J. (1993). The experience of emotional well-being. In M. Lewis & J. M. Haviland (Eds.), *Handbook of emotions* (pp. 405–415). New York: Guilford Press.

Diener, E., Sandvik, E., Seidlitz, L., & Diener, M. (1993). The relationship between income and subjective well-being: Relative or absolute? *Social Indicators Research, 28,* 195–223.

Diener, E., Smith, H., & Fujita, F. (1995). The personality structure of affect. *Journal of Personality and Social Psychology, 69,* 130–141.

Digman, J. M. (1990). Personality structure: Emergence of the five-factor model. *Annual Review of Psychology, 41,* 417–440.

Digman, J. M. (1997). Higher-order factors of the Big Five. *Journal of Personality and Social Psychology, 73,* 1246–1256.

Digman, J. M., & Inouye, J. (1986). Further specification of five robust factors of personality. *Journal of Personality and Social Psychology, 50,* 116–123.

Dyck, M. J., Jolly, J. B., & Kramer, T. (1994). An evaluation of positive affectivity, negative affectivity, and hyperarousal as markers for assessing between syndrome relationships. *Personality and Individual Differences, 17,* 637–646.

Eaves, L. J., Eysenck, H. J., & Martin, N. G. (1989). *Genes, culture and personality: An empirical approach.* San Diego, CA: Academic Press.

Egloff, B., Tausch, A., Kohlmann, C-W., & Krohne, H. W. (1995). Relationships between time of day, day of the week, and positive mood: Exploring the role of the mood measure. *Motivation and Emotion, 19,* 99–110.

Ekman, P. (1982). *Emotion in the human face* (2nd ed.). Cambridge, UK: Cambridge University Press.

Ekman, P. (1994). Strong evidence for universals in facial expressions: A reply to Russell's mistaken critique. *Psychological Bulletin, 115,* 268–287.

Ekman, P., & Davidson, R. J. (Eds.). (1994). *The nature of emotion: Fundamental questions.* New York: Oxford University Press.

Ekman, P., & Friesen, W. V. (1975). *Unmasking the face.* Englewood Cliffs, NJ: Prentice-Hall.

Ekman, P., Friesen, W. V., O'Sullivan, M., Chan, A., Diacoyanni-Tarlatzis, I., Heider, K., Krause, R., LeCompte, W. A., Pitcairn, T., Ricci-Bitti, P. E., Scherer, K., Tomita, M., & Tzavaras, A. (1987). Universals and cultural differences in the judgments of facial expressions of emotion. *Journal of Personality and Social Psychology, 53,* 712–717.

Ekman, P., Levenson, R. W., & Friesen, W. V. (1983). Autonomic nervous system activity distinguishes between emotions. *Science, 221,* 1208–1210.

Elkin, I., Shea, M. T., Watkins, J. T., Imber, S. D., Sotsky, S. M., Collins, J. F., Glass, D. R., Pilkonis, P. A., Leber, W. R., Docherty, J. P., Fiester, S. J., & Parloff, M. B. (1989). NIMH Treatment of Depression Collaborative Research Program: I. General effectiveness of treatments. *Archives of General Psychiatry, 46,* 971–983.

Ellis, A. (1962). *Reason and emotion in psychotherapy.* Secaucus, NJ: Citadel Press.

Ellis, A. (1987). The impossibility of achieving consistently good mental health. *American Psychologist, 42,* 364–375.

Ellison, C. G. (1991). Religious involvement and subjective well-being. *Journal of Health and Social Behavior, 32,* 80–99.

Emmons, R. A. (1986). Personal strivings: An approach to personality and subjective well-being. *Journal of Personality and Social Psychology, 51,* 1058–1068.

Emmons, R. A., & Diener, E. (1985). Personality correlates of subjective well-being. *Personality and Social Psychology Bulletin, 11,* 89–97.

Emmons, R. A., & Diener, E. (1986). Influence of impulsivity and sociability on subjective well-being. *Journal of Personality and Social Psychology, 50,* 1211–1215.

Emmons, R. A., & King, L. A. (1989). Personal striving differentiation and affective reactivity. *Journal of Personality and Social Psychology, 56,* 478–484.

Epstein, S. (1980). The stability of behavior: II. Implications for psychological research. *American Psychologist, 35,* 790–806.

Ewart, C. K., & Kolodner, K. B. (1994). Negative affect, gender, and expressive style predict elevated ambulatory blood pressure in adolescents. *Journal of Personality and Social Psychology, 66,* 596–605.

Eysenck, H. J. (1967). *The biological basis of personality.* Springfield, IL: C. C. Thomas.

Eysenck, H. J. (1980). Personality, marital satisfaction, and divorce. *Psychological Reports, 47,* 1235–1238.

Eysenck, H. J. (1983). Cicero and the state-trait theory of anxiety: Another case of delayed recognition. *American Psychologist, 38,* 114–115.

Eysenck, H. J. (1992). Four ways five factors are *not* basic. *Personality and Individual Differences, 6,* 667–673.

Eysenck, H. J. (1994). Cancer, personality and stress: Prediction and prevention. *Advances in Behaviour Research and Therapy, 16,* 167–215.

Eysenck, H. J., & Eysenck, S. B. G. (1968). *Manual of the Eysenck Personality Inventory.* San Diego, CA: Educational and Industrial Testing Service.

Eysenck, H. J., & Eysenck, S. B. G. (1975). *Manual of the Eysenck Personality Questionnaire.* San Diego, CA: Educational and Industrial Testing Service.

Eysenck, H. J., & Wakefield, J. A. (1981). Psychological factors as predictors of marital satisfaction. *Advances in Behavior Research and Therapy, 3,* 151–192.

Eysenck, M. W. (1990). *Happiness: Facts and myths.* East Sussex, UK: Erlbaum.

Falconer, D. S. (1960). *Introduction to quantitative genetics.* New York: Ronald Press.

Farber, M. L. (1953). Time-perspective and feeling-tone: A study in the perception of the days. *Journal of Psychology, 35,* 253–257.

Feldman, L. A. (1993). Distinguishing depression from anxiety in self-report: Evidence from confirmatory factor analysis on nonclinical and clinical samples. *Journal of Consulting and Clinical Psychology, 61,* 631–638.

Feldman Barrett, L., & Russell, J. A. (1998). Independence and bipolarity in the structure of current affect. *Journal of Personality and Social Psychology, 74,* 967–984.

Festinger, L. (1954). A theory of social comparison processes. *Human Relations, 7,* 117–140.

Fibiger, H. C., & Phillips, A. G. (1986). Reward, motivation, cognition: Psychobiology of mesotelencephalic dopamine systems. In F. E. Bloom (Ed.), *Handbook of physiology I: The nervous system* (Vol. 4, pp. 647–675). Bethesda, MD: American Physiological Society.

Fillingim, R. B., & Fine, M. A. (1986). The effects of internal versus external information processing on symptom perception in an exercise setting. *Health Psychology, 5,* 115–123.

Finn, S. E. (1986). Stability of personality self-ratings over 30 years: Evidence for an age/cohort interaction. *Journal of Personality and Social Psychology, 50,* 813–818.

Fiske, D. W. (1949). Consistency of the factorial structures of personality ratings from different sources. *Journal of Abnormal and Social Psychology, 44,* 329–344.

Folkard, S. (1975). Diurnal variation in logical reasoning. *British Journal of Psychology, 66,* 1–8.

Follick, M. J., Gorkin, L., Capone, R. J., Smith, T. W., Ahern, D. K., Stablein, D., Niaura, R., & Visco, J. (1988). Psychological distress as predictor of ventricular arrhythmias in a post-myocardial infarction population. *American Heart Journal, 116,* 32–36.

Fowles, D. C. (1980). The three arousal model: Implications of Gray's two-factor learning theory for heart rate, electrodermal activity, and psychopathy. *Psychophysiology, 17,* 87–104.

Fowles, D. C. (1987). Application of a behavioral theory of motivation to the concepts of anxiety and impulsivity. *Journal of Research in Personality, 21,* 417–435.

Fowles, D. C. (1992). Schizophrenia: Diathesis-stress revisited. *Annual Review of Psychology, 43,* 303–336.

Fowles, D. C. (1994). A motivational theory of psychopathology. In W. Spaulding (Ed.), *Nebraska symposium on motivation: Integrated views of motivation, cognition and emotion* (Vol. 41, pp. 181–238). Lincoln: University of Nebraska Press.

Frasure-Smith, N. (1991). In-hospital symptoms of psychological stress as predictors of long-term outcome after acute myocardial infarction in men. *American Journal of Cardiology, 67,* 121–127.

Frasure-Smith, N., Lespérance, F., & Talajic, M. (1993). Depression following myocardial infarction: Impact on 6–month survival. *Journal of the American Medical Association, 270,* 1819–1825.

Frasure-Smith, N., Lespérance, F., & Talajic, M. (1995). The impact of negative emotions on prognosis following myocardial infarction: Is it more than depression? *Health Psychology, 14,* 388–398.

Freedman, J. L. (1978). *Happy people.* New York: Harcourt Brace Jovanovich.

Freud, S. (1961). *Civilization and its discontents* (J. Strachey, Ed. and Trans). New York: Norton. (Original work published 1930)

Friedman, H. S., & Booth-Kewley, S. (1987). The "disease-prone personality": A meta-analytic view of the construct. *American Psychologist, 42,* 539–555.

Friedman, H. S., Tucker, J. S., Tomlinson-Keasey, C., Schwartz, J. E., Wingard, D. L., & Criqui, M. H. (1993). Does childhood personality predict longevity? *Journal of Personality and Social Psychology, 65,* 176–185.

Frijda, N. (1988). The laws of emotion. *American Psychologist, 43,* 349–358.

Froberg, J. (1977). Twenty-four hour patterns in human performance, subjective and physiological variables and differences between morning and evening active subjects. *Biological Psychology, 5,* 119–134.

Froberg, J., Karlsson, C. G., Levi, L., & Lidberg, L. (1972). Circadian variations in performance, psychological ratings, catecholamine excretion, and diuresis during prolonged sleep deprivation. *International Journal of Psychobiology, 2,* 23–36.

Froberg, J., Karlsson, C. G., Levi, L., & Lidberg, L. (1975). Circadian rhythms of catecholamine excretion, shooting range performance and self-ratings of fatigue during sleep deprivation. *Biological Psychology, 2,* 175–188.

Fuchs, C. Z., & Zaichkowsky, L. D. (1983). Psychological characteristics of male and female bodybuilders: The iceberg profile. *Journal of Sport Behavior, 6,* 136–145.

Fujita, F., Diener, E., & Sandvik, E. (1991). Gender differences in dysphoria and well-being: The case for emotional intensity. *Journal of Personality and Social Psychology, 61,* 427–434.

Funder, D. C., & Colvin, C. R. (1988). Friends and strangers: Acquaintanceship, agreement, and the accuracy of personality judgment. *Journal of Personality and Social Psychology, 55,* 149–158.

Funder, D. C., & Dobroth, K. M. (1987). Differences between traits: Properties associated with interjudge agreement. *Journal of Personality and Social Psychology, 52,* 409–418.

Futterman, A. D., Kemeny, M. E., Shapiro, D., Polonsky, W., & Fahey, J. (1992). Immunological variability associated with experimentally-induced positive and negative affective states. *Psychological Medicine, 22,* 231–238.

Gainotti, G., Caltagirone, C., & Zoccolotti, P. (1993). Left/right and cortical/

subcortical dichotomies in the neuropsychological study of human emotions. *Cognition and Emotion, 7,* 71–93.

Gallup, G., Jr. (1984). *Religion in America* [Gallup report].

Gayton, W. F., Bassett, J. E., Tavormina, J., & Ozmon, K. L. (1978). Repression-sensitization and health behavior. *Journal of Consulting and Clinical Psychology, 46,* 1542–1544.

George, J. M. (1989). Mood and absence. *Journal of Applied Psychology, 74,* 317–324.

Gerhart, B. (1987). How important are dispositional factors as determinants of job satisfaction? Implications for job design and other personnel programs. *Journal of Applied Psychology, 72,* 366–373.

Glenn, N. D., & Weaver, C. N. (1981). Education's effects on psychological well-being. *Public Opinion Quarterly, 45,* 22–39.

Goldberg, L. R. (1983, June). *The magical number five, plus or minus two: Some conjectures on the dimensionality of personality descriptions.* Paper presented at a research seminar, Gerontology Research Center, Baltimore.

Goldberg, L. R. (1993). The structure of phenotypic personality traits. *American Psychologist, 48,* 26–34.

Goldman-Rakic, P. S., Lidow, M. S., & Gallagher, D. W. (1990). Overlap of dopaminergic, adrenergic, and serotoninergic receptors and complementarity of their subtypes in primate prefrontal cortex. *Journal of Neuroscience, 10,* 2125–2138.

Goldstein, K. M. (1972). Weather, mood, and internal–external control. *Perceptual and Motor Skills, 35,* 786.

Goldstein, M. D., & Strube, M. J. (1994). Independence revisited: The relation between Positive and Negative Affect in a naturalistic setting. *Personality and Social Psychology Bulletin, 20,* 57–64.

Gotlib, I. H. (1984). Depression and general psychopathology in university students. *Journal of Abnormal Psychology, 93,* 19–30.

Gottesman, I. I. (1963). Genetic aspects of intelligent behavior. In N. Ellis (Ed.), *The handbook of mental deficiency: Psychological theory and research* (pp. 253–296). New York: McGraw-Hill.

Gottesman, I. I. (1974). Developmental genetics and ontogenetic psychology: Overdue detente and propositions from a matchmaker. In A. Pick (Ed.), *Minnesota symposium on child psychology* (Vol. 6, pp. 55–80). Minneapolis: University of Minnesota Press.

Gottesman, I. I., & Goldsmith, H. H. (1994). Developmental psychopathology of antisocial behavior: Inserting genes into its ontogenesis and epigenesis. In C. A. Nelson (Ed.), *Threats to optimal development: Integrating biological, psychological, and social risk factors* (pp. 69–104). Hillsdale, NJ: Erlbaum.

Gough, H. G. (1987). *California Psychological Inventory* [Administrator's guide]. Palo Alto, CA: Consulting Psychologists Press.

Gray, J. A. (1981). The psychophysiology of anxiety. In R. Lynn (Ed.), *Dimensions of personality: Papers in honor of H. J. Eysenck* (pp. 233–252). New York: Pergamon Press.

Gray, J. A. (1982). *The neuropsychology of anxiety: An enquiry into the functions of the septo-hippocampal system.* New York: Oxford University Press.

Gray, J. A. (1985). Issues in the neuropsychology of anxiety. In A. H. Tuma & J. D. Maser (Eds.), *Anxiety and the anxiety disorders* (pp. 5–25). Hillsdale, NJ: Erlbaum.

Green, D. P., Goldman, S. L., & Salovey, P. (1993). Measurement error masks bipolarity in affect ratings. *Journal of Personality and Social Psychology, 64,* 1029–1041.

Gregory, T. (1994, October 2). Monday blues are almost tolerable compared to the Sunday night blahs. *Chicago Tribune,* pp. 1, 3.

Gross, J. J., Sutton, S. K., & Ketelaar, T. (1998). Relations between affect and personality: Support for the affect-level and affective-reactivity views. *Personality and Social Psychology Bulletin, 24,* 279–288.

Haan, N., Millsap, R., & Hartka, E. (1986). As time goes by: Change and stability in personality over fifty years. *Psychology and Aging, 1,* 220–232.

Hackman, J. R., & Oldham, G. R. (1975). Development of the Job Diagnostic Survey. *Journal of Applied Psychology, 60,* 159–170.

Halberg, F. (1983). Quo vadis basic and clinical chronobiology: Promise for health maintenance. *American Journal of Anatomy, 168,* 545–594.

Hall, E. (1987). *Growing and changing: What the experts say.* New York: Random House.

Hamilton, M. (1960). A rating scale for depression. *Journal of Neurology, Neurosurgery and Psychiatry, 23,* 56–62.

Hamilton, W. D. (1964). The genetical evolution of social behavior. *Journal of Theoretical Biology, 7,* 1–52.

Hampson, S. E., John, O. P., & Goldberg, L. R. (1986). Category breadth and hierarchical structure in personality: Studies of asymmetries in judgments of trait implications. *Journal of Personality and Social Psychology, 51,* 37–54.

Haring, M. J., Stock, W. A., & Okun, M. A. (1984). A research synthesis of gender and social class as correlates of subjective well-being. *Human Relations, 37,* 645–657.

Haring-Hidore, M., Stock, W. A., Okun, M. A., & Witter, R. A. (1985). Marital status and subjective well-being: A research synthesis. *Journal of Marriage and the Family, 47,* 947–953.

Harrell, J. P. (1980). Psychological factors and hypertension: A status report. *Psychological Bulletin, 87,* 482–501.

Harris, D. V. (1987). Comparative effectiveness of running therapy and psychotherapy. In W. P. Morgan & S. E. Goldston (Eds.), *Exercise and mental health* (pp. 123–130). Washington, DC: Hemisphere.

Harris, S., & Dawson-Hughes, B. (1993). Seasonal mood changes in 250 normal women. *Psychiatry Research, 49,* 77–87.

Hartmann, G. W. (1934). Personality traits associated with variations in happiness. *Journal of Abnormal and Social Psychology, 29,* 202–212.

Hathaway, S. R., & McKinley, J. C. (1943). *The Minnesota Multiphasic Personality Inventory* (rev. ed.). Minneapolis: University of Minnesota Press.

Haus, E., Lakatua, D. J., Swoyer, J., & Sackett-Lundeen, L. (1983). Chronobiology in hematology and immunology. *American Journal of Anatomy, 168,* 467–517.

Hayden, R. M., & Allen, G. J. (1984). Relationship between aerobic exercise, anxiety, and depression: Convergent validation by knowledgeable informants. *Journal of Sports Medicine, 24,* 69–74.

Headey, B., Holmstrom, E., & Wearing, A. (1984). The impact of life events and changes in domain satisfaction on well-being. *Social Indicators Research, 15,* 203–227.

Headey, B., & Wearing, A. (1989). Personality, life events, and subjective well-being: Toward a dynamic equilibrium model. *Journal of Personality and Social Psychology, 57,* 731–739.

Headey, B., & Wearing, A. (1991). Subjective well-being: A stocks and flows framework. In F. Strack, M. Argyle, & N. Schwarz (Eds.), *Subjective well-being: An interdisciplinary perspective* (pp. 49–73). New York: Pergamon Press.

Headey, B., & Wearing, A. (1992). *Understanding happiness: A theory of well-being.* Melbourne, Australia: Longman Cheshire.

Healy, D., & Williams, J. M. G. (1988). Dysrhythmia, dysphoria, and depression: The interaction of learned helplessness and circadian dysrhythmia in the pathogenesis of depression. *Psychological Bulletin, 103,* 163–178.

Heath, A. C., Cloninger, C. R., & Martin, N. G. (1994). Testing a model for the genetic structure of personality: A comparison of the personality systems of Cloninger and Eysenck. *Journal of Personality and Social Psychology, 66,* 762–775.

Heller, W. (1993). Neuropsychological mechanisms of individual differences in emotion, personality, and arousal. *Neuropsychology, 7,* 476–489.

Heller, W., Etienne, M. A., & Miller, G. A. (1995). Patterns of perceptual asymmetry in depression and anxiety: Implications for neuropsychological models of emotion and psychopathology. *Journal of Abnormal Psychology, 104,* 327–333.

Hellmich, N. (1995, June 9). Optimism often survives spinal cord injuries. *USA Today,* p. 4D.

Helson, R., & Klohnen, E. C. (1998). Affective coloring of personality from young adulthood to midlife. *Personality and Social Psychology Bulletin, 24,* 241–252.

Helson, R., & Moane, G. (1987). Personality change in women from college to midlife. *Journal of Personality and Social Psychology, 53,* 176–186.

Hendrick, C., & Lilly, R. S. (1970). The structure of mood: A comparison between sleep deprivation and normal wakefulness conditions. *Journal of Personality, 38,* 453–465.

Henriques, J. B., & Davidson, R. J. (1990). Regional brain electrical asymmetries discriminate between previously depressed subjects and healthy controls. *Journal of Abnormal Psychology, 99,* 22–31.

Henriques, J. B., & Davidson, R. J. (1991). Left frontal hypoactivation in depression. *Journal of Abnormal Psychology, 100,* 535–545.

Henriques, J. B., Glowacki, J. M., & Davidson, R. J. (1994). Reward fails to alter response bias in depression. *Journal of Abnormal Psychology, 103,* 460–466.

Herberman, R. (Ed.). (1982). *NK cells and other natural effector cells.* New York: Academic Press.

Herberman, R., & Ortaldo, J. (1981). Natural killer cells: Their role in defenses against disease. *Science, 214,* 24–30.

Herbert, T. B., & Cohen, S. (1993). Depression and immunity: A meta-analytic review. *Psychological Bulletin, 113,* 472–486.

Hildebrandt, G., & Geyer, F. (1984). Adaptive significance of circaseptum reactive periods. *Journal of Interdisciplinary Cycle Research, 15,* 109–117.

Hinden, B. R., Compas, B. E., Howell, D. C., & Achenbach, T. M. (1997). Covariation of the anxious-depressed syndrome during adolescence: Separating fact from artifact. *Journal of Consulting and Clinical Psychology, 65,* 6–14.

Hodges, W. F., & Spielberger, C. D. (1966). The effects of threat of shock on heart rate for subjects who differ in manifest anxiety and fear of shock. *Psychophysiology, 2,* 287–294.

Hogan, R. T. (1983). A socioanalytic theory of personality. In M. Page (Ed.), *1982 Nebraska symposium on motivation* (pp. 55–89). Lincoln: University of Nebraska Press.

Hope, D. A., & Heimberg, R. G. (1985). *Public and private self-consciousness in a social phobic sample.* Paper presented at the meeting of the Association for the Advancement of Behavior Therapy, Houston.

Hope, D. A., Heimberg, R. G., Zollo, L. G., Nyman, D. J., & O'Brien, G. T. (1987). *Thought listing in the natural environment: Valence and focus of listed thoughts among socially anxious and nonanxious subjects.* Paper presented at the meeting of the Association for the Advancement of Behavior Therapy, Boston.

Horne, J. A., & Ostberg, O. (1976). A self-assessment questionnaire to determine morningness–eveningness in human circadian rhythms. *International Journal of Chronobiology, 4,* 97–110.

Howarth, E., & Hoffman, M. S. (1984). A multidimensional approach to the relationship between mood and weather. *British Journal of Psychology, 75,* 15–23.

Inglehart, R. (1990). *Culture shift in advanced industrialized society.* Princeton, NJ: Princeton University Press.

Ingram, R. E. (1990). Self-focused attention in clinical disorders: Review and a conceptual model. *Psychological Bulletin, 107,* 156–176.

Iverson, R. D., Olekalns, M., & Erwin, P. J. (1998). Affectivity, organizational stressors, and absenteeism: A causal model of burnout and its consequences. *Journal of Vocational Behavior, 52,* 1–23.

Izard. C. E. (1971). *The face of emotion.* New York: Appleton-Century-Crofts.

Izard, C. E. (1972). *Patterns of emotions: A new analysis of anxiety and depression.* San Diego, CA: Academic Press.

Izard, C. E. (1977). *Human emotions.* New York: Plenum.

Izard, C. E. (1991). *The psychology of emotions.* New York: Plenum.

Izard, C. E. (1994). Innate and universal facial expressions: Evidence from developmental and cross-cultural research. *Psychological Bulletin, 115,* 288–299.

Izard, C. E., Dougherty, F. E., Bloxom, B. M., & Kotsch, W. E. (1974). *The differential emotions scale: A method of measuring the subjective experience of discrete emotions.* Unpublished manuscript, Vanderbilt University, Nashville, TN.

Izard, C. E., Libero, D. Z., Putnam, P., & Haynes, O. M. (1993). Stability of emotion experiences and their relations to traits of personality. *Journal of Personality and Social Psychology, 64,* 847–860.

James, W. (1884). What is an emotion? *Mind, 9,* 188–205.

Jamner, L. D., & Schwartz, G. E. (1986). Self-deception predicts self-report and endurance of pain. *Psychosomatic Medicine, 48,* 211–223.

Jardine, R., Martin, N. G., & Henderson, A. S. (1984). Genetic covariation between neuroticism and the symptoms of anxiety and depression. *Genetic Epidemiology, 1,* 89–107.

Jensen, M. R. (1984). *Psychobiological factors in the prognosis and treatment of neoplastic disorders.* Unpublished doctoral dissertation, Yale University.

John, O. P. (1990). The "Big Five" factor taxonomy: Dimensions of personality in the natural language and in questionnaires. In L. A. Pervin (Ed.), *Handbook of personality: Theory and research* (pp. 66–100). New York: Guilford Press.

John, O. P., Donahue, E. M., & Kentle, R. L. (1991). *The Big Five Inventory—Versions 4a and 54* [Technical report]. University of California, Institute of Personality and Social Research, Berkeley.

John, O. P., Goldberg, L. R., & Angleitner, A. (1984). Better than the alphabet: Taxonomies of personality-descriptive terms in English, Dutch, and German. In H. C. J. Bonarius, G. L. M. van Heck, & N. G. Smid (Eds.), *Personality psychology in Europe: Theoretical and empirical development* (Vol. 1, pp. 83–100). Lisse, The Netherlands: Swets & Zeitlinger.

Johnson, C., & Mullen, B. (1994). Evidence for the accessibility of paired distinctiveness in distinctiveness-based illusory correlation in stereotyping. *Personality and Social Psychology Bulletin, 20,* 65–70.

Johnson, D. T. (1968). Effects of interview stress on measures of state and trait anxiety. *Journal of Abnormal Psychology, 73,* 245–251.

Joiner, T. E. (1996). A confirmatory factor-analytic investigation of the tripartite model of depression and anxiety in college students. *Cognitive Therapy and Research, 20,* 521–539.

Joiner, T. E., Catanzaro, S. J., & Laurent, J. (1996). Tripartite structure of positive and negative affect, depression, and anxiety in child and adolescent psychiatric inpatients. *Journal of Abnormal Psychology, 105,* 401–409.

Joiner, T. E., & Metalsky, G. I. (1995). A prospective test of an integrative interpersonal theory of depression: A naturalistic study of college roommates. *Journal of Personality and Social Psychology, 69,* 778–788.

Jolly, J. B., Dyck, M. J., Kramer, T. A., & Wherry, J. N. (1994). Integration of positive and negative affectivity and cognitive content–specificity: Improved discrimination of anxious and depressive symptoms. *Journal of Abnormal Psychology, 103,* 544–552.

Jolly, J. B., & Dykman, R. A. (1994). Using self-report data to differentiate anxious and depressive symptoms in adolescents: Cognitive content specificity *and* global distress? *Cognitive Therapy and Research, 18,* 25–37.

Jolly, J. B., & Kramer, T. A. (1994). The hierarchical arrangement of internalizing cognitions. *Cognitive Therapy and Research, 18,* 1–14.

Judge, T. A., & Hulin, C. L. (1993). Job satisfaction as a reflection of disposition: A multiple source causal analysis. *Organizational Behavior and Human Decision Processes, 56,* 388–421.

Kammann, R. (1983). Objective circumstances, life satisfactions, and sense of well-being: Consistencies across time and place. *New Zealand Journal of Psychology, 12*, 14–22.

Kammann, R., Smith, R., Martin, C., & McQueen, M. (1984). Low accuracy in judgments of others' psychological well-being as seen from a phenomenological perspective. *Journal of Personality, 52*, 107–123.

Kaplan, G. A., & Camacho, T. (1983). Perceived health and mortality: A nine-year follow-up of the Human Population Laboratory cohort. *American Journal of Epidemiology, 117*, 292–304.

Kaplan, G. A., & Kotler, P. L. (1985). Self-reports predictive of mortality from ischemic heart disease: A nine-year follow-up of the Human Population Laboratory cohort. *Journal of Chronic Diseases, 38*, 195–201.

Kaplan, G. A., & Reynolds, P. (1988). Depression and cancer mortality and morbidity: Prospective evidence from the Alameda County study. *Journal of Behavioral Medicine, 11*, 1–13.

Karney, B. R., Bradbury, T. N., Fincham, F. D., & Sullivan, K. T. (1994). The role of negative affectivity in the association between attributions and marital satisfaction. *Journal of Personality and Social Psychology, 66*, 413–424.

Kasl, S. V., Cobb, S., & Brooks, G. W. (1968). Changes in serum uric acid and cholesterol level in men undergoing job stress. *Journal of the American Medical Association, 206*, 1500–1507.

Kasper, S., & Rosenthal, N. E. (1989). Anxiety and depression in seasonal affective disorders. In P. C. Kendall & D. Watson (Eds.), *Anxiety and depression: Distinctive and overlapping features* (pp. 341–375). San Diego, CA: Academic Press.

Katon, W., & Roy-Byrne, P. P. (1991). Mixed anxiety and depression. *Journal of Abnormal Psychology, 100*, 337–345.

Keehn, R. J., Goldberg, I. D., & Beebe, G. W. (1974). Twenty-four year mortality follow-up of army veterans with disability separations for psychoneurosis in 1944. *Psychosomatic Medicine, 36*, 27–46.

Kelly, E. L., & Conley, J. J. (1987). Personality and compatibility: A prospective analysis of marital stability and marital satisfaction. *Journal of Personality and Social Psychology, 52*, 27–40.

Kendall, P. C. (1978). Anxiety: States, traits—situations? *Journal of Consulting and Clinical Psychology, 46*, 280–287.

Kendall, P. C., Finch, A. J., Jr., Auerbach, S. M., Hooke, J. F., & Mikulka, P. J. (1976). The State–Trait Anxiety Inventory: A systematic investigation. *Journal of Consulting and Clinical Psychology, 44*, 406–412.

Kendall, P. C., Finch, A. J., Jr., & Montgomery, L. E. (1978). Vicarious anxiety: A systematic evaluation of a vicarious threat to self-esteem. *Journal of Consulting and Clinical Psychology, 46*, 997–1008.

Kendall, P. C., & Watson, D. (Eds.). (1989). *Anxiety and depression: Distinctive and overlapping features.* San Diego, CA: Academic Press.

Kendler, K. S. (1996). Major depression and generalised anxiety disorder: Same genes, (partly) different environments—Revisited. *British Journal of Psychiatry, 168*(Suppl. 30), 68–75.

Kendler, K. S., Heath, A. C., Martin, N. G., & Eaves, L. J. (1987). Symptoms of anxiety and symptoms of depression: Same genes, different environments? *Archives of General Psychiatry, 44,* 451–457.

Kendler, K. S., Neale, M. C., Kessler, R. C., Heath, A. C., & Eaves, L. J. (1992). Major depression and generalized anxiety disorder: Same genes, (partly) different environments? *Archives of General Psychiatry, 49,* 716–722.

Kendler, K. S., Neale, M. C., Kessler, R. C., Heath, A. C., & Eaves, L. J. (1993a). A longitudinal twin study of personality and major depression in women. *Archives of General Psychiatry, 50,* 853–862.

Kendler, K. S., Neale, M. C., Kessler, R. C., Heath, A. C., & Eaves, L. J. (1993b). Major depression and phobias: The genetic and environmental sources of comorbidity. *Psychological Medicine, 23,* 361–371.

Kendler, K. S., Walters, E. E., Neale, M. C., Kessler, R. C., Heath, A. C., & Eaves, L. J. (1995). The structure of the genetic and environmental risk factors for six major psychiatric disorders in women: Phobia, generalized anxiety disorder, panic disorder, bulimia, major depression, and alcoholism. *Archives of General Psychiatry, 52,* 374–383.

Kennedy-Moore, E., Greenberg, M. A., Newman, M. G., & Stone, A. A. (1992). The relationship between daily events and mood: The mood measure may matter. *Motivation and Emotion, 16,* 143–155.

Kenrick, D. T., & Funder, D. C. (1988). Profiting from controversy: Lessons from the person–situation debate. *American Psychologist, 43,* 23–34.

Kessler, R. C., McGonagle, K. A., Zhao, S., Nelson, C. B., Hughes, M., Eshelman, S., Wittchen, H., & Kendler, K. S. (1994). Lifetime and 12 month prevalence of *DSM-III-R* psychiatric disorders in the United States: Results from the National Comorbidity Study. *Archives of General Psychiatry, 51,* 8–19.

Kessler, R. C., Nelson, C. B., McGonagle, K. A., Liu, J., Swartz, M., & Blazer, D. G. (1996). Comorbidity of *DSM-III-R* major depressive disorder in the general population: Results from the US National Comorbidity Survey. *British Journal of Psychiatry, 168*(Suppl. 30), 17–30.

Kidson, M. A. (1973). Personality and hypertension. *Journal of Psychosomatic Research, 17,* 35–41.

King, A. C., Taylor, C. B., Albright, C. A., & Haskell, W. L. (1990). The relationship between repressive and defensive coping styles and blood pressure responses in healthy, middle-aged men and women. *Journal of Psychosomatic Research, 34,* 461–471.

Kirmayer, L. J., Robbins, J. M., & Paris, J. (1994). Somatoform disorders: Personality and the social matrix of somatic distress. *Journal of Abnormal Psychology, 103,* 125–136.

Kissen, D. M. (1964). Relationship between lung cancer, cigarette smoking, inhalation, and personality. *British Journal of Medical Psychology, 37,* 203–216.

Kissen, D. M., & Eysenck, H. J. (1962). Personality in male lung cancer patients. *Journal of Psychosomatic Research, 6,* 123–127.

Knapp, P. H., Levy, E. M., Giorgi, R. G., Black, P. H., Fox, B. H., & Heeren, T. C. (1992). Short-term immunological effects of induced emotion. *Psychosomatic Medicine, 54,* 133–148.

Krueger, R. F., Caspi, A., Moffitt, T. E., Silva, P. A., & McGee, R. (1996). Personality traits are differentially linked to mental disorders: A multitrait–multi-diagnosis study of an adolescent birth cohort. *Journal of Abnormal Psychology, 105,* 299–312.

Kupfer, D. J. (1976). REM latency: A psychobiologic marker for primary depressive disease. *Biological Psychiatry, 11,* 159–174.

Kupfer, D. J. (1995). Sleep research in depressive illness: Clinical implications—A tasting menu. *Biological Psychiatry, 36,* 391–403.

Kurdek, L. A. (1991). Predictors of increases in marital distress in newlywed couples: A 3-year prospective longitudinal study. *Developmental Psychology, 27,* 627–636.

Kurdek, L. A. (1993). Predicting marital dissolution: A 5-year prospective longitudinal study of newlywed couples. *Journal of Personality and Social Psychology, 64,* 221–242.

Lafer, B., Sachs, G. S., Labbate, L. A., & Thibault, A. (1994). Phototherapy for seasonal affective disorder: A blind comparison of three different schedules. *American Journal of Psychiatry, 151,* 1081–1083.

LaForge, R., & Suczek, R. (1955). The interpersonal dimension of personality: III. An interpersonal check list. *Journal of Personality, 24,* 94–112.

Lamb, D. H. (1972). Speech anxiety: Towards a theoretical conceptualization and preliminary scale development. *Speech Monographs, 39,* 62–67.

Lamb, D. H. (1976). On the distinction between psychological and physical stressors. *Psychological Reports, 38,* 797–798.

Lang, P. J., Bradley, M. M., & Cuthbert, B. N. (1992). A motivational analysis of emotion: Reflex-cortex connections. *Psychological Science, 3,* 44–49.

Lang, P. J., Bradley, M. M., Cuthbert, B. N., & Patrick, C. J. (1993). Emotion and psychopathology: A startle probe analysis. In L. J. Chapman, J. P. Chapman, & D. C. Fowles (Eds.), *Progress in experimental personality and psychopathology research* (Vol. 16, pp. 163–199). New York: Springer.

Larsen, C. L., Davidson, R. J., & Abercrombie, H. C. (1995). Prefrontal brain function and depression severity: EEG differences in melancholic and nonmelancholic depressives. *Psychophysiology, 32,* S49.

Larsen, R. J. (1985). Individual differences in circadian activity rhythm and personality. *Personality and Individual Differences, 6,* 305–311.

Larsen, R. J. (1987). The stability of mood variability: A spectral analytic approach to daily mood assessments. *Journal of Personality and Social Psychology, 52,* 1195–1204.

Larsen, R. J. (1992). Neuroticism and selective encoding and recall of symptoms: Evidence from a combined concurrent-retrospective study. *Journal of Personality and Social Psychology, 62,* 480–488.

Larsen, R. J., & Diener, E. (1992). Promises and problems with the circumplex model of emotion. *Review of Personality and Social Psychology, 13,* 25–59.

Larsen, R. J., & Kasimatis, M. (1990). Individual differences in entrainment of mood to the weekly calendar. *Journal of Personality and Social Psychology, 58,* 164–171.

Larsen, R. J., & Ketelaar, T. (1991). Personality and susceptibility to positive and negative emotional states. *Journal of Personality and Social Psychology, 61,* 132–140.

LaRue, A., Bank, L., Jarvik, L., & Hetland, M. (1979). Health in old age: How do physicians' ratings and self-ratings compare? *Journal of Gerontology, 34,* 687–691.

Lazarus, R. S. (1982). Thoughts on the relation between emotion and cognition. *American Psychologist, 37,* 1019–1024.

Lazarus, R. S. (1984). On the primacy of cognition. *American Psychologist, 39,* 124–129.

Lazarus, R. S. (1991a). *Emotion and adaptation.* New York: Oxford University Press.

Lazarus, R. S. (1991b). Progress on a cognitive–motivational–relational theory of emotion. *American Psychologist, 46,* 819–834.

Lee, G. R., Seccombe, K., & Shehan, C. L. (1991). Marital status and personal happiness: An analysis of trend data. *Journal of Marriage and the Family, 53,* 839–844.

Le Moal, M., & Simon, M. (1991). Mesocorticolimbic dopaminergic network: Functional and regulatory roles. *Physiological Reviews, 71,* 155–234.

Lester, D., Haig, C., & Monello, R. (1989). Spouses' personality and marital satisfaction. *Personality and Individual Differences, 10,* 253–254.

Levenson, R. W., Ekman, P., & Friesen, W. V. (1990). Voluntary facial action generates emotion-specific autonomic nervous system activity. *Psychophysiology, 27,* 363–384.

Leventhal, E. A., Hansell, M., Diefenbach, M., Leventhal, H., & Glass, D. C. (1996). Negative affect and self-report of physical symptoms: Two longitudinal studies of older adults. *Health Psychology, 15,* 193–199.

Levi, F., & Halberg, F. (1982). Circaseptum (about 7 day) bioperiodicity—spontaneous and reactive—and the search for pacemakers. *La Ricera, 12,* 323–370.

Levin, I., & Stokes, J. P. (1989). Dispositional approach to job satisfaction: Role of negative affectivity. *Journal of Applied Psychology, 74,* 752–758.

Levy, S. M., Herberman, R. B., Maluish, A. M., Schlien, B., & Lippman, M. (1985). Prognostic risk assessment in primary breast cancer by behavioral and immunological parameters. *Health Psychology, 4,* 99–113.

Lewinsohn, P. M., Redner, J. E., & Seeley, J. R. (1991). The relationship between life satisfaction and psychosocial variables: New perspectives. In F. Strack, M. Argyle, & N. Schwarz (Eds.), *Subjective well-being: An interdisciplinary perspective* (pp. 141–169). New York: Pergamon Press.

Lichtman, S., & Poser, E. G. (1983). The effects of exercise on mood and cognitive functioning. *Journal of Psychosomatic Research, 27,* 43–52.

Linn, B. S., & Linn, M. W. (1980). Objective and self-assessed health in the old and very old. *Social Science and Medicine, 14,* 311–315.

Locke, E. A. (1976). The nature and causes of job satisfaction. In M. D. Dunnette (Ed.), *Handbook of industrial and organizational psychology* (pp. 1297–1349). Chicago: Rand McNally.

Locke, H., & Wallace, K. (1959). Short marital-adjustment and prediction tests: Their reliability and validity. *Marriage and Family Living, 21,* 251–255.

Loehlin, J. C. (1992). *Genes and environment in personality development.* Newbury Park, CA: Sage.

Loevinger, J. (1957). Objective tests as instruments of psychological theory. *Psychological Reports, 3,* 635–694.

Loevinger, J. (1987). *Paradigms of personality.* New York: Freeman.

Long, B. C. (1984). Aerobic conditioning and stress inoculation: A comparison of stress-management interventions. *Cognitive Therapy and Research, 8,* 517–541.

Long, B. C. (1985). Stress-management interventions: A 15-month follow-up of aerobic conditioning and stress inoculation training. *Cognitive Therapy and Research, 9,* 471–478.

Lonigan, C. J., Carey, M. P., & Finch, A. J., Jr. (1994). Anxiety and depression in children and adolescents: Negative affectivity and the utility of self-reports. *Journal of Consulting and Clinical Psychology, 62,* 1000–1008.

Lubin, B., Zuckerman, M., & Woodward, L. (1985). *Bibliography for the Multiple Affect Adjective Check List.* San Diego, CA: Educational and Industrial Testing Service.

Lykken, D., & Tellegen, A. (1996). Happiness is a stochastic phenomenon. *Psychological Science, 7,* 186–189.

Lynn, R., & Eysenck, H. J. (1961). Tolerance for pain, extraversion and neuroticism. *Perceptual and Motor Skills, 12,* 161–162.

Lyubomirsky, S., & Nolen-Hoeksema, S. (1993). Self-perpetuating properties of dysphoric rumination. *Journal of Personality and Social Psychology, 65,* 339–349.

Magnus, K., & Diener, E. (1991, May). *A longitudinal analysis of personality, life events, and subjective well-being.* Paper presented at the 63rd annual meeting of the Midwestern Psychological Association, Chicago.

Mansfield, P. K., Hood, K. E., & Henderson, J. (1989). Women and their husbands: Mood and arousal fluctuations across the menstrual cycle and days of the week. *Psychosomatic Medicine, 51,* 66–80.

Markovitz, J. H., Matthews, K. A., Kannel, W. B., Cobb, J. L., & D'Agostino, R. B. (1993). Psychological predictors of hypertension in the Framingham Study: Is there tension in hypertension? *Journal of the American Medical Association, 270,* 2439–2443.

Martin, L. R., Friedman, H. S., Tucker, J. S., Schwartz, J. E., Criqui, M. H., Wingard, D. L., & Tomlinson-Keasey, C. (1995). An archival prospective study of mental health and longevity. *Health Psychology, 14,* 381–387.

Martin, N. G., Jardine, R., Andrews, G., & Heath, A. C. (1988). Anxiety disorders and neuroticism: Anxiety disorders and neuroticism: Are there genetic factors specific to panic? *Acta Psychiatrica Scandinavica, 77,* 698–706.

Martinez-Urrutia, A. (1975). Anxiety and pain in surgical patients. *Journal of Consulting and Clinical Psychology, 43,* 437–442.

Martinsen, E. W. (1993). Therapeutic implications of exercise for clinically anxious and depressed patients. *International Journal of Sport Psychology, 24,* 185–199.

Maser, J., & Cloninger, C. R. (Eds.). (1990). *Comorbidity in anxiety and mood disorders.* Washington, DC: American Psychiatric Press.

Mastekaasa, A. (1992). Marriage and psychological well-being: Some evidence on selection into marriage. *Journal of Marriage and the Family, 54,* 901–911.

May, R. R. (1976). Mood shifts and the menstrual cycle. *Journal of Psychosomatic Research, 20,* 125–130.

Mayer, J. D., & Gaschke, Y. N. (1988). The experience and meta-experience of mood. *Journal of Personality and Social Psychology, 55,* 102–111.

McAdams, D. P. (1992). The five-factor model in personality: A critical appraisal. *Journal of Personality, 60,* 329–361.

McCartney, K., Harris, M. J., & Bernieri, F. (1990). Growing up and growing apart: A developmental meta-analysis of twin studies. *Psychological Bulletin, 107,* 226–237.

McCrae, R. R. (1982). Consensual validation of personality traits: Evidence from self-reports and ratings. *Journal of Personality and Social Psychology, 43,* 293–303.

McCrae, R. R., & Costa, P. T., Jr. (1985). Updating Norman's "adequate taxonomy": Intelligence and personality dimensions in natural language and in questionnaires. *Journal of Personality and Social Psychology, 49,* 710–721.

McCrae, R. R., & Costa, P. T., Jr. (1986). Clinical assessment can benefit from recent advances in personality psychology. *American Psychologist, 41,* 1001–1003.

McCrae, R. R., & Costa, P. T., Jr. (1987). Validation of a five-factor model of personality across instruments and observers. *Journal of Personality and Social Psychology, 52,* 81–90.

McCrae, R. R., & Costa, P. T., Jr. (1990). *Personality in adulthood.* New York: Guilford Press.

McCrae, R. R., & Costa, P. T., Jr. (1991). Adding *Liebe und Arbeit:* The full five-factor model and well-being. *Personality and Social Psychology Bulletin, 17,* 227–232.

McCrae, R. R., & Costa, P. T., Jr. (1997). Personality trait structure as a human universal. *American Psychologist, 52,* 509–516.

McFarland, C., Ross, M., & DeCourville, N. (1989). Women's theories of menstruation and biases in recall of menstrual symptoms. *Journal of Personality and Social Psychology, 57,* 522–531.

McFarlane, J., Martin, C. L., & Williams, T. M. (1988). Mood fluctuations: Women versus men and menstrual versus other cycles. *Psychology of Women Quarterly, 12,* 201–223.

McGrath, J. E., & Kelly, J. R. (1986). *Time and human interaction: Toward a social psychology of time.* New York: Guilford Press.

McGue, M., Bacon, S., & Lykken, D. T. (1993). Personality stability and change in early adulthood: A behavioral genetic analysis. *Developmental Psychology, 29,* 96–109.

McIntosh, D. N., Silver, R. C., & Wortman, C. B. (1993). Religion's role in adjustment to a negative life event: Coping with the loss of a child. *Journal of Personality and Social Psychology, 65,* 812–821.

McIntyre, C. W., & Watson, D. (1991). [Effects of test stress, exercise, and social interaction on general and specific mood measures]. Unpublished raw data.

McIntyre, C. W., Watson, D., Clark, L. A., & Cross, S. A. (1991). The effect of induced social interaction on positive and negative affect. *Bulletin of the Psychonomic Society, 29,* 67–70.

McIntyre, C. W., Watson, D., & Cunningham, A. C. (1990). The effects of social interaction, exercise, and test stress on positive and negative affect. *Bulletin of the Psychonomic Society, 28,* 141–143.

McNair, D. M., Lorr, M., & Droppleman, L. F. (1971). *Manual: Profile of Mood States.* San Diego, CA: Educational and Industrial Testing Service.

Mechanic, D. (1979). Correlates of physician utilization: Why do major multivariate studies of physician utilization find trivial psychosocial and organizational effects? *Journal of Health and Social Behavior, 20,* 387–396.

Mechanic, D. (1980). The experience and reporting of common physical complaints. *Journal of Health and Social Behavior, 21,* 146–155.

Mechanic, D., & Hansell, S. (1989). Divorce, family conflict, and adolescents' well-being. *Journal of Health and Social Behavior, 30,* 105–116.

Meddis, R. (1972). Bipolar factors in mood adjective checklists. *British Journal of Social and Clinical Psychology, 11,* 178–184.

Meehl, P. E. (1975). Hedonic capacity: Some conjectures. *Bulletin of the Menninger Clinic, 39,* 295–307.

Mehnert, T., Krauss, H. H., Nadler, R., & Boyd, M. (1990). Correlates of life satisfaction in those with disabling conditions. *Rehabilitation Psychology, 35,* 3–17.

Meyer, G. J., & Shack, J. R. (1989). Structural convergence of mood and personality: Evidence for old and new directions. *Journal of Personality and Social Psychology, 57,* 691–706.

Michalos, A. C. (1985). Multiple discrepancies theory (MDT). *Social Indicator Research, 16,* 347–413.

Michalos, A. C. (1991). *Global report on student well-being. Vol. I: Life satisfaction and happiness.* New York: Springer-Verlag.

Mineka, S., Watson, D., & Clark, L. A. (1998). Comorbidity of anxiety and unipolar mood disorders. *Annual Review of Psychology, 49,* 377–412.

Monk, T. H., Leng, V. C., Folkard, S., & Weitzman, E. D. (1983). Circadian rhythms in subjective alertness and core body temperature. *Chronobiologica, 10,* 49–55.

Moore, R. Y., & Eichler, V. B. (1972). Loss of a circadian adrenal corticosterone rhythm following suprachiasmic lesions in the rat. *Brain Research, 42,* 201–206.

Moore-Ede, M. C., Czeisler, C. A., & Richardson, G. S. (1983a). Circadian time-keeping in health and disease. *New England Journal of Medicine, 309,* 469–476.

Moore-Ede, M. C., Czeisler, C. A., & Richardson, G. S. (1983b). Circadian time-keeping in health and disease. Part 2. Clinical implications of circadian rhythmicity. *New England Journal of Medicine, 309,* 530–536.

Moos, R. H. (1968). Development of a Menstrual Distress Questionnaire. *Psychosomatic Medicine, 30,* 853–867.

Moos, R. H. (1969). Typology of menstrual cycle symptoms. *American Journal of Obstetrics and Gynecology, 103,* 390–402.

Morgan, R. L., & Heise, D. (1988). Structure of emotions. *Social Psychology Quarterly, 51,* 19–31.

Morgan, W. P. (1982). Psychological effects of exercise. *Behavioral Medicine Update, 4,* 25–30.

Morgan, W. P., & Horstman, D. H. (1978). Psychometric correlates of pain perception. *Perceptual and Motor Skills, 47,* 27–39.

Morgan, W. P., & Johnson, R. W. (1978). Psychological characterization of national level oarsmen differing in level of ability. *International Journal of Sport Psychology, 9,* 119–133.

Morgan, W. P., O'Connor, P. J., Sparling, P. B., & Pate, R. R. (1987). Psychological characterization of the elite female distance runner. *International Journal of Sports Medicine, 8,* 124–131.

Mrosovsky, N. (1988). Seasonal affective disorder, hibernation, and annual cycles in animals: Chipmunks in the sky. *Journal of Biological Rhythms, 3,* 189–207.

Murrell, S. A., Norris, F. H., & Chipley, Q. T. (1992). Functional vs. structural social support, desirable events, and positive affect in older adults. *Psychology and Aging, 7,* 562–570.

Musante, L., MacDougall, J. M., Dembroski, T. M., & Costa, P. T., Jr. (1989). Potential for hostility and dimensions of anger. *Health Psychology, 8,* 343–354.

Myers, D. G., & Diener, E. (1995). Who is happy? *Psychological Science, 6,* 10–19.

Nagle, F. J., Morgan, W. P., Hellickson, R. O., Serfass, R. C., & Alexander, J. F. (1975). Sporting success traits in Olympic contenders. *Physician Sports Medicine, 3,* 31–34.

Nelson, G. (1990). Women's life strains, social support, coping, and positive and negative affect: Cross-sectional and longitudinal tests of the two-factor theory of emotional well-being. *Journal of Community Psychology, 18,* 239–263.

Nesse, R. M. (1991, November/December). What good is feeling bad? The evolutionary benefits of psychic pain. *The Sciences,* pp. 30–37.

Newman, W. P., III, Freedman, D. S., Voors, A. W., Gard, P. D., Srinivasan, S. R., Cresanta, J. L., Williamson, G. D., Webber, L. S., & Berenson, G. S. (1986). Relation of serum lipoprotein levels and systolic blood pressure to early atherosclerosis: The Bogalusa Heart study. *New England Journal of Medicine, 314,* 138–144.

Newton, T., & Keenan, T. (1991). Further analyses of the dispositional argument in organizational behavior. *Journal of Applied Psychology, 76,* 781–787.

Nitschke, J. B., Heller, W., Imig, J. C., & Miller, G. A. (1997). *Distinguishing dimensions of anxiety and depression.* Manuscript submitted for publication.

Nolen-Hoeksema, S. (1987). Sex differences in unipolar depression: Evidence and theory. *Psychological Bulletin, 101,* 259–282.

Nolen-Hoeksema, S. (1990). *Sex differences in depression.* Stanford, CA: Stanford University Press.

Norman, W. T. (1963). Toward an adequate taxonomy of personality attributes: Replicated factor structure in peer nomination personality ratings. *Journal of Abnormal and Social Psychology, 66,* 574–583.

Norman, W. T. (1969). "To see oursels as ithers see us!" Relations among self-perceptions, peer-perceptions, and expected peer-perceptions of personality attributes. *Multivariate Behavioral Research, 4,* 417–433.

Norman, W. T., & Goldberg, L. R. (1966). Raters, ratees, and randomness in personality structure. *Journal of Personality and Social Psychology, 4,* 681–691.

Norton, R. (1983). Measuring marital quality: A critical look at the dependent variable. *Journal of Marriage and the Family, 45,* 141–151.

Norvell, N., & Belles, D. (1993). Psychological and physical benefits of circuit weight training in law enforcement personnel. *Journal of Consulting and Clinical Psychology, 61,* 520–527.

Nowlis, V. (1965). Research with the Mood Adjective Checklist. In S. S. Tomkins & C. E. Izard (Eds.), *Affect, cognition, and personality* (pp. 352–389). New York: Springer.

Okun, M. A., & Stock, W. A. (1987). Correlates and components of subjective well-being among the elderly. *Journal of Applied Gerontology, 6,* 95–112.

Orme, J. G., Reis, J., & Herz, E. J. (1986). Factorial and discriminant validity of the Center for Epidemiological Studies Depression (CES-D) Scale. *Journal of Clinical Psychology, 42,* 28–33.

Ormel, J., & Schaufeli, W. B. (1991). Stability and change in psychological distress and their relationship with self-esteem and locus of control: A dynamic equilibrium model. *Journal of Personality and Social Psychology, 60,* 288–299.

Ormel, J., & Wohlfarth, T. (1991). How neuroticism, long-term difficulties, and life situation change influence psychological distress: A longitudinal model. *Journal of Personality and Social Psychology, 60,* 744–755.

Ortony, A., Clore, G. L., & Collins, A. (1988). *The cognitive structure of emotions.* New York: Cambridge University Press.

Ortony, A., Clore, G. L., & Foss, M. A. (1987). The referential structure of the affective lexicon. *Cognitive Science, 11,* 341–364.

Ortony, A., & Turner, T. J. (1990). What's basic about basic emotions? *Psychological Review, 97,* 315–331.

Ostfeld, A. M., Lebovits, B. Z., Shekelle, R. B., & Paul, O. (1964). A prospective study of the relationship between personality and coronary heart disease. *Journal of Chronic Diseases, 17,* 265–276.

Paige, K. E. (1971). Effects of oral contraceptives on affective fluctuations associated with the menstrual cycle. *Psychosomatic Medicine, 33,* 515–537.

Paloutzian, R. F., & Ellison, C. W. (1982). Loneliness, spiritual well-being and the quality of life. In L. A. Peplau & D. Perlman (Eds.), *Loneliness: A sourcebook of current theory, research and therapy* (pp. 224–237). New York: Wiley.

Parlee, M. B. (1974). Stereotypic beliefs about menstruation: A methodological note on the MDQ and some new data. *Psychosomatic Medicine, 36,* 229–240.

Parrott, W. G., & Sabini, J. (1990). Mood and memory under natural conditions: Evidence for mood incongruent recall. *Journal of Personality and Social Psychology, 59,* 321–336.

Patkai, P. (1971). Interindividual differences in diurnal variations in alertness, performance, and adrenaline excretion. *Acta Physiologica Scandinavica, 81,* 35–46.

Paulhus, D. L., & Reynolds, S. (1995). Enhancing target variance in personality impressions: Highlighting the person in person perception. *Journal of Personality and Social Psychology, 69,* 1233–1242.

Pauls, D. L. (1992). The genetics of obsessive compulsive disorder and Gilles de la Tourette's syndrome. *Psychiatric Clinics of North America, 15,* 759–766.

Pauls, D. L., Alsobrook, J. P., II, Goodman, W., Rasmussen, S., & Leckman, J. F. (1995). A family study of obsessive–compulsive disorder. *American Journal of Psychiatry, 152,* 76–84.

Pauls, D. L., Leckman, J. F., & Cohen, D. J. (1994). Evidence against a genetic relationship between Tourette's syndrome and anxiety, depression, panic and phobic disorders. *British Journal of Psychiatry, 164,* 215–221.

Pedersen, N. L., Plomin, R., McClearn, G. E., & Friberg, L. (1988). Neuroticism, extraversion, and related traits in adult twins reared apart and reared together. *Journal of Personality and Social Psychology, 55,* 950–957.

Pennebaker, J. W. (1980). Perceptual and environmental determinants of coughing. *Basic and Applied Social Psychology, 1,* 83–91.

Pennebaker, J. W. (1982) *The psychology of physical symptoms.* New York: Springer-Verlag.

Pennebaker, J. W., & Brittingham, G. L. (1982). Environmental and sensory cues affecting the perception of physical symptoms. In A. Baum & J. Singer (Eds.), *Advances in environmental psychology* (Vol. 4, pp. 115–136). Hillsdale, NJ: Erlbaum.

Pennebaker, J. W., & Lightner, J. M. (1980). Competition of internal and external information in an exercise setting. *Journal of Personality and Social Psychology, 39,* 165–174.

Penner, L. A., Shiffman, S., Paty, J. A., & Fritzsche, B. A. (1994). Individual differences in intraperson variability in mood. *Journal of Personality and Social Psychology, 66,* 712–721.

Phifer, J. F., & Norris, F. H. (1989). Psychological symptoms in older adults following natural disaster: Timing, duration, and course. *Journals of Gerontology, 44,* S207–S217.

Phillips, D. L. (1967). Social participation and happiness. *American Journal of Sociology, 72,* 472–488.

Plomin, R., & Daniels, D. (1987). Why are children in the same family so different from one another? *Behavioral and Brain Sciences, 10,* 1–60.

Plutchik, R. (1962). *The emotions: Facts, theories, and a new model.* New York: Random House.

Plutchick, R. (1980). *Emotion: A psychoevolutionary synthesis.* New York: Harper & Row.

Polivy, J. (1981). On the induction of emotion in the laboratory: Discrete moods or multiple affect states? *Journal of Personality and Social Psychology, 41,* 803–817.

Pyszczynski, T., & Greenberg, J. (1987). Self-regulatory perseveration and the depressive self-focusing style: A self-awareness theory of reactive depression. *Psychological Bulletin, 102,* 122–138.

Radloff, L. S. (1977). The CES-D Scale: A new self-report depression scale for research in the general population. *Applied Psychological Measurement, 1,* 385–401.

Raglin, J. S., & Morgan, W. P. (1987). Influence of exercise and quiet rest on state anxiety and blood pressure. *Medicine and Science in Sports, 19,* 456–463.

Reich, J. (1993). Distinguishing mixed anxiety/depression from anxiety and depressive groups using the family history method. *Comprehensive Psychiatry, 34,* 285–290.

Reme, C., Terman, M., & Wirz-Justice, A. (1990). Are deficient retinal photoreceptor renewal mechanisms involved in the pathogenesis of winter depression? *Archives of General Psychiatry, 47,* 878–879.

Robbins, A. S., Spence, J. T., & Clark, H. (1991). Psychological determinants of health and performance: The tangled web of desirable and undesirable characteristics. *Journal of Personality and Social Psychology, 61,* 755–765.

Robins, L. N., Helzer, J. E., Croughan, I., & Ratcliff, K. S. (1981). The NIMH Diagnostic Interview Schedule: Its history, characteristics, and validity. *Archives of General Psychiatry, 38,* 381–389.

Robins, L. N., & Regier D. A. (Eds.). (1991). *Psychiatric disorders in America: The Epidemiologic Catchment Area study.* New York: Free Press.

Robinson, J. O. (1962). A study of neuroticism and casual arterial blood pressure. *British Journal of Social and Clinical Psychology, 2,* 56–61.

Rogentine, G. N., Fox, B. H., VanKammen, D. P., Rosenblatt, J., Docherty, J. P., & Bunney, W. E. (1979). Psychological and biological factors in the short-term prognosis of malignant melanoma. *Psychosomatic Medicine, 41,* 647–655.

Rook, K. S. (1984). The negative side of social interaction: Impact on psychological well-being. *Journal of Personality and Social Psychology, 46,* 1097–1108.

Rosen, L. N., Targum, S. D., Terman, M., & Bryant, M. J. (1990). Prevalence of seasonal affective disorder at four latitudes. *Psychiatry Research, 31,* 131–144.

Rosenthal, N. E., Sack, D. A., Gillin, J. C., Lewy, A. J., Goodwin, F. K., Davenport, Y., & Mueller, P. S. (1984). Seasonal affective disorder: A description of the syndrome and preliminary findings with light therapy. *Archives of General Psychiatry, 41,* 72–80.

Rossi, A. S., & Rossi, P. E. (1977). Body time and social time: Mood patterns by menstrual cycle phase and day of the week. *Social Science Research, 6,* 273–308.

Roy, M.-A., Neale, M. C., Pedersen, N. L., Mathé, A. A., & Kendler, K. S. (1995). A twin study of generalized anxiety disorder and major depression. *Psychological Medicine, 25,* 1037–1049.

Roy-Byrne, P. P. (1996). Generalized anxiety and mixed anxiety–depression: Association with disability and health care utilization. *Journal of Clinical Psychiatry, 57*(Suppl. 7), 86–91.

Ruble, D. N. (1977). Premenstrual symptoms: A reinterpretation. *Science, 197,* 291–292.

Ruffner, J. A., & Blair, F. E. (Eds.). (1977). *The weather almanac* (2nd ed.). New York: Avon Books.

Runciman, W. G. (1966). *Relative deprivation and social justice.* London: Routledge & Kegan Paul.

Rushton, J. P., Brainerd, C. J., & Pressley, M. (1983). Behavioral development and construct validity: The principle of aggregation. *Psychological Bulletin, 94,* 18–38.

Russell, J. A. (1979). Affective space is bipolar. *Journal of Personality and Social Psychology, 37,* 345–356.

Russell, J. A. (1980). A circumplex model of affect. *Journal of Personality and Social Psychology, 39,* 1161–1178.

Russell, J. A. (1994). Is there universal recognition of emotion from facial expression? A review of the cross-cultural studies. *Psychological Bulletin, 115,* 102–141.

Russell, J. A., & Carroll, J. M. (1999). On the bipolarity of positive and negative affect. *Psychological Bulletin, 125,* 3–30.

Russell, J. A., Weiss, A., & Mendelsohn, G. A. (1989). Affect Grid: A single-item scale of pleasure and arousal. *Journal of Personality and Social Psychology, 57,* 493–502.

Rusting, C. L., & Larsen, R. J. (1997). Extraversion, Neuroticism, and susceptibility to Positive and Negative affect: A test of two theoretical models. *Personality and Individual Differences, 22,* 607–612.

Sainsbury, P. (1964). Neuroticism and hypertension in an out-patient population. *Journal of Psychosomatic Research, 8,* 235–238.

Saklofske, D. H., Blomme, G. C., & Kelly, I. W. (1992). The effects of exercise and relaxation on energetic and tense arousal. *Personality and Individual Differences, 13,* 623–625.

Salovey, P., & Birnbaum, D. (1989). Influence of mood on health-relevant cognitions. *Journal of Personality and Social Psychology, 57,* 539–551.

Salovey, P., O'Leary, A., Stretton, M. S., Fishkin, S. A., & Drake, C. A. (1991). Influence of mood on judgments about health and illness. In J. P. Forgas (Ed.), *Emotion and social judgments* (pp. 241–262). Oxford, UK: Pergamon Press.

Sanders, J. L., & Brizzolara, M. S. (1982). Relationships between weather and mood. *Journal of General Psychology, 107,* 155–156.

Sapolsky, R. (1996). Why stress is bad for your brain. *Science, 273,* 749–750.

Sartorius, N., Üstün, B., Korten, A., Cooper, J. E., & van Drimmelen, J. (1995). Progress toward achieving a common language in psychiatry, II: Results from the International Field Trials of the ICD-10 diagnostic criteria for research for mental and behavioral disorders. *American Journal of Psychiatry, 152,* 1427–1437.

Saudino, K. J., Pedersen, N. L., Lichtenstein, P., McClearn, G. E., & Plomin, R. (1997). Can personality explain genetic influences on life events? *Journal of Personality and Social Psychology, 72,* 196–206.

Scarpetti, W. L. (1973). The repression–sensitization dimension in relation to impending painful stimulation. *Journal of Consulting and Clinical Psychology, 40,* 377–382.

Scarr, S., Webber, P. L., Weinberg, R. A., & Wittig, M. A. (1981). Personality resemblance among adolescents and their parents in biologically related and adoptive families. *Journal of Personality and Social Psychology, 40,* 885–898.

Schmitt, N., & Bedeian, A. G. (1982). A comparison of LISREL and two-stage least squares analysis of a hypothesized life-job satisfaction reciprocal relationship. *Journal of Applied Psychology, 67,* 806–817.

Schmitt, N., & Pulakos, E. D. (1985). Predicting job satisfaction from life satisfaction: Is there a general satisfaction factor? *International Journal of Psychology, 20,* 155–167.

Schneider, B. (1976). *Staffing organizations.* Santa Monica, CA: Goodyear.

Schneider, B., & Dachler, H. P. (1978). A note on the stability of the Job Descriptive Index. *Journal of Applied Psychology, 63,* 650–653.

Schneider, K. (1986). *The effects of varying levels of exercise on depression and its mood components.* Unpublished master's thesis, Southern Methodist University, Dallas, TX.

Schroeder, E. D. (1972). Relationship between A-Trait scores and use of a student health center. *Dissertation Abstracts International, 33,* 921B-922B.

Schwarz, N., & Clore, G. L. (1983). Mood, misattribution, and judgments of well-being: Informative and directive functions of affective states. *Journal of Personality and Social Psychology, 45,* 513–523.

Scott, C. (1992). *Personality versus the situational effect in the relation between marriage and subjective well-being.* Unpublished doctoral dissertation, University of Illinois, Champaign.

Seligman, M. E. P. (1971). Phobias and preparedness. *Behaviour Therapy, 2,* 307–320.

Seligman, M. E. P. (1991). *Learned optimism.* New York: Random House.

Selye, H. (1936). A syndrome produced by diverse nocuous agents. *Nature, 138,* 32.

Selye, H. (1956). *The stress of life.* New York: McGraw-Hill.

Selye, H. (1976). *The stress of life* (2nd ed.). New York: McGraw-Hill.

Shaffer, D. R., & Smith, J. (1985). Effects of preexisting moods on observers' reactions to helpful and nonhelpful models. *Motivation and Emotion, 9,* 101–122.

Shanahan, M. J., Finch, M., Mortimer, J. T., & Ryu, S. (1991). Adolescent work experience and depressive affect. *Social Psychology Quarterly, 54,* 299–317.

Shekelle, R. B., Raynor, W. J., Jr., Ostfeld, A. M., Garron, D. C., Bieliauskas, L. A., Liu, S. C., Maliza, C., & Paul, O. (1981). Psychological depression and 17–year risk of death from cancer. *Psychosomatic Medicine, 43,* 117–125.

Shekelle, R. B., Vernon, S. W., & Ostfeld, A. M. (1991). Personality and coronary heart disease. *Psychosomatic Medicine, 53,* 176–184.

Sher, K. J., & Trull, T. J. (1994). Personality and disinhibitory psychopathology: Alcoholism and antisocial personality disorder. *Journal of Abnormal Psychology, 103,* 92–102.

Siegman, A. W., Dembroski, T. M., & Ringel, N. (1987). Components of hostility and severity of coronary artery disease. *Psychosomatic Medicine, 49,* 127–135.

Siever, L. J., & Davis, K. L. (1991). A psychobiological perspective on the personality disorders. *American Journal of Psychiatry, 148,* 1647–1658.

Silver, R. L. (1982). *Coping with an undesirable life event: A study of early reactions to physical disability.* Unpublished doctoral dissertation, Northwestern University, Evanston, IL.

Sime, W. E. (1977). A comparison of exercise and meditation in reducing physiological response to stress. *Medicine and Science in Sports, 9,* 55.

Simons, A. D., McGowan, C. R., Epstein, L. H., Kupfer, D. J., & Robertson, R. J. (1985). Exercise as a treatment for depression: An update. *Clinical Psychology Review, 5,* 553–568.

Sinclair, R. C., Mark, M. M., & Clore, G. L. (1994). Mood-related persuasion depends on (mis)attributions. *Social Cognition, 12,* 309–326.

Singer, J. A., & Salovey, P. (1996). Motivated memory: Self-defining memories, goals, and affect regulation. In L. L. Martin & A. Tesser (Eds.), *Striving and feeling: Interactions among goals, affect, and self-regulation* (pp. 229–250). Mahwah, NJ: Erlbaum.

Skinner, B. F. (1971). *Beyond freedom and dignity.* New York: Bantom Books.

Slade, P. (1984). Premenstrual emotional changes in normal women: Fact or fiction? *Journal of Psychosomatic Research, 28,* 1–7.

Smith, P. C., Kendall, L. M., & Hulin, C. L. (1969). *The measurement of satisfaction in work and retirement: A strategy for the study of attitudes.* Chicago: Rand McNally.

Smith, S., & Razzell, P. (1975). *The pools winners.* London: Caliban Books.

Smith, T. W. (1979). Happiness: Time trends, seasonal variations, intersurvey differences, and other mysteries. *Social Psychology Quarterly, 42,* 18–30.

Smith, T. W., & Williams, P. G. (1992). Personality and health: Advantages and limitations of the five-factor model. *Journal of Personality, 60,* 395–423.

Spanier, G. B. (1976). Measuring dyadic adjustment: New scales for assessing the quality of marriage and similar dyads. *Journal of Marriage and the Family, 38*, 15–28.

Spence, S. H. (1997). Structure of anxiety symptoms among children: A confirmatory factor-analytic study. *Journal of Abnormal Psychology, 106*, 280–297.

Spielberger, C. D. (1983). *State–Trait Anxiety Inventory: A comprehensive bibliography.* Palo Alto, CA: Consulting Psychologists Press.

Spielberger, C. D., Gorsuch, R. L., Lushene, R., Vagg, P. R., & Jacobs, G. A. (1983). *Manual for the State–Trait Anxiety Inventory (Form Y).* Palo Alto, CA: Consulting Psychologists Press.

Spielberger, C. D., Jacobs, G. A., Russell, S., & Crane, R. S. (1983). Assessment of anger: The State–Trait Anger Scale. In J. N. Butcher & C. D. Spielberger (Eds.), *Advances in personality assessment* (Vol. 2., pp. 52–76). Hillsdale, NJ: Erlbaum.

Spiro, A., III, Aldwin, C. M., Ward, K. D., & Mroczek, D. K. (1995). Personality and the incidence of hypertension among older men: Longitudinal findings from the Normative Aging Study. *Health Psychology, 14*, 563–569.

Stacey, C. A., & Gatz, M. (1991). Cross-sectional age differences and longitudinal change on the Bradburn Affect Balance Scale. *Journals of Gerontology, 46*, P76–P78.

Stagner, R. (1988). *A history of psychological theories.* New York: Macmillan.

Starkstein, S. E., & Robinson, R. G. (1989). Affective disorders and cerebral vascular disease. *British Journal of Psychiatry, 154*, 170–182.

Staw, B., Bell, N. E., & Clausen, J. A. (1986). The dispositional approach to job attitudes: A lifetime longitudinal test. *Administrative Science Quarterly, 31*, 56–77.

Staw, B., & Ross, J. (1985). Stability in the midst of change: A dispositional approach to job attitudes. *Journal of Applied Psychology, 70*, 469–480.

Steer, R. A., Clark, D. A., Beck, A. T., & Ranieri, W. F. (1995). Common and specific dimensions of self-reported anxiety and depression: A replication. *Journal of Abnormal Psychology, 104*, 542–545.

Steer, R. A., Clark, D. A., & Ranieri, W. F. (1994). Symptom dimensions of the SCL-90–R: A test of the tripartite model of anxiety and depression. *Journal of Personality Assessment, 62*, 525–536.

Steinberg, D. (Chair). (1985). Statement on lowering blood cholesterol to reduce coronary heart disease. *Journal of the American Medical Association, 253*, 2080–2086.

Stellar, J. R., & Stellar, E. (1985). *The neurobiology of motivation and reward.* New York: Springer-Verlag.

Sternbach, R. A. (Ed.). (1978). *The psychology of pain.* New York: Raven Press.

Stock, W. A., Okun, M. A., Haring, M. J., & Witter, R. A. (1983). Age and subjective well-being: A meta-analysis. In R. J. Light (Ed.), *Evaluation studies: Review annual* (Vol. 8, pp. 279–302). Beverly Hills, CA: Sage.

Stone, A. A. (1981). The association between perceptions of daily experiences and self- and spouse-rated mood. *Journal of Research in Personality, 15*, 510–522.

Stone, A. A., Cox, D. S., Valdimarsdottir, H., Jandorf, L., & Neale, J. M. (1987). Evidence that secretory IgA antibody is associated with daily mood. *Journal of Personality and Social Psychology, 52*, 988–993.

Stone, A. A., Hedges, S. M., Neale, J. M., & Satin, M. S. (1985). Prospective and cross-sectional mood reports offer no evidence of a "blue-Monday" phenomenon. *Journal of Personality and Social Psychology, 49,* 129–134.

Stone, A. A., Kessler, R. C., & Haythornwaite, J. A. (1991). Measuring daily events and experiences: Decisions for the researcher. *Journal of Personality, 59,* 575–607.

Stone, A. A., & Neale, J. M. (1984). Effects of severe daily events on mood. *Journal of Personality and Social Psychology, 46,* 137–144.

Strickland, B. R., Hale, W. D., & Anderson, L. K. (1975). Effect of induced mood states on activity and self-reported affect. *Journal of Consulting and Clinical Psychology, 43,* 587.

Stroebel, C. F. (1985). Biological rhythms in psychiatry. In H. I. Kaplan & B. J. Sadock (Eds.), *Comprehensive textbook in psychiatry* (4th ed., pp. 67–70). Baltimore: Williams & Wilkins.

Stroessner, S. J., Hamilton, D. L., & Mackie, D. M. (1992). Affect and stereotyping: The effect of induced mood on distinctiveness-based illusory correlations. *Journal of Personality and Social Psychology, 62,* 564–576.

Suh, E., Diener, E., & Fujita, F. (1996). Events and subjective well-being: Only recent events matter. *Journal of Personality and Social Psychology, 70,* 1091–1102.

Susman, E. J., Dorn, L. D., & Chrousos, G. P. (1991). Negative affect and hormone levels in young adolescents: Concurrent and predictive perspectives. *Journal of Youth and Adolescence, 20,* 167–190.

Tamarkin, L., Baird, C. J., & Almeida, O. F. (1985). Melatonin: A coordinating signal for mammalian reproduction. *Science, 227,* 714–720.

Taub, J. M., & Berger, R. J. (1974). Diurnal variations in mood as asserted by self-report and verbal content analysis. *Journal of Psychiatry Research, 10,* 83–88.

Taylor, J. A. (1953). A personality scale of manifest anxiety. *Journal of Abnormal and Social Psychology, 48,* 285–290.

Taylor, M. C. (1982). Improved conditions, rising expectations, and dissatisfaction: A test of the past/present relative deprivation hypothesis. *Social Psychology Quarterly, 45,* 24–33.

Taylor, S. E. (1989). *Positive illusions.* New York: Basic Books.

Taylor, S. E., & Brown, J. D. (1988). Illusion and well-being: A social psychological perspective on mental health. *Psychological Bulletin, 103,* 193–210.

Tellegen, A. (1982). *Brief manual for the Differential Personality Questionnaire.* Unpublished manuscript, University of Minnesota, Minneapolis.

Tellegen, A. (1985). Structures of mood and personality and their relevance to assessing anxiety, with an emphasis on self-report. In A. H. Tuma & J. D. Maser (Eds.), *Anxiety and the anxiety disorders* (pp. 681–706). Hillsdale, NJ: Erlbaum.

Tellegen, A. (1993). Folk concepts and psychological concepts of personality and personality disorder. *Psychological Inquiry, 4,* 122–130.

Tellegen, A. (in press). *Multidimensional personality questionnaire.* Minneapolis, MN: University of Minnesota Press.

Tellegen, A., Lykken, D. T., Bouchard, T. J., Jr., Wilcox, K. J., Segal, N. L., & Rich. S. (1988). Personality similarity in twins reared apart and together. *Journal of Personality and Social Psychology, 54,* 1031–1039.

Tellegen, A., Watson, D., & Clark, L. A. (1994, August). Modeling dimensions of mood. In L. A. Feldman (Chair), *Mood: Consensus and controversy.* Symposium presented at the 102nd annual convention of the American Psychological Association, Los Angeles.

Tellegen, A., Watson, D., & Clark, L. A. (1999). On the dimensional and hierarchical structure of affect. *Psychological Science, 10,* 297–303.

Tessler, R., Mechanic, D., & Dimond, M. (1976). The effect of psychological distress on physician utilization: A prospective study. *Journal of Health and Social Behavior, 17,* 353–364.

Thayer, R. E. (1978a). Factor analytic and reliability studies on the Activation-Deactivation Adjective Check List. *Psychological Reports, 42,* 747–756.

Thayer, R. E. (1978b). Toward a psychological theory of multidimensional activation (arousal). *Motivation and Emotion, 2,* 1–34.

Thayer, R. E. (1986). Activation-Deactivation Adjective Check List: Current overview and structural analysis. *Psychological Reports, 58,* 607–614.

Thayer, R. E. (1987a). Energy, tiredness, and tension effects of a sugar snack versus moderate exercise. *Journal of Personality and Social Psychology, 52,* 119–125.

Thayer, R. E. (1987b). Problem perception, optimism, and related states as a function of time of day (diurnal rhythm) and moderate exercise: Two arousal systems in interaction. *Motivation and Emotion, 11,* 19–36.

Thayer, R. E. (1989). *The biopsychology of mood and arousal.* New York: Oxford University Press.

Thayer, R. E., & Cheatle, M. (1976). *The effect of treadmill walking on energy and tension.* Unpublished manuscript, California State University at Long Beach.

Thayer, R. E., Peters, D. P., Takahashi, P. J., & Birkhead-Flight, A. M. (1993). Mood and behavior (smoking and sugar snacking) following moderate exercise: A partial test of self-regulation theory. *Personality and Individual Differences, 14,* 97–104.

Thayer, R. E., Takahashi, P. J., & Pauli, J. A. (1988). Multidimensional arousal states, diurnal rhythms, cognitive and social processes, and extraversion. *Personality and Individual Differences, 9,* 15–24.

Thompson, S. C., Sobolew-Shubin, A., Galbraith, M. E., Schwankovsky, L., & Cruzen, D. (1993). Maintaining perceptions of control: Finding perceived control in low-control circumstances. *Journal of Personality and Social Psychology, 64,* 293–304.

Tiggemann, M., Winefield, A. H., Winefield, H. R., & Goldney, R. D. (1991). The stability of attributional style and its relation to psychological distress. *British Journal of Clinical Psychology, 30,* 247–255.

Tomarken, A. J., Davidson, R. J., Wheeler, R. E., & Doss, R. C. (1992). Individual differences in anterior brain asymmetry and fundamental dimensions of emotion. *Journal of Personality and Social Psychology, 62,* 676–687.

Tomarken, A. J., & Keener, A. D. (1998). Frontal brain asymmetry and depression: A self-regulatory perspective. *Cognition and Emotion, 12,* 387–420.

Tomkins, S. S. (1962). *Affect, imagery, and consciousness. Vol 1. The positive affects.* New York: Springer.

Tomkins, S. S. (1963). *Affect, imagery, and consciousness. Vol 1. The negative affects.* New York: Springer.

Townsend, A., Noelker, L., Deimling, G., & Bass, D. (1989). Longitudinal impact of interhousehold caregiving on adult children's mental health. *Psychology and Aging, 4,* 393–401.

Trull, T. J., & Sher, K. J. (1994). Relationship between the five-factor model of personality and Axis I disorders in a nonclinical sample. *Journal of Abnormal Psychology, 103,* 350–360.

Tucker, D. M., & Williamson, P. A. (1984). Asymmetric neural control systems in human self-regulation. *Psychological Review, 91,* 185–215.

Tupes, E. C., & Christal, R. E. (1992). Recurrent personality factors based on trait ratings. *Journal of Personality, 60,* 225–251.

Turkheimer, E., & Gottesman, I. I. (1991). Individual differences and the canalization of human behavior. *Developmental Psychology, 27,* 18–22.

Turner, T. J., & Ortony, A. (1992). Basic emotions: Can conflicting criteria converge? *Psychological Review, 99,* 566–571.

Ulrich-Jakubowski, D., Russell, D. W., & O'Hara, M. W. (1988). Marital adjustment difficulties: Cause or consequence of depressive symptomatology? *Journal of Social and Clinical Psychology, 7,* 312–318.

Veenhoven, R. (1991). Questions on happiness: Classical topics, modern answers, blind spots. In F. Strack, M. Argyle, & N. Schwarz (Eds.), *Subjective well-being: An interdisciplinary perspective* (pp. 7–26). New York: Pergamon.

Veenhoven, R. (1994). Is happiness a trait? Tests of the theory that a better society does not make people any happier. *Social Indicators Research, 32,* 101–160.

Veroff, J., Douvan, E., & Kulka, R. A. (1981). *The inner American.* New York: Basic Books.

Viken, R. J., Rose, R. J., Kaprio, J., & Koskenvuo, M. (1994). A developmental genetic analysis of adult personality: Extraversion and neuroticism from 18 to 59 years of age. *Journal of Personality and Social Psychology, 66,* 722–730.

Vitousek, K., & Manke, F. (1994). Personality variables and disorders in anorexia nervosa and bulimia nervosa. *Journal of Abnormal Psychology, 103,* 137–147.

Vogel, G. W., Buffenstein, A., Minter, K., & Hennessey, A. (1990). Drug effects on REM sleep and on endogenous depression. *Neuroscience and Biobehavioral Reviews, 14,* 49–63.

Vogel, G. W., Neill, D., Hagler, M., & Kors, D. (1990). A new animal model of endogenous depression: A summary of present findings. *Neuroscience and Biobehavioral Reviews, 14,* 85–91.

Vogel, G. W., Vogel, F., McAbee, R. S., & Thurmond, A. J. (1980). Improvement of depression by REM sleep deprivation: New findings and a theory. *Archives of General Psychiatry, 37,* 247–253.

Walker, J. M., Garber, A., Berger, R. J., & Heller, H. C. (1979). Sleep and estivation (shallow torpor): Continuous processes of energy conservation. *Science, 204,* 1098–1100.

Waller, N., Kojetin, B., Lykken, D., Tellegen, A., & Bouchard, T. (1990). Religious interests, personality, and genetics: A study of twins reared together and apart. *Psychological Science, 1,* 138–142.

Waltz, M., & Badura, B. (1988). Subjective health, intimacy, and perceived self-efficacy after heart attack: Predicting life quality five years afterward. *Social Indicators Research, 20,* 303–332.

Warr, P., Barter, J., & Brownbridge, G. (1983). On the independence of positive and negative affect. *Journal of Personality and Social Psychology, 44*, 644–651.

Warr, P., & Jackson, P. (1984). Men without jobs: Some correlations of age and length of employment. *Journal of Occupational Psychology, 57*, 77–85.

Warr, P., & Payne, R. (1982). Experience of strain and pleasure among British adults. *Social Science and Medicine, 16*, 1691–1697.

Watson, D. (1988a). Intraindividual and interindividual analyses of Positive and Negative Affect: Their relation to health complaints, perceived stress, and daily activities. *Journal of Personality and Social Psychology, 54*, 1020–1030.

Watson, D. (1988b). The vicissitudes of mood measurement: Effects of varying descriptors, time frames, and response formats on measures of positive and negative affect. *Journal of Personality and Social Psychology, 55*, 128–141.

Watson, D. (1989). Strangers' ratings of the five robust personality factors: Evidence of a surprising convergence with self-report. *Journal of Personality and Social Psychology, 57*, 120–128.

Watson, D., & Clark, L. A. (1984). Negative Affectivity: The disposition to experience aversive emotional states. *Psychological Bulletin, 96*, 465–490.

Watson, D., & Clark, L. A. (1991a). *The Mood and Anxiety Symptom Questionnaire.* Unpublished manuscript, University of Iowa, Iowa City.

Watson, D., & Clark, L. A. (1991b). Self- versus peer-ratings of specific emotional traits: Evidence of convergent and discriminant validity. *Journal of Personality and Social Psychology, 60*, 927–940.

Watson, D., & Clark, L. A. (1992a). Affects separable and inseparable: On the hierarchical arrangement of the negative affects. *Journal of Personality and Social Psychology, 62*, 489–505.

Watson, D., & Clark, L. A. (1992b). On traits and temperament: General and specific factors of emotional experience and their relation to the five-factor model. *Journal of Personality, 60*, 441–476.

Watson, D., & Clark, L. A. (1993). Behavioral disinhibition versus constraint: A dispositional perspective. In D. M. Wegner & J. W. Pennebaker (Eds.), *Handbook of mental control* (pp. 506–527). New York: Prentice-Hall.

Watson, D., & Clark, L. A. (1994a). Emotions, moods, traits, and temperaments: Conceptual distinctions and empirical findings. In P. Ekman & R. J. Davidson (Eds.), *The nature of emotion: Fundamental questions* (pp. 89–93). New York: Oxford University Press.

Watson, D., & Clark, L. A. (1994b). *The PANAS-X: Manual for the Positive and Negative Affect Schedule—Expanded Form.* Unpublished manuscript, University of Iowa, Iowa City.

Watson, D., & Clark, L. A. (1994c). The vicissitudes of mood: A schematic model. In P. Ekman & R. J. Davidson (Eds.), *The nature of emotion: Fundamental questions* (pp. 400–405). New York: Oxford University Press.

Watson, D., & Clark, L. A. (1995). Depression and the melancholic temperament. *European Journal of Personality, 9*, 351–366.

Watson, D., & Clark, L. A. (1997a). Extraversion and its positive emotional core. In R. Hogan, J. Johnson, & S. Briggs (Eds.), *Handbook of personality psychology* (pp. 767–793). San Diego, CA: Academic Press.

Watson, D., & Clark, L. A. (1997b). Measurement and mismeasurement of mood: Recurrent and emergent issues. *Journal of Personality Assessment, 68,* 267–296.

Watson, D., Clark, L. A., & Carey, G. (1988). Positive and Negative Affectivity and their relation to anxiety and depressive disorders. *Journal of Abnormal Psychology, 97,* 346–353.

Watson, D., Clark, L. A., & Harkness, A. R. (1994). Structures of personality and their relevance to psychopathology. *Journal of Abnormal Psychology, 103,* 18–31.

Watson, D., Clark, L. A., McIntyre, C. W., & Hamaker, S. (1992). Affect, personality, and social activity. *Journal of Personality and Social Psychology, 63,* 1011–1025.

Watson, D., Clark, L. A., & Tellegen, A. (1984). Cross-cultural convergence in the structure of mood: A Japanese replication and a comparison with U.S. findings. *Journal of Personality and Social Psychology, 47,* 127–144.

Watson, D., Clark, L. A., & Tellegen, A. (1988). Development and validation of brief measures of positive and negative affect: The PANAS scales. *Journal of Personality and Social Psychology, 54,* 1063–1070.

Watson, D., Clark, L. A., Weber, K., Assenheimer, J. S., Strauss, M. E., & McCormick, R. A. (1995). Testing a tripartite model: II. Exploring the symptom structure of anxiety and depression in student, adult, and patient samples. *Journal of Abnormal Psychology, 104,* 15–25.

Watson, D., Hubbard, B., & Wiese, D. (in press-a). General traits of personality and affectivity as predictors of satisfaction in intimate relationships: Evidence from self- and partner-ratings. *Journal of Personality.*

Watson, D., Hubbard, B., & Wiese, D. (in press-b). Self–other agreement in personality and affectivity: The role of acquaintanceship, trait visibility, and assumed similarity. *Journal of Personality and Social Psychology.*

Watson, D., & Kendall, P. C. (1983). Methodological issues in research on coping with chronic disease. In T. G. Burish & L. A. Bradley (Eds.), *Coping with chronic disease: Research and applications* (pp. 39–81). New York: Academic Press.

Watson, D., & Kendall, P. C. (1989). Understanding anxiety and depression: Their relation to negative and positive affective states. In P. C. Kendall & D. Watson (Eds.), *Anxiety and depression: Distinctive and overlapping features* (pp. 3–26). San Diego, CA: Academic Press.

Watson, D., & Pennebaker, J. W. (1989). Health complaints, stress, and distress: Exploring the central role of Negative Affectivity. *Psychological Review, 96,* 234–254.

Watson, D., & Pennebaker, J. W. (1991). Situational, dispositional, and genetic bases of symptom reporting. In J. A. Skelton & R. T. Croyle (Eds.), *Mental representations in health and illness* (pp. 60–84). New York: Springer-Verlag.

Watson, D., & Slack, A. K. (1993). General factors of affective temperament and their relation to job satisfaction over time. *Organizational Behavior and Human Decision Processes, 54,* 181–202.

Watson, D., & Tellegen, A. (1985). Toward a consensual structure of mood. *Psychological Bulletin, 98,* 219–235.

Watson, D., & Walker, L. M. (1996). The long-term temporal stability and predictive validity of trait measures of affect. *Journal of Personality and Social Psychology, 70,* 567–577.

Watson, D., Weber, K., Assenheimer, J. S., Clark, L. A., Strauss, M. E., & McCormick, R. A. (1995). Testing a tripartite model: I. Evaluating the convergent and discriminant validity of anxiety and depression symptom scales. *Journal of Abnormal Psychology, 104,* 3–14.

Watson, D., Wiese, D., Vaidya, J., & Tellegen, A. (1999). The two general activation systems of affect: Structural findings, evolutionary considerations, and psychobiological evidence. *Journal of Personality and Social Psychology, 76,* 820–838.

Watts, C., Cox, T., & Robson, J. (1983). Morningness–eveningness and diurnal variations in self-reported mood. *Journal of Psychology, 113,* 251–256.

Webb, W. B. (1979). Theories of sleep functions and some clinical implications. In R. Drucker-Colin, M. Shkurovich, & M. B. Sterman (Eds.), *The functions of sleep* (pp. 19–35). San Diego, CA: Academic Press.

Weerasinghe, J., & Tepperman, L. (1994). Suicide and happiness: Seven tests of the connection. *Social Indicators Research, 32,* 199–233.

Wegner, D. M., & Vallacher, R. (Eds.). (1980). *The self in social psychology.* New York: Oxford University Press.

Wehr, T. A., Jacobsen, F. M., Sack, D. A., Arendt, J., Tarmarkin, L., & Rosenthal, N. E. (1986). Phototherapy of seasonal affective disorder: Time of day and suppression of melatonin are not critical for antidepressant effects. *Archives of General Psychiatry, 43,* 870–875.

Wehr, T. A., & Rosenthal, N. E. (1989). Seasonality and affective illness. *American Journal of Psychiatry, 146,* 829–839.

Wehr, T. A., & Wirz-Justice, A. (1982). Circadian rhythm mechanisms in affective illness and in antidepressant drug action. *Pharmacopsychiatria, 15,* 31–39.

Weinberg, R. A. (1989). Intelligence and IQ: Landmark issues and great debates. *American Psychologist, 44,* 98–104.

Weinberger, D. A. (1990). The construct validity of the repressive coping style. In J. L. Singer (Ed.), *Repression and dissociation: Implications for personality theory, psychopathology, and health* (pp. 337–386). Chicago: University of Chicago Press.

Weinberger, D. A., Schwartz, G. E., & Davidson, R. J. (1979). Low-anxious, high-anxious, and repressive coping styles: Psychometric patterns and behavioral and physiological responses to stress. *Journal of Abnormal Psychology, 88,* 369–380.

Weiss, D. J., Dawis, R. V., England, G. W., & Lofquist, L. H. (1967). *Manual for the Minnesota Satisfaction Questionnaire.* Minneapolis, MN: University of Minnesota Press.

Weiss, R. L., & Aved, B. M. (1978). Marital satisfaction and depression as predictors of physical health state. *Journal of Consulting and Clinical Psychology, 46,* 1379–1384.

Weissman, M. M. (1993). Family genetic studies of panic disorder. *Journal of Psychiatric Research, 27*(Suppl. 1), 69–78.

Wicklund, R. A. (1975). Objective self-awareness. In L. Berkowitz (Ed.), *Advances in experimental social psychology* (Vol. 8, pp. 233–275). New York: Academic Press.

Widiger, T. A., & Costa, P. T., Jr. (1994). Personality and the personality disorders. *Journal of Abnormal Psychology, 103*, 78–91.

Widiger, T. A., & Trull, T. J. (1992). Personality and psychopathology: An application of the five-factor model. *Journal of Personality, 60*, 363–393.

Wiggins, J. S. (1973). *Personality and prediction: Principles of personality assessment.* Reading, MA: Addison-Wesley.

Wiggins, J. S. (1979). A psychological taxonomy of trait-descriptive terms: The interpersonal domain. *Journal of Personality and Social Psychology, 37*, 395–412.

Wiggins, J. S. (1982). Circumplex models of interpersonal behavior in clinical psychology. In P. C. Kendall & J. N. Butcher (Eds.), *Handbook of research methods in clinical psychology* (pp. 183–221). New York: Wiley.

Wiggins, J. S., & Pincus, A. L. (1989). Conceptions of personality disorders and dimensions of personality. *Psychological Assessment: A Journal of Consulting and Clinical Psychology, 1*, 305–316.

Wiggins, J. S., & Trapnell, P. D. (1997). Personality structure: The return of the Big Five. In R. Hogan, J. Johnson, & S. Briggs (Eds.), *Handbook of personality psychology* (pp. 737–765). San Diego, CA: Academic Press.

Willner, P. (1985). *Depression: A psychobiological synthesis.* New York: Wiley.

Wirz-Justice, A., Graw, P., Krauchi, K., & Gisin, B. (1993). Light therapy in seasonal affective disorder is independent of time of day or circadian phase. *Archives of General Psychiatry, 50*, 929–937.

Wise, R. A., & Rompre, P.-P. (1989). Brain dopamine and reward. *Annual Review of Psychology, 40*, 191–225.

Wistow, D. J. (1990). The relationship between personality, health symptoms and disease. *Personality and Individual Differences, 11*, 717–723.

Witter, R. A., Stock, W. A., Okun, M. A., & Haring, M. J. (1985). Religion and subjective well-being in adulthood: A quantitative synthesis. *Review of Religious Research, 26*, 332–342.

Wolfe, V. V., Finch, A. J., Jr., Saylor, C. F., Blount, R. L., Pallmeyer, T. P., & Carek, D. J. (1987). Negative affectivity in children: A multitrait/multimethod investigation. *Journal of Consulting and Clinical Psychology, 55*, 245–250.

Wolpe, J. (1961). The systematic desensitization treatment of neuroses. *Journal of Nervous and Mental Disease, 132*, 189–203.

Wood, D. T. (1977). The relationship between state anxiety and acute physical activity. *American Corrective Therapy Journal, 31*, 67–69.

Wood, W., Rhodes, N., & Whelan, M. (1989). Sex differences in positive well-being: A consideration of emotional style and marital status. *Psychological Bulletin, 106*, 249–264.

Woodman, C. L. (1993). The genetics of panic disorder and generalized anxiety disorder. *Annals of Clinical Psychiatry, 5*, 231–240.

World Health Organization. (1992). *International classification of diseases* (10th ed.). Geneva: Author.

Wortman, C. B., & Silver, R. C. (1987). Coping with irrevocable loss. In G. R. VandenBos & B. K. Bryant (Eds.), *Cataclysms, crises, and catastrophes: Psychology in action* (pp. 185–235). Washington, DC: American Psychological Association.

Wu, J. C., & Bunney, W. E. (1990). The biological basis of an antidepressant response to sleep deprivation and relapse: Review and hypothesis. *American Journal of Psychiatry, 147,* 14–21.

Zajonc, R. B. (1980). Feeling and thinking: Preferences need no inferences. *American Psychologist, 35,* 151–175.

Zajonc, R. B. (1984). On the primacy of affect. *American Psychologist, 39,* 117–123.

Zautra, A. J., & Reich, J. W. (1983). Life events and perceptions of life quality: Developments in a two-factor approach. *Journal of Community Psychology, 11,* 121–132.

Zerubavel, E. (1985). *The seven day circle: The history and meaning of the week.* New York: Free Press.

Zevon, M. A., & Tellegen, A. (1982). The structure of mood change: An idiographic/nomothetic analysis. *Journal of Personality and Social Psychology, 43,* 111–122.

Zinbarg, R. E., & Barlow, D. H. (1991). Mixed anxiety–depression: A new diagnostic category? In R. M. Rapee & D. H. Barlow (Eds.), *Chronic anxiety: Generalized anxiety disorder and mixed anxiety–depression* (pp. 136–152). New York: Guilford Press.

Zinbarg, R., E., & Barlow, D. H. (1996). Structure of anxiety and the anxiety disorders: A hierarchical model. *Journal of Abnormal Psychology, 105,* 181–193.

Zinbarg, R. E., Barlow, D. H., Liebowitz, M., Street, L., Broadhead, E., Katon, W., Roy-Byrne, P., Lepine, J.-P., Teherani, M., Richards, J., Brantley, P. J., & Kraemer, H. (1994). The *DSM-IV* Field Trial for mixed anxiety–depression. *American Journal of Psychiatry, 151,* 1153–1162.

Zuckerman, M. (1987). A critical look at three arousal constructs in personality theories: Optimal levels of arousal, strength of the nervous system, and sensitivities to signals of reward and punishment. In J. Strelau & H. J. Eysenck (Eds.), *Personality dimensions and arousal* (pp. 217–232). New York: Plenum.

Zuckerman, M., & Lubin, B. (1965). *Manual for the Multiple Affect Adjective Check List.* San Diego, CA: Educational and Industrial Testing Service.

Zuckerman, M., & Lubin, B. (1985). *Manual for the MAACL-R: The Multiple Affect Adjective Check List Revised.* San Diego, CA: Educational and Industrial Testing Service.

Zuckerman, M., Lubin, B., & Rinck, C. M. (1983). Construction of new scales for the Multiple Affect Adjective Check List. *Journal of Behavioral Assessment, 5,* 119–129.

Zung, W. W. K. (1965). A self-rating depression scale. *Archives of General Psychiatry, 13,* 508–516.

Zung, W. W. K. (1971). A rating instrument for anxiety disorders. *Psychosomatics, 12,* 371–379.

INDEX

"f" indicates a figure; "t" indicates a table